DROWNING

New Perspectives on
Intervention and Prevention

DROWNING

New Perspectives on Intervention and Prevention

Edited by

John R. Fletemeyer
Samuel J. Freas

International Swimming Hall of Fame, Inc.
Fort Lauderdale, Florida

with the assistance of
Sports-Aid International, Inc.

informa

healthcare

New York London

First published in 1999 by CRC Press, Inc.

This edition published in 2011 by Informa Healthcare, Telephone House, 69-77 Paul Street, London EC2A 4LQ, UK.

Simultaneously published in the USA by Informa Healthcare, 52 Vanderbilt Avenue, 7th Floor, New York, NY 10017, USA.

Informa Healthcare is a trading division of Informa UK Ltd. Registered Office: 37–41 Mortimer Street, London W1T 3JH, UK. Registered in England and Wales number 1072954.

A CIP record for this book is available from the Library of Congress.

ISBN-13: 9781574442236

Orders may be sent to: Informa Healthcare, Sheepen Place, Colchester, Essex CO3 3LP, UK
Telephone: +44 (0)20 7017 5540
Email: CSDhealthcarebooks@informa.com
Website: http://informahealthcarebooks.com/

For corporate sales please contact: CorporateBooksIHC@informa.com
For foreign rights please contact: RightsIHC@informa.com
For reprint permissions please contact: PermissionsIHC@informa.com

The Editors

John R. Fletemeyer, Ph.D., has postgraduate degrees in anthropology and education from the University of Cape Town, the University of Wisconsin, and Florida International University. He is currently vice president of the International Swimming Hall of Fame, Fort Lauderdale, Florida, and director of beach safety operations for Palm Beach, Florida.

Dr. Fletemeyer serves as editor-in-chief of the *World of Aquatics.* He has more than 100 publications to his credit, on topics ranging from beach and aquatic safety to wildlife ecology, conservation, and archaeology. Over the past two decades, he has served on various professional committees and as a consultant to numerous organizations, including the National Oceanographic and Atmospheric Administration, the United States Lifesaving Association, the YMCA of the USA, the U.S. Army Corps of Engineers, and the Centers for Disease Control and Prevention.

Samuel James Freas, Ed.D., is one of the world's foremost authorities on aquatics. As president of the International Swimming Hall of Fame in Fort Lauderdale, Florida, he consults on all phases of aquatics both nationally and internationally. He has written eight aquatics-related books on competitive swimming, recreation, safety, and facility utilization.

Dr. Freas has been a teacher, coach, and administrator at the State University of New York at Potsdam, Allegheny College, the University of Arkansas, Louisiana State University, and Kenyon College. He is past president and executive director of the College Swimming Coaches Association of America and served as national team swimming coach 1980–1989. He was voted National Swim Coach of the Year in 1976, SEC Conference Coach of the Year in 1985, and SWC Coach of the Year in 1980, 1981, and 1984. His teams produced 115 collegiate All-Americans, five Olympic medalists, three world records, and five American records. He has been president of the International Swimming Hall of Fame since 1989.

As a beach lifeguard in Wildwood, New Jersey, from 1959 to 1971, Dr. Freas was credited with over 100 rescues. He was among the first lifesavers to use mouth-to-mouth resuscitation and was an early proponent of resuscitation while the victim was still in the water. He was a high school All-American swimmer, a national prep school record holder, and a collegiate All-American and New England Champion swimmer at Springfield College, Massachusetts.

As president of the International Swimming Hall of Fame, Dr. Freas is aware of the high rate of drowning and the apparent shift away from teaching swimming and water safety. The May 1996 International Drowning Symposium was the catalyst for this collaborative effort to call attention to the problem of drowning. As this book demonstrates, Dr. Freas, Dr. Fletemeyer, and their eighteen contributors believe this situation could be greatly improved by teaching children and adults to swim and by teaching home, water, and boating safety.

The Editors

John R. Fletemeyer, Ph.D., has postgraduate degrees in anthropology and education from the University of Cape Town, the University of Wisconsin, and Florida International University. He is currently vice president of the International Swimming Hall of Fame, Fort Lauderdale, Florida, and director of beach safety operations for Palm Beach, Florida.

Dr. Fletemeyer serves as editor-in-chief of the *World of Aquatics*. He has more than 100 publications to his credit, on topics ranging from beach and aquatic safety to wildlife ecology, conservation, and archaeology. Over the past two decades, he has served on various professional committees and as a consultant to numerous organizations, including the National Oceanographic and Atmospheric Administration, the United States Lifesaving Association, the YMCA of the USA, the U.S. Army Corps of Engineers, and the Centers for Disease Control and Prevention.

Samuel James Freas, Ed.D., is one of the world's foremost authorities on aquatics. As president of the International Swimming Hall of Fame in Fort Lauderdale, Florida, he consults on all phases of aquatics both nationally and internationally. He has written eight aquatics-related books on competitive swimming, recreation, safety, and facility utilization.

Dr. Freas has been a teacher, coach, and administrator at the State University of New York at Potsdam, Allegheny College, the University of Arkansas, Louisiana State University, and Kenyon College. He is past president and executive director of the College Swimming Coaches Association of America and served as national team swimming coach 1980–1989. He was voted National Swim Coach of the Year in 1976, SEC Conference Coach of the Year in 1985, and SWC Coach of the Year in 1980, 1981, and 1984. His teams produced 115 collegiate All-Americans, five Olympic medalists, three world records, and five American records. He has been president of the International Swimming Hall of Fame since 1989.

As a beach lifeguard in Wildwood, New Jersey, from 1959 to 1971, Dr. Freas was credited with over 100 rescues. He was among the first lifesavers to use mouth-to-mouth resuscitation and was an early proponent of resuscitation while the victim was still in the water. He was a high school All-American swimmer, a national prep school record holder, and a collegiate All-American and New England Champion swimmer at Springfield College, Massachusetts.

As president of the International Swimming Hall of Fame, Dr. Freas is aware of the high rate of drowning and the apparent shift away from teaching swimming and water safety. The May 1996 International Drowning Symposium was the catalyst for this collaborative effort to call attention to the problem of drowning. As this book demonstrates, Dr. Freas, Dr. Fletemeyer, and their eighteen contributors believe this situation could be greatly improved by teaching children and adults to swim and by teaching home, water, and boating safety.

Contributors

Desmond Bohn
Department of Critical Care
  Medicine
The Hospital for Sick Children
Toronto, Ontario, Canada

Christine M. Branche
Centers for Disease Control
  and Prevention
Chamblee, GA

Robert G. Dean
Department of Oceanography
  and Engineering
University of Florida
Gainesville, FL

John R. Fletemeyer
International Swimming
  Hall of Fame
Fort Lauderdale, FL

Samuel J. Freas
International Swimming
  Hall of Fame
Fort Lauderdale, FL

Ralph S. Goto
Director of Beach Safety
Honolulu, HI

Tom Griffiths
Aquatics Department
The Pennsylvania State University
University Park, PA

Henry J. Heimlich
The Heimlich Institute
Cinncinati, OH

Brad Keshlear
U.S. Army Corps of Engineers
South Atlantic Division
Atlanta, GA

James B. Lushine
National Oceanographic and
  Atmospheric Administration
Weather and Forecasting
Miami, FL

Fred A. Mael
U.S. Army Research Institute
Alexandria, VA

Jerome H. Modell
Health Science Center
University of Florida
Gainesville, FL

Frank Pia
Pia Enterprises
Larchmont, NY

E. Louise Priest
American Red Cross
Kingwood, TX

Bruce Schmidt
U.S. Coast Guard
Washington, DC

Laura Slane
YMCA of the USA
Chicago, IL

Eric Spletzer
The Heimlich Institute
Cincinnati, OH

Don Steel
University of Maryland
College Park, MD

David Szpilman
Barra da Tijuca
Rio de Janeiro, Brazil

Hans Vogelsong
The Pennsylvania State University
College Park, PA

Introduction

In May 1996, the International Swimming Hall of Fame hosted a tremendously successful international drowning symposium, which provided a forum to compile expert up-to-date information, data, and statistics on drowning and water safety issues. The result of this compilation is *Drowning: New Perspectives on Intervention and Prevention*, a quintessential information source that enables us to better understand and prevent drowning. The editors hope this book will stimulate additional research in the area of drowning and drowning prevention.

Drowning represents the third-leading cause of accidental death in America and the second-leading cause of accidental death in Americans ages 5–44. Although such statistical data does not exist, there is little doubt that drownings and near-drownings have a major social and economic impact on our society and on our healthcare system. Emergency room care for drowning victims accounts for millions of dollars in annual expenditures that could be spent on other positive endeavors.

Dr. Christine M. Branche of the Centers for Disease Control and Prevention challenges reports that drowning rates have decreased slightly in recent years. In Chapter 3, Dr. Branche maintains that when data on America's drowning rate is subjected to scientific scrutiny and analyzed according to specific categories such as age, sex, race, and socio-economic position, a different conclusion emerges. For example, the drowning rate is increasing among certain races and age groups. In recent years, however, some have used the overall reduction in the drowning rate as proof of the success of many drowning prevention programs developed by private and public organizations. Because of the lack of statistical data to support this proof, considerable caution is necessary before a causal relationship between the two can be established. The reduction in the drowning rate may only be a statistical anomaly.

The definition of drowning has changed over the years. The general public probably believes death from immersion in the water is considered a drowning. In some states, if someone dies more than 24 hours after being immersed in water that is considered a resuscitative death, not a drowning. In some states, a death from falling into the water from a dock or boat is considered a marine or boating accident. These varying methods of maintaining statistics prompted the editors to seek public awareness and help in redefining this tragic loss of life known to the public as drowning. A uniform definition of drowning is a step toward manifest change in understanding the magnitude of this problem.

Many aquatics professionals believe it is only a matter of time before we begin to see a rise in the number of drownings in America, largely due to the de-emphasis on aquatics in our educational system. Many "learn-to-swim" programs that were once an integral part of our secondary school, college, and university curricula have been cut or eliminated altogether. This problem has been exacerbated by the fact that swimming, together with sports such as golf and tennis, has often been considered a country club activity that offers little or nothing for the so-called masses.

Consequently, for many, access to swimming programs is limited. The efforts of public service-oriented organizations such as the YMCA and the Red Cross to offer learn-to-swim lessons mainly to young people are commendable, but they are band-aid remedies at best. Until government at all levels commits to making every child and adult a swimmer, drowning will continue to be one of America's major public health and safety problems — perhaps our most preventable problem.

The situation in other countries, especially those labeled as Third World, is even worse. Funds and expertise for learn-to-swim and other aquatics-related safety programs tend to be in short supply, and the emphasis on drowning prevention is virtually nonexistent. It is indeed unfortunate that we have no statistics for drowning in these countries; if we had statistics, it would be possible to demonstrate on a global basis the terrible impact of drowning on the human population. Hopefully, this book will help put drowning in the proper perspective and encourage intervention and prevention programs that can be expanded into a national program that can ultimately be adopted and supported by all governments.

Aspects of drowning have traditionally been studied as three — often mutually exclusive — categories: medical, prevention, and intervention. *Drowning: New Perspectives on Intervention and Prevention* represents a significant departure from this approach. As the editors reviewed the materials and assimilated the chapters of this text, it became obvious these categories overlap to a considerable degree. As you read this material, you will realize that drowning is more a predictable, preventable process rather than simply an uncontrollable, tragic event.

This unique book will benefit both individuals directly employed in aquatics and "outsiders" with more than just a cursory interest in drowning, such as risk managers, lawyers, public safety officers, members of the medical profession, and perhaps even social scientists.

Identifying topics appropriate to the theme of this book was not a simple undertaking. Even more difficult was identifying contributors considered by their peers to be leaders in their respective fields. The impressive academic backgrounds, research credentials, and the positions they hold distinguish the respected contributors to this book.

The editors extend sincere thanks to the contributing authors who gave their time, expertise, and talent to make this book a reality. We also thank those who helped put the book together and make it available to the public. In every regard, this book represents a team effort to advance drowning prevention.

John Fletemeyer, Ph.D.
Samuel James Freas, Ed.D.

Contents

1 A History of Drowning and Resuscitation

Samuel J. Freas

The histories of swimming, drowning, and resuscitation techniques are inextricably intertwined. Since the earth is more than two thirds water, people have always been challenged by the need to traverse water for transportation, recreational, and commercial reasons. Because water has always been important to mankind's basic needs and sustenance, the ability of an individual to swim has been a challenge since the beginning of mankind. As people used water more and more, drowning and the need for resuscitative techniques became greater concerns. The history of swimming, drowning, and resuscitation techniques will help the reader understand and appreciate the magnitude of these problems and how people have attempted to resolve them over the ages.

Ironically, the earliest known pictorial record of swimming is wall carvings of the Wadi Sori tribe found in the Libyan Desert. These carvings, which date from 9000 B.C., are the only known pictures of swimmers in prehistoric art.[1] One can deduce that prehistoric man had to negotiate water using some means of primitive swimming, but the first written record of swimming dates from ca. 2160–1780 B.C. This account, from the Middle Kingdom of Egypt, states that children of the king and noblemen took swimming lessons together. Swimming was part of the required curriculum for Greek and Roman boys as well, and the educational organizations of these peoples strongly indicate that swimming was part of their instructional programs.[2]

Egyptian wall reliefs depict the route of the Hittites across the Orontes River in Northern Syria during the reign of Ramses II, ca. 1292–1225 B.C. (Figure 1). Two Assyrian reliefs show soldiers in the act of swimming, one using breaststroke, the other a stroke with overarm action. Another relief, depicting the battle of Kadesh, pictures a primitive method of resuscitation. It shows soldiers grasping King Aleppo by the ankles and supporting him with his head down to hasten his recovery. Perhaps the earliest known rescue method is also pictured here: men on shore extend their hands to comrades in the water.

In II Kings 4:32–37, the Bible provides the earliest known written account of artificial respiration using a mouth-to-mouth technique (ca. 852–841 B.C.). It is interesting to note that some historians believe mouth-to-mouth resuscitation to be a 19th- or 20th-century phenomenon, but in reality it was utilized 2000–3000 years earlier. A painting by Lord Frederick Leighton depicts the Prophet Elisha applying a mouth-to-mouth method to a Shunammite child (Figure 2). The Bible records the event:

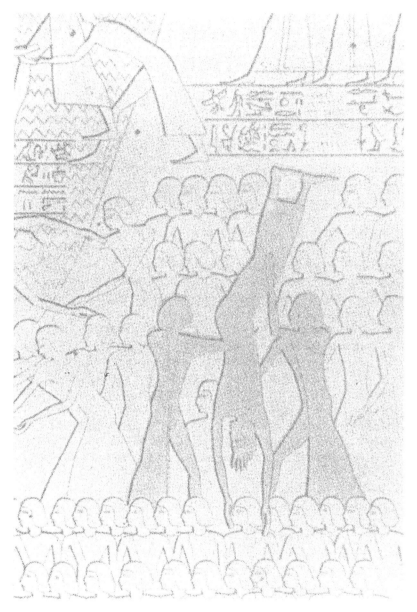

FIGURE 1   Relief from the Battle of Kadesh: An ancient depiction of the inversion method of resuscitation (University of Chicago Press, 1904).

When Elisha reached the house there was a boy lying dead on his couch. He went in, shut the door on the two of them (the boy's mother and Gehazi) and prayed to the Lord. Then he got on the bed and lay upon the boy, mouth to mouth, eyes to eyes, hands to hands. As he stretched himself out upon him, the boy's body grew warm. Elisha turned away and walked back and forth in the room and then got on the bed, and stretched upon him once more. The boy sneezed seven times and opened his eyes.[3]

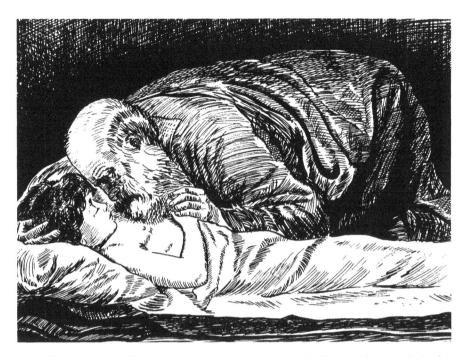

FIGURE 2   Drawing of Prophet Elisha and Shunammite child (Redrawn from a painting by Lord Frederick Leighton).

Some say this story is the basis of the saying "God bless you" when someone sneezes. One historian has reduced the miracle to the following: "By Elisha throwing himself several times on the child, caused a few respirations by compression and depression of the chest. Moreover, Elisha's beard and mustache tickled the child's nose and caused subsequent sneezing."[4] Clearly Elisha prayed to the Lord, and the first known written record of mouth-to-mouth resuscitation was more of a miracle than a technique. For many, mouth-to-mouth remains a lifesaving miracle today.

In 1538, Nicholas Winman wrote the first book on swimming. He advocated that a swimming rescuer should have (1) a real presence of mind; (2) the ability to avoid being seized by the victim; (3) a cord or floating device; and (4) the ability to swim with one hand. Swimming with one hand is the basis of most lifesaving strokes we know of today.[5] In 1555, Olaus Magnus emphasized the importance of lifesaving devices in the rescue of nonswimmers.[6] The ancient Greeks and Romans wrote of swimmers using an alternating arm action, but, during the Middle Ages, breaststroke swimming and swimming with the head out of the water were preferred methods because of the fear of spreading diseases. Swimming fell out of favor throughout Europe because of the belief that outdoor bathing spread the epidemics of the Middle Ages.[7] Even Shakespeare made reference to water rescue, although not factual, when he had Caesar cry, "Help me Cassius, ere I sink." Caesar actually decreed that every soldier in his army be able to swim and pass a swimming test.

A variety of practices to revive drowning persons were recorded after the invention of the printing press. There is evidence that placing burning coals, shaking, slapping, and yelling were primitive techniques used to revive drowning persons. Some methods may seem bizarre, but because they are part of the history of resuscitation, it is important to chronicle them. Hippocrates recorded the importance of keeping a victim's body warm to increase chances of revival. He also recommended assisting an unconscious person by tickling the throat to induce vomiting and stimulation.[8]

Almost a thousand years later, Bagellardus, a contemporary of Christopher Columbus, suggested blowing air into the mouth and rectum.[9] For obvious reasons, his technique did not endure. Since drowning was second to stillbirth as the leading cause of asphyxia death, the same revival techniques were sometimes used for both. L. Bourgeois, midwife to Marie de Medici, suggested inserting urine into the mouth of a newborn to stimulate breathing, and there were reports that this technique was used in drowning cases.[10] Many paintings from the 15th to 18th centuries show sailors being placed over barrels and rolled back and forth in apparent efforts to resuscitate them (Figure 3). In 1766, a pamphlet was printed in Zurich, Switzerland with instructions for resuscitation utilizing a barrel in a different manner: "Lay the victim with their belly over a round piece of wood or barrel so that the head lies flat in front and the feet hang down in back; if the head is held in this position and the body is shaken water, mucous and froth usually pass off."[11]

In 1752, Louis attempted to scientifically analyze the nature of drowning by drowning several animals in colored water and observing the presence of water in the lungs.[12] Profound interest in drowning developed when Amsterdam, Holland, a city surrounded by water, became the leader in water safety and resuscitative techniques. The Society for Recovery of the Apparently Drowned, organized in Amsterdam in 1767, published instructions for resuscitation:

> (1) Victim was laid on a table or bench in a sloping position, head higher than the feet, victim was stripped, put in a blanket and examined. (2) To combat hypothermia rub body dry with warm hands. If dry rubbing is not effective, spirit of sal amoniac, or hartshorn or eau-de-luce mixed with white brandy, rum or malt spirits is used. Backbone, sides of body, abdomen and breast, palms of the hands, soles of the feet, temples, ears and neck are to be chaffed with the above mentioned mixture. (3) Mouth and nose are to be cleared of foreign matter with a goose feather or repeated injections of luke warm water, tea or another aromatic infusion. (4) Introduction of air into the body to blow up the lungs, to renew the circulation, or to swell the intestines to produce motion.[13]

This society also recommended use of both internal and external emetics and stimulants to aid in resuscitation. Suspension by the heels and inversion of the body were other methods occasionally employed by the society.

The work of the Amsterdam society spread to other countries. In 1768, the Imperial Academy of Sciences at St. Petersburg translated the society's writings into

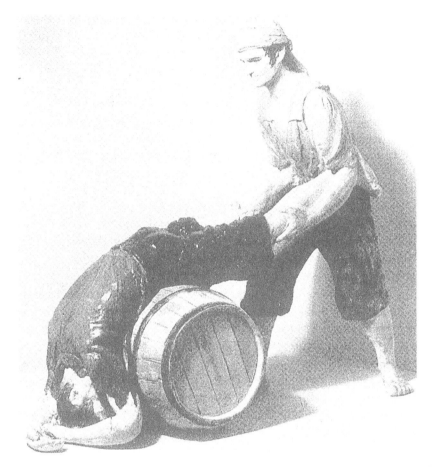

FIGURE 3 Rolling a victim over a barrel was an early method of resuscitation (Public Service Co. of Northern Illinois).

Russian. As these concepts were translated into more languages, Societies for the Apparently Drowned were created in Naples, Florence, Genoa, Hamburg, and Hungary. In Hamburg, The Society for the Encouragement of Useful Arts distributed directions for lifesaving and offered a reward for every successful rescue reported.[14] Research in drowning continued. In 1772, A. de Haen, a professor of medicine in Vienna, found that water entered the lungs during drowning and strongly advocated inversion of the drowning victim for successful revival.

In Ireland and other countries in Europe the superstition persisted that it was unlucky to rescue and revive a drowned person. In England, this myth prevented people from engaging in lifesaving attempts. In 1782, the efforts of Dr. Hawes of London to dispel these fears resulted in passage of the first Good Samaritan type law, making it legal to resuscitate or assist in resuscitating a drowning person.[15] By 1804, the Royal Humane Society, organized by Drs. Cogan and Hawes, was credited with saving 2,859 lives and awarded 4,587 people merits of heroism for preserving the lives of drowning people. The society was also responsible for introducing various methods of resuscitation, particularly the use of fireplace bellows. A positive result of the interest in bellows was E. Goodwun's discovery, around 1782, that the tongue might fall back, occluding the opening into the larynx and rendering the bellows ineffective until the tongue was repositioned.

In 1781, Dr. A. Fothergill suggested the use of oxygen in resuscitation was more efficient than the air we breathe. Fothergill was also an early advocate of electrical stimulation in all methods of revival.[16] The use of bellows to revive a drowning victim was widespread until the 1820s, when Dr. Leroy d'Etiolles of France demonstrated that it was possible to kill an animal by suddenly inflating the lungs with bellows, and that emphysema and pneumothorax of the lungs often resulted. He found 20–80 millimeters of mercury pressure from the use of bellows was sufficient to create these problems (Figure 3).[17] It was not until the late 1800s that emphysema was acknowledged to be a recognized consequence of drowning. Dr. d'Etiolles' work precipitated greater interest in the manual methods of resuscitation.

The American colonies experienced problems similar to their European counterparts. In an effort to resolve drowning problems, the Humane Society of Philadelphia and the Massachusetts Humane Society were formed in the 1780s. Members distributed handbills at tavern gates about the dangers of cold water and brought lifesaving and learn-to-swim campaigns to the colonies.[18] Fumigation or the strong infusion of tobacco smoke, reportedly the favorite technique of Native Americans to revive drowning victims, fell out of favor in the early 1800s as colonial drowning societies became more active. The Massachusetts Society, in Cohasset, provided a significant piece of lifesaving equipment to the Americas by constructing the first lifeboat in 1807.

In 1815, J. Curry, in the book *Observations on Apparent Death from Drowning, Hanging, etc.*, observed very little water entered the lungs during drowning, which conflicted with Louis' 1752 finding that indicated water definitely entered the lungs. The medical professionals of this era disagreed. There were three schools of thought in regard to water penetrating the lungs during drowning: (1) no water in the lungs; (2) water in the lungs; (3) sometimes water appears in the lungs and sometimes it does not.[19] As the medical debate continued, lifesavers were challenged to find more effective ways to resuscitate victims.

The Europeans discovered that manual manipulation of the chest cavity appeared to be the most successful method of resuscitating a drowning victim. The first systematic attempt at manual artificial respiration was advocated by Dr. Marshall Hall, a learned English physiologist who published a paper in 1857 entitled *Prone and Postural Respiration in Drowning*. In analyzing this method, the patient's position was altered from a lateral to a prone position. These positional changes produced alterations in the capacity of the thorax, theoretically inducing the breathing cycle.[20] This early research resulted in the method of resuscitation used during the first half of the 20th century (Figure 4).

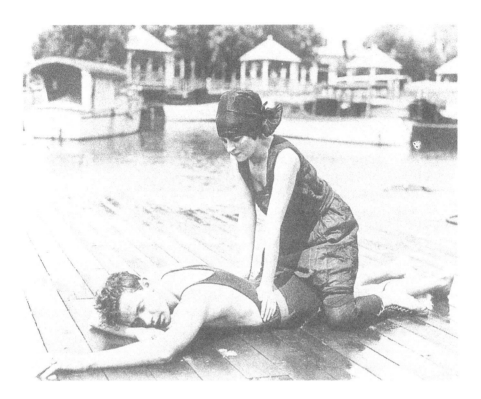

FIGURE 4   An early manual on resuscitation methodology shows a method used during the first half of the 20th century.

In 1858, Dr. Silvester devised a method of artificial respiration using a different principle. He tried to imitate as closely as possible the natural movements of breathing through elevation of the ribs. He selected the supine position for the resuscitative effort and advocated pulling the arms forcibly above the head, thereby dragging upon the ribs and causing an enlargement of the thoracic cavity. Expiration was brought about by lowering the arms again to the sides and compressing the thorax laterally.[21]

In 1869, Dr. Benjamin Howard of New York published a description of another method that depended on pressure alone. Dr. Howard's instructions were: (1) turn the patient face downward and press two or three times with all your weight upon the back; (2) then turn the patient face upward, creating a hyperextension of the spine by placing a support under the patient; (3) pressure is then applied by a triple movement: first the lower six ribs are depressed; second, the abdominal contents, especially the liver and spleen, are compressed to force the diaphragm upward and empty the lungs; and third, the extension of the spine is partly undone. The pressure is relieved by a sudden jerk backward. Inspiration is effected by the rebound. This procedure should be repeated 10–12 times per minute.[22]

About this same time, Dalziel of Drumlanrig suggested an innovative idea.[23] He built an airtight box that engulfed the victim's body, except for the head. The box was connected to a large hand pump, which created pressure on the patient's body and caused the patient to breathe. This idea underlies when Dr. M. Woilly's spirophere machine, an award winner at the Exposition of Lifesaving Equipment in Le Havre, France, in 1876. These two innovative men are credited with developing the basis for the iron lung.

In 1889, French researchers Barouardel and Loye demonstrated that water enters the lungs during drowning and quantified the amount and how it entered. This fueled the debate on the nature of drowning because Barouardel and Loye had anesthetized their dogs, blocking the laryngeal spasm reflex that would have prevented water from entering the lungs.

In 1882, Flaschar reintroduced a manual method of resuscitation that originated in 1831 with Dalrymple. This method entailed wrapping a shawl around the patient's chest and pulling the ends to cause compression and expiration of the chest. This technique was most effective when partners took opposite ends of the shawl.[24]

The U.S. Volunteer Life Saving Corps, the foundation of the American Red Cross Water Safety section in which Commodore W. E. Longfellow played a leadership role, was founded in 1890. The mission of the U.S. Volunteer Life Saving Corps was to (1) rescue the drowning; (2) aid the injured; (3) safeguard the public; (4) teach swimming; and (5) reward bravery.

Until the late 1800s, swimming and lifesaving were usually done in a traditional manner, with arms underwater, pulling out and back from the chest, coordinated with a frog kicking motion. In their travels, J. Arthur Trudgen and Captain Cook observed Pacific Islanders and South American Indians who swam with alternating arms and kicks.[25]

In the late 1800s, competitive water sports had a profound effect on lifesaving and swimming. When Captain Matthew Webb successfully swam the English Channel on August 24, 1875, the news captivated the world and created more interest in swimming.[26] The Trudgen stroke, a modified side stroke that utilized an overarm recovery, emerged shortly before the 1896 Olympic Games in Athens. When Alex Wickham, a native of the Solomon Islands, migrated to Australia in 1898,[27] he brought the alternating arm and kicking stroke he saw the islanders use, as Captain Cook previously reported. This stroke, known as the Australian crawl, might have been more correctly called the Hawaiian crawl because Captain Cook initially reported it after visiting the Sandwich Islands. When Australian swimmer Richard Cavill utilized this stroke to set a world record for the 100-meter freestyle (58.6 seconds) in 1902, the stroke was known forever more as the Australian crawl. This stroke rapidly became the preferred stroke of lifesavers when approaching a victim because it was much faster.

Water polo also had a tremendous effect on lifesaving, largely because of its extremely combative nature (Figure 5). A player could legally hold, sink, and nearly drown opponents, resulting in the invention of escapes and releases from opponents. Many lifesaving techniques were created by water polo players trying to survive their matches.

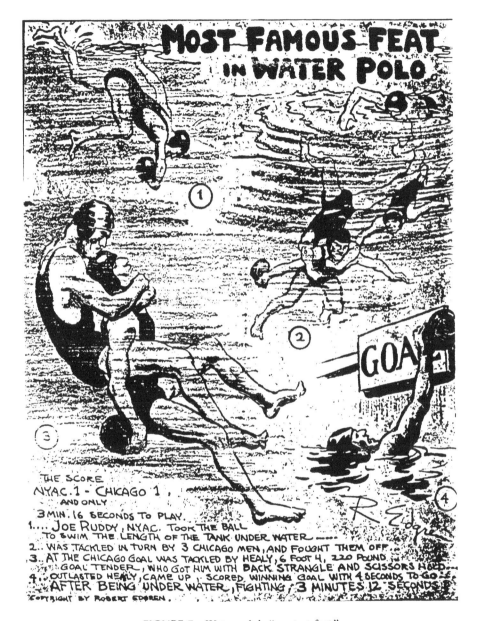

FIGURE 5   Water polo's "greatest feat."

The modern Olympics also played a role in the revival of society's interest in water. In 1896, the first swimming events of the modern Olympic Games were held outdoors in Athens, in and around the Bay of Phaleron, where 40,000 people watched from shore and boats (Figure 6). The weather turned cold, and the water temperature was reported at 13°C or 15°F. Alfred Hajos of Hungary won the 100-meter freestyle with a time of 1:22.2. His father's death by drowning motivated Hajos to become an accomplished swimmer.

During this era, the Royal Life Saving Society was organized to supplement the work of the Royal Humane Society in England. The aims and objectives of the society were: (1) to promote education in lifesaving and resuscitation; (2) to stimulate public opinion in favor of general education and lifesaving in schools; (3) to encourage floating, diving, and plunging that would be of assistance to a person endeavoring to save a life; and (4) to arrange and promote public lectures, demonstrations, and competitions, and to form classes of instruction.[28] The organization had profound worldwide influence. Its techniques included: (1) the lifesaver's frontal approach to the victim; (2) the lifesaver's releases from the clutches of the drowning victim; (3) the lifesaver's towing or transporting of the victim; (4) recovery from the bottom; (5) lifts and carries out of the water; (6) the Schafer method of artificial respiration.[29] The Schafer method of resuscitation, introduced by Professor E. A. Schafer in 1903, advocated prone pressure arm lift. This was the preferred method until 1932, when Holger Nielson of the Danish Red Cross advocated the back pressure arm lift.

In the early 1900s, the Australians organized the Surf Lifesaving Association of Australia, which remains one of the world's foremost surf rescue organizations. In its first 30 years of existence, the association made over 39,000 rescues. During this period, lifeguard equipment also changed significantly. In 1897, Capt. Harry Sheffield developed the first formally designed rescue flotation device (RFD) for a lifesaving club in South Africa. Olympic swimming champion Duke Kahanamoku introduced his redwood surfboard (Figure 7) to the United States during a visit to California. American lifeguards found his "toy" an important lifesaving tool (Figure 8).[30]

In the Americas, the YMCA was the first organization to employ field representatives to promote a national swimming and lifesaving education program. Indoor swimming pool construction received impetus from the YMCA's building program. The first "Y" pool was constructed in Brooklyn, New York, in 1885.[31] In 1909, the American Red Cross and the YMCA entered into an agreement to promote first aid training, which included lifesaving — part of Commodore Longfellow's great lasting contribution to the national and international lifesaving scene.

Nineteenth-century America emerged as the world leader in competitive swimming and water polo. Johnny Weissmuller set 52 world records and won five gold medals, but his greatest exploit was as Tarzan on the movie screen (Figure 9). The boom in swimming during this era was largely due to the press glorification of Weissmuller, Buster Crabbe, Duke Kahanamoku, Eleanor Holm, and others. Every mother wanted her child to look great and be safe. The sport of swimming seemed to provide this.

In 1924, Dr. James E. West started the "Every Scout A Swimmer" program. That same year, Commodore Longfellow wrote the *Boy Scout Guide: Swimming,*

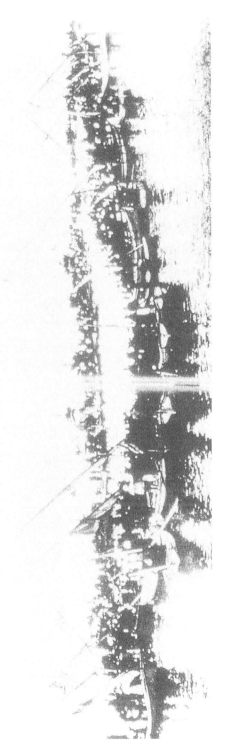

FIGURE 6   Swimming venue of the Athens Olympic Games of 1896.

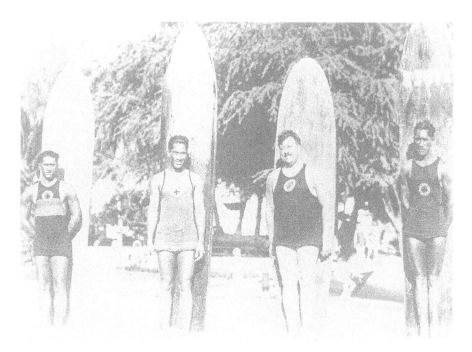

FIGURE 7   Duke Kahanamoku, Olympic swimmer, water polo player, and father of surfing (center left), pictured with Commodore Longfellow (center right).

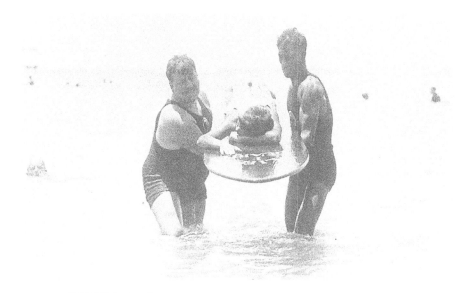

FIGURE 8   Surfboards were used to carry victims to shore (ca. 1920).

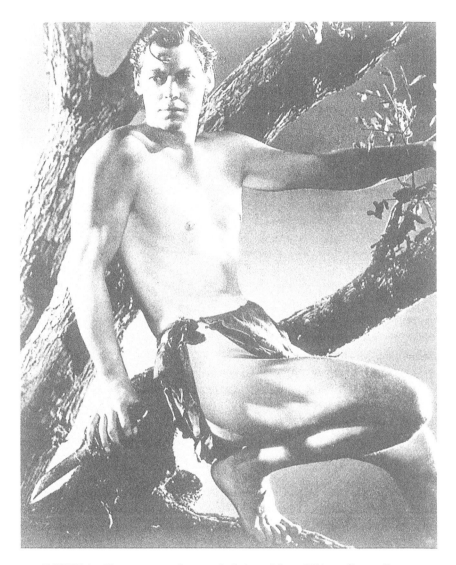

FIGURE 9   The greatest swimmer of all time, Johnny Weissmuller, as Tarzan.

Water Sports and Safety, helping yet another organization establish a learn-to-swim campaign. Inspired by the deaths of U.S. aviators and Navy personnel during World War I, Fred R. Lanoue introduced the survival technique of drownproofing in 1936.[32] Drownproofing, which taught individuals how best to stay alive when alone in the water, had a profound impact on both civilian lifesavers and the military.

As interest in water safety and swimming peaked during the two world wars, mothers told their children not to go swimming right after they ate or they could drown. This advice demonstrates the overall safety consciousness of the era, resulting from two wars and the tremendous efforts of Longfellow and others to elevate the importance of water safety in the thought process of families. In 1935, Thompson advocated yet another lifesaving technique, the back pressure hip lift. In 1948, Emerson proposed a slightly different prone pressure hip lift. Gordon then advocated the back pressure hip roll. In 1949, the YMCA was the first to advocate mouth-to-mouth resuscitation, the primary resuscitation method currently utilized by lifesavers.

A closer analysis of mouth-to-mouth vs. manual respiration methods is useful. Safar stated:

> The size of an average breath for an adult is 500cc. Only 350cc of this breath gets into the air spaces of the lungs. 150cc remain in dead spaces where oxygen nor CO_2 is processed. Resuscitation, therefore, must move at least 150cc with each breath in order to penetrate the lungs. Mouth to mouth with untrained resuscitators moved 1000cc and 2000cc on most victims. With experts using manual methods could not move much more than 150cc of air into the lungs.[33]

The air we breathe contains 21% oxygen. A person's exhalation is still 16% oxygen during the resuscitation process, but, with deep breathing, exhalation has approached 18% oxygen. Mouth-to-mouth has been adopted as primary life support care and continues to be the preferred method, but researchers discovered the simultaneous stimulation of respiratory and circulatory systems are essential to resuscitation. In the late 1940s, Thompson and Rockey reported that the two principal functions of resuscitation are oxygenation of the blood and the circulation of the oxygenated blood to the vital centers. As outlined in this chapter, man had been consumed with the restoration of breath and it soon became apparent that the newly oxygenated blood of mouth-to-mouth had little or no value unless this blood was moved to the vital centers and distributed over the body.

In 1961, stimulated by Safar's research, Charles E. Silvia, another pioneer in lifesaving, introduced closed chest cardiac massage in *Life Saving and Water Safety Today*. Silvia indicated that external heart massage can be combined with mouth-to-nose or mouth-to-mouth resuscitation when there is no discernible heart action or respiration. Heart massage should be used to restart the heart if it stops for a short time. If a radial (wrist) or carotid (neck) check indicates no pulse, the heart is to be massaged as follows: Place the victim on his back and if assistance is available, have him prepare the airway and start mouth-to-mouth while the rescuer places the heel of one hand on the sternum just above the bottom end and the heel of the other hand on the top of it. Alternate pushes down after each lung inflation (12 times per minute) to squeeze the heart with controlled force, keeping in mind the age and size of the rescuer and victim. Release pressure to allow the heart to fill at one second intervals about 48 times per minute. Duration of massage has varied from one to 65 minutes.[34]

As previously stated, large volumes of research on drowning occurred as a result of the two world wars and in the interest of keeping troops out of harm's way in the water. Unfortunately, the Nazi regime did most of the research on drowning during World War II. For ethical reasons, all available information will not be reported. One piece of pertinent information from that era is research confirming that drowning can result from a perforation of the eardrum. The invasion of water into the lungs through the Eustachian tube was found to cause asphyxiation. This had many implications for the military, particularly for aviators who "ditched" in the oceans.

Despite the tremendous success of Mark Spitz in the 1972 Olympic Games, interest in swimming began dissipating as the American Red Cross and other agencies started addressing other issues, thus reducing interest in and money spent on water safety (Figure 10). The net effect from the 1960s to the 1990s was that a lower percentage of the human population learned swimming and water safety. While water safety diminished in priority, competitive swimming, water polo, synchronized swimming, and diving in the Olympics rekindled world interest in aquatics every four years. Knowing how to swim as part of a lifetime activity that began as the first step of a water safety initiative started to decline. As the fitness craze developed throughout the 1970s to the 1990s, water sports were left behind. In a 1996 survey of American colleges and universities to examine this decline as it relates to higher education, the International Swimming Hall of Fame determined the following: (1) There has been a great reduction in aquatic courses taught at the collegiate level; (2) There has been a significant drop in colleges requiring a minimum swimming requirement for graduation; (3) Only water exercise and scuba classes have grown in number and participants since the 1960s.

Unlike the United States, many countries have maintained their water safety initiatives. In 1997, Saddam Hussein highlighted Iraq's national learn-to-swim campaign by swimming in the Tigris River to promote the Iraqi goal that everyone learn to swim. In the 1990s, in an effort to keep its children fit and safe, Great Britain initiated a goal that every 11-year-old be able to swim at least 25 meters.

Aquatics is largely dependent on leadership and the forum these leaders impact. Since the U.S. no longer has leaders such as Commodore Longfellow, Charles E. Silvia, and T. K. Cureton, water safety has taken a back seat to gun, boating, and fire safety. Initiative was taken in 1995 with the formation of the National Aquatic Summit, a coalition of aquatics-related organizations pursuing common goals. The most important theme of the Summit's representative organizations was that the coalition needed to work toward the goal of "Every American a Swimmer for Life." "Life" has the dual meaning of ensuring the safety of life by learning to swim and living an enjoyable and fit existence through swimming.

Competitive water sports, scuba diving, and fitness swimming have not grown proportionately to the increase in population. The aquatic groups perform better now than ever before in history, but they lack industry growth due to contemporary's society lack of orientation to water. Water safety at pools and beaches has

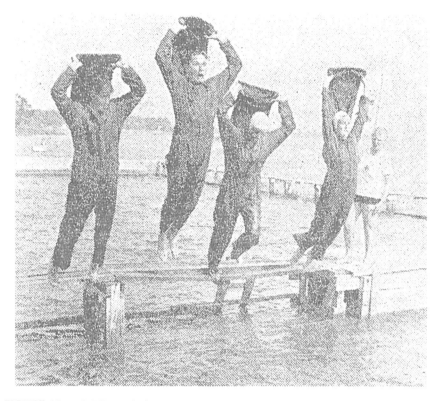

FIGURE 10   ARC Water Safety School (1960s).

advanced tremendously, but drowning remains one of the leading causes of accidental death in the United States. Families who lose loved ones to drowning often blame themselves. These families usually feel very guilty for not ensuring that their family members were water safe. They cannot accept drowning as an act of God. They have no one to cry out to or to blame. Government insensitivity to the problem contributes to the lack of interest in and attention to drowning in today's society.

The understanding of the "physiology of drowning" is somewhat more scientific today compared to 50 years ago. The humanitarian efforts of animal activists to stop the use of animals in scientific experimentation have had a negative effect on providing continued information about drowning. Today it is generally accepted that there are distinct stages of drowning: distress, panic, and submersion. The inhalation of water into the lungs is known as aspiration, and swallowing of water into the stomach is ingestion.

Four types of drowning are generally accepted among the aquatic safety community.[35] Wet drownings account for more than 80% of all drownings where water enters the lungs upon relaxation of the larynx. Osmosis and acidosis of salt or fresh water, respectively, in the drowning victim further complicate the ability of oxygen to penetrate the blood stream and necessary tissues. These processes, by themselves,

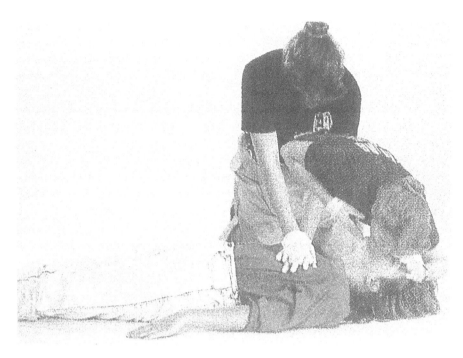

FIGURE 11   CPR can be used in all types of drowning.

known to render the victim unconscious, can further complicate the analysis of drowning. Dry drownings, which make up approximately 10% of all drownings, result when the laryngeal spasm fails to allow water to penetrate the lungs and asphyxia occurs. Secondary drowning takes place when a victim is saved from the water and delayed physiological complications occur. The fourth type of drowning, sudden drowning syndrome, refers to the death of a victim in the water from heart attack, stroke, epileptic seizure, or other problems that can also occur on land.[36]

Cardiopulmonary resuscitation (CPR) can be used in all types of drowning (Figure 11). The American Red Cross and the American Heart Association have formulated techniques that are currently used in resuscitation methods. CPR is a widely accepted technique for the layman to initiate on a drowning victim. The CPR taught today in most water safety programs represents an evolution from the 1949 version Silvia first wrote about in a lifesaving text.

The American Red Cross, in its text *CPR For The Professional Rescuer*, advocates the following steps to CPR. First, the preliminary survey is done by executing the ABCs:

"A" means airway, and is a reminder of the importance of the rescuer to insure that the airway is open from mouth and nose to the lungs. To open an unconscious victim's airway the rescuer is told to tilt the head back and lift the chin. "B" is for breathing. If the victim is breathing the chest will rise and fall upon inspection. Look, listen and feel for breathing for five seconds. "C" is for circulation. To assess the circulation check at the carotid artery for a pulse for five to 10 seconds.[37]

CPR for the rescuer also calls for the following actions: (1) Check for consciousness; (2) Check for breathing; (3) If not breathing, keep the head tilted back, pinch the nose shut, seal the rescuer's lips around the victim's mouth, give two slow breaths, each lasting one and one half seconds, and check to see if the breaths are entering the lungs; (4) Check for pulse; if none begin chest compression with the heel of the hand located two fingers higher than the zyphoid process on the sternum; position the shoulders over the hands and compress the sternum one and one half to two inches; do 15 compressions in 10 seconds; (5) Repeat the cycle of 15 compressions and two breaths; after one minute feel for a pulse and continue the process until the victim is resuscitated. Slight but significant modifications for children and infants are prescribed, as are modified techniques when two or more rescuers work on the same victim.[38]

A major obstacle to understanding the magnitude of drowning is statistical irregularities. Drowning statistics should be uniform and consistent. Many states in the United States and many countries of the world vary their definition and classifications of drowning. Generally, those in aquatics agree that death due to immersion in water should be considered a drowning, but many government agencies label cause of death due to immersion in different ways. For example, if one drowns while boating, many groups label this as a boating accident. If someone falls off a dock and drowns, many label this as a marine accident. If someone dies after 24 hours of immersion, it is labeled death due to asphyxiation or some other complication. Even with the lack of uniformity in drowning statistics, drowning is usually the third leading cause of accidental death in the United States and the second leading cause of accidental death for persons ages 5–44.[39] In warm weather states like California, Florida, and Hawaii, drowning is the leading cause of injury death in youth. Even more alarming, for every person that drowns, 14 people are treated as outpatients and 3.6 people are admitted to hospitals for treatment.[40] This translates into millions of dollars that we spend each year to treat a largely preventable problem.

From the earliest time of recorded history, societies have been preoccupied with water, swimming, and resuscitation. Mankind has attempted to reduce the frequent, often fatal, incidence of drowning. Although science has advanced the understanding of the causes and effects of drowning, governments have retreated from addressing the problem. The early lifesaving societies had the answer: lifesaving and resuscitation techniques were a partial solution, but education of the populace was the key. It is ironic that although our techniques and organizations committed to lifesaving are better than ever, drowning remains a leading cause of accidental death, particularly of children. The public must demand that governments assist in education and public awareness campaigns. When the nations of the world adopt aggressive policies of education, the tragedy of drowning will be greatly reduced as all citizens learn how to swim, water safety, how to perform water rescue, and how to resuscitate their fellow human beings. Then, and only then, will mankind finally adapt to its world of two thirds water.

REFERENCES

1. Office of Naval Operations, *Swimming*, U.S. Naval Institute, 1944, p. 3.
2. Office of Naval Operations, p. 3.
3. Kenneth Barker, ed., *NIV Study Bible*, Zondervan Publishing, Grand Rapids, MI, 1984, p. 524
4. Peter V. Karpovich, *Adventures in Artificial Respiration*, Association Press, New York, 1953, p. 9.
5. Ralph Thomas, *Swimming*, Samson, Law, Marston & Co., London, 1904.
6. Thomas.
7. Cecil M. Colwin, *Swimming into the 21st Century*, Human Kinetics, Champaign, IL, 1993, p. 5.
8. Karpovich, p. 4.
9. Karpovich, p. 11.
10. Karpovich, p. 12.
11. Karpovich, p. 18.
12. Karpovich, p. 117.
13. Charles E. Silvia, *Lifesaving and Water Safety Today*, Association Press, New York, 1974, p. 134.
14. Karpovich, p. 17.
15. Silvia, p. 134.
16. Karpovich, p. 21.
17. Karpovich, p. 15.
18. M. A. Howe, *The Humane Society of the Commonwealth of Massachusetts*, Riverside Press, 1918.
19. Karpovich, p. 117.
20. Silvia, p. 134.
21. Silvia, p. 135.
22. Silvia.
23. Karpovich.
24. Karpovich, p. 28.
25. Buck Dawson, *Weissmuller to Spitz*, 1972, p. 12.
26. Dawson, p. 20.
27. Colwin, p. 6.
28. Silvia.
29. Silvia.
30. Chris Brewster, ed., *USLA Manual of Open Water Lifesaving*, p. 11.
31. Silvia, p. 19.
32. Silvia.
33. Peter Safar and Martin C. McMahan, *Resuscitation of an Unconscious Victim*, Springfield, IL, 1959.
34. Silvia.
35. Brewster, p. 75.
36. American Red Cross, *CPR for the Professional Rescuer*, Human Kinetics, Champaign, IL, p. 52.
37. *CPR for the Professional Rescuer.*
38. *CPR for the Professional Rescuer*, p. 142.
39. Brewster, p. 72.
40. Brewster.

2 Etiology and Treatment of Drowning

Jerome H. Modell

A treatise, published in Scandinavia in 1796, describes a method for resuscitating drowned persons by placing the tip of a hand-operated bellows into the patient's mouth and then squeezing the bellows rhythmically.[1] If the victim did not respond appropriately, pushing on the middle of the victim's chest was recommended. This maneuver, supposedly, is to expel air from the chest, and the purpose of the bellows is to inflate the chest. This method, crude as it may sound, is similar in principle to the mouth-to-mouth ventilation and closed-chest cardiac massage described in 1960 by Kouwenhoven, Jude, and Knickerbocker.[2] Between the publications of these two methods other techniques were advocated, including blowing smoke into the rectum of the victim to stimulate breathing,[1] rolling the victim over a barrel in a rocking motion, and the external chest compression method of artificial respiration.

Among the many descriptions of what occurs when a person drowns is Lowson's account. Lowson, a physician, survived a shipwreck in 1892, and later published his very vivid description of awakening underwater with a crushing, burning sensation in his chest, and swallowing what he thought were large amounts of water in order to avoid the urge to breathe while submerged.[3] After losing consciousness, Lowson apparently surfaced, began breathing, and thus survived the episode. In 1933, Karpovich described what he believed to be the stages of drowning, based in part on his observations of animals.[4] Karpovich reported an immediate struggle for freedom, suspension of movement, exhalation of a little air, frequent swallowing, and then a violent physical attempt at freedom by the victim, using arms and legs to stay at the surface or remove himself from the water, during which time fear and panic are elicited. He then postulated that the victim suffers convulsions, exhalation of air and spasmodic inspiratory efforts, disappearance of reflexes, and death. The vocal cords, reflexly, go into laryngospasm to protect the airway from aspiration of water. Finally, after the victim loses consciousness, the laryngospasm relents, and the victim breathes water, prior to suffering cessation of respiration and cardiac activity.

In my experience treating and/or consulting on over 100 near-drowning cases, I have interviewed several persons at the scene of drowning accidents. Karpovich's description of events rarely applies. Observers more often report that they just observed the victims motionless underwater, observed them to jump or dive into the water never to resurface, or observed the victim hyperventilating and then swimming underwater only to become suddenly motionless and seem to be floating while submerged. There is, then, no "classic" description of a drowning or near-drowning episode. Some persons, indeed, do find themselves suddenly in an aqueous environment when they cannot swim and appear to panic or struggle in what is termed the "fight for survival." More often than not, however, the victim does not fit into this category. Some victims dive into shallow bodies of water and hit their heads on the bottom of the pool or some other hard object, suffer a concussion, lose consciousness, are unable to help themselves, and aspirate water. Others suffer severe injury to their cervical spinal cords, resulting in paralysis of their arms and legs. Others become disoriented while submerged in muddy or unclear water and swim in the wrong direction until they no longer can remain conscious. Still others hyperventilate, hold their breath, and then attempt to swim for long periods of time underwater. In this latter case, arterial carbon dioxide tension is decreased to very low levels, thus prolonging the interval from beginning of breath-holding until the irresistible urge to breathe.[5–8] Since there is no significant increase in arterial oxygenation during hyperventilation, the victims' ability to maintain an adequate amount of oxygen in the blood that can perfuse and oxygenate the brain is not prolonged commensurate with their breath-holding or ability to suppress the carbon dioxide-induced drive to breathe. These individuals then lose consciousness, after which they breathe underwater and aspirate water into their lungs, what many term the "hyperventilation syndrome" or "shallow water blackout."

A significant number of teenagers and adults show evidence of having ingested alcoholic beverages, which likely compromised their ability to perform swimming maneuvers in an effective manner.[9] Still others suffer a medical event, such as a seizure, syncope, or heart attack, and become submerged and then asphyxiate, unable to protect themselves in an aqueous environment. Finally, victims of foul play are found in the water, although they may have been unconscious or deceased prior to entering the water. A myriad of environmental situations may result in drownings or near-drownings.

The terminology surrounding this tragedy can also be confusing. By definition, "drowned" means the individual died secondary to being submerged in an aqueous environment.[10–11] It is possible to drown without aspiration, in which case water is not aspirated into the lungs. This can occur if the patient undergoes laryngospasm while submerged, and cardiac arrest occurs without the victim taking an intervening breath. Approximately 10% of drowned victims are thought to have drowned without aspiration.[12] The real incidence of drowning without aspiration actually may be lower since such a diagnosis can be confused with that of someone who suffers foul play and then enters the water or someone who suffers sudden cardiac death. The remaining victims are those who drown with aspiration, i.e., water actively enters the lungs. This occurs when the individual breathes while submerged. Although some have postulated that the lungs may become "filled" with water after death,[13] this is not compatible with autopsy findings in drowned victims where very little evidence of water may be seen in the lungs. I believe, therefore, that for water to enter the lungs in more than insignificant quantities, active breathing must have occurred while the victim was submerged.

The term "near-drowning" refers to one who has survived, at least for a time, after a submersion episode.[10-11] Near-drowning can occur both with and without aspiration of water in approximately the same percentage as drowned victims for each category.

Animal studies of Swann and associates in the 1940s suggest that severe electrolyte changes occur during submersion and that those changes are directly related to the cause of death.[14-15] Experience in treating human near-drowning victims suggests that this is not the case; very few of those individuals demonstrate significant abnormalities in serum electrolyte concentration as measured in the emergency room of the hospital.[16] Subsequent studies suggest that the volume of water aspirated by humans is relatively small compared to the animals that Swann studied under conditions of total immersion. These studies have clearly demonstrated that the electrolyte changes that might occur with the aspiration of water are directly proportional to the amount of water aspirated.[17-18] Further, when we compared serum electrolyte changes after aspiration of water in an anesthetized animal model with those seen at autopsy in humans, 85% of human drowning victims aspirated only 22 ml/kg of water or less.[19] Thus, serum electrolyte changes are not an important factor in determining survival after submersion. Based on evaluations of serum electrolyte and blood gas analyses of near-drowned patients, the same statistics apply to them as well.

The foremost problems confronting both the drowned and the near-drowned victim are the consequences of hypoxemia and the resulting metabolic acidosis that occurs secondary to a submersion event. Through correlation of observations in humans and results obtained in anesthetized animal models, it is believed that, based on arterial oxygen levels, unless there are other complicating medical factors, it would be unusual for humans submerged for a minute or less not to survive spontaneously with normal cerebral function if they are removed from the water by that time. Likewise, in the event that they have suffered apnea, the prognosis is excellent if respiration is restored immediately. By three minutes of submersion, arterial oxygen tension falls to a level that is incompatible with the normal individual maintaining consciousness.[20] These individuals may also suffer respiratory and cardiac arrest. Prompt restoration of spontaneous ventilation and circulation using basic cardiopulmonary resuscitation usually results in survival if appropriate and definitive therapy is made available in a timely fashion. Those rescued after a submersion episode of three to five minutes are subject to a more severe degree of cerebral hypoxia. In these individuals, although cardiopulmonary resuscitation is often effective at re-establishing spontaneous ventilation and circulation, there is considerable likelihood that these individuals may suffer some type of permanent neurologic impairment. The incidence of such complications usually is directly related to the length of submersion.[21]

Recovery has been reported in persons submerged for from five to ten minutes; however, in this group, more likely than not, normal neurologic function will not return completely. With resuscitation after a submersion episode of at least ten minutes, complete restoration of normal brain function is very uncommon unless the submersion episode has occurred in very cold water.

During submersion in very cold water, if the victim aspirates water or if a significant portion of the body surface area is in contact with the water, very rapid body cooling will occur and tolerance to hypoxia will be significantly prolonged.[22] Remember, it is not the temperature of the water alone, but the resulting temperature of the victim that is important in determining whether survival with normal brain function will occur after prolonged submersion in cold water because hypothermia decreases the requirement for oxygen. For every degree Centigrade that body temperature drops, there is approximately a 7–9% decrease in oxygen required. Thus, when profound, rapid cooling occurs, it protects the brain and other vital organs from hypoxic injury. Hypothermia is a double-edged sword, however, since, as the heart cools, it is more subject to fatal arrhythmias. Once a body temperature below 28°C occurs, for example, ventricular arrhythmia resulting in an inadequate cardiac output is quite common.

It should be obvious that normal survival should be expected if effective cardiopulmonary resuscitation is performed prior to the time the patient suffers irreversible neurologic hypoxic damage and if the patient has not aspirated water in amounts that alter lung function.

It is well known that drowning and near-drowning victims frequently experience apnea or cessation of respiration before they suffer cardiac arrest. They also frequently display a severe bradycardia, or slowed heartbeat, and peripheral vasoconstriction. Thus, if effective mouth-to-mouth ventilation is performed, the heart may become reoxygenated, pulse rate will increase, and there will be better tissue perfusion. In this situation, closed-chest cardiac massage is not necessary.

After freshwater aspiration, the water is absorbed very rapidly from the alveoli into the circulation because the water is hypotonic. However, the surface tension of pulmonary surfactant, which is a material lining the alveoli of the lungs, is significantly altered so that those alveoli are less likely to remain open upon exhalation.[23] Thus, there is a decrease in the ventilation-perfusion ratio or even atelectasis, which results in "shunting" of blood past alveoli that are poorly ventilated, or not ventilated, but perfused. Because these alveoli cannot effectively participate in gas exchange, the victim is unable to oxygenate his/her blood in those areas of the lung. This results in arterial hypoxemia, which may compromise the viability of the individual. After seawater aspiration, arterial hypoxemia also occurs secondary to intrapulmonary shunting, although the mechanism is different. Seawater, being hypertonic, draws fluid from the circulation into the lung, and results in fluid-filled but perfused alveoli, which are incapable of normal gas exchange.[17,24]

Understanding these physiologic changes in the lung is important so that the physician is able to apply the proper methods of intensive pulmonary care necessary to restore more normal pulmonary function. Such care includes the administration of oxygen, mechanical support of ventilation, and the application of positive pressure to the airway, either as positive end-expiratory pressure in persons who require mechanical ventilation, or as continuous positive airway pressure in persons who are permitted to breathe spontaneously for a portion of the respiratory cycle. Application of positive pressure to the airway is aimed at increasing functional residual capacity, better matching ventilation-to-perfusion ratios,[24–28] decreasing the amount of intrapulmonary shunting, and, thus, improving arterial oxygenation. The exact pattern of mechanical ventilatory support and the duration it is required will be judged by the treating physician based on the patient's response to therapy. The patient should be able to oxygenate his or her blood and to eliminate the carbon dioxide.

Because of the fluid shifts that occur across the alveolar-capillary interface in the lung, persons who aspirate substantial amounts of freshwater will usually develop acute hypervolemia.[18] However, within an hour there is redistribution of fluid and pulmonary edema occurs, which results in a decreased circulating blood volume.[28] After seawater aspiration, because of the hypertonic effect of the seawater, pulmonary edema occurs rapidly, usually within three minutes, and results in decreased circulating blood volume.[17] For both freshwater- and seawater-aspiration patients, it may be necessary to intravenously replace substantial volumes of fluid, while the effective circulating blood volume and resulting cardiac output are monitored. Treating the lungs may result in good arterial oxygenation of blood, but, without adequate cardiac output, the blood cannot reach the peripheral tissues to provide them with nutrients.[28]

Even if the patient regains consciousness, this is not a guarantee that the patient will recover completely. Some patients suffer significant pulmonary infection or sufficient damage to the lung to cause adult respiratory distress syndrome (ARDS), which further complicates pulmonary therapy. Such individuals may die of pulmonary insufficiency, regardless of the level and type of therapy applied. At one time it was considered therapeutic to administer intravenous corticosteroids to decrease the inflammation caused by the aspirated liquid.[29] This has been shown to be ineffective,[30] however, and may result in an altered ability of the body to isolate areas of infection in the lung.[31] Hemolysis of red blood cells and changes in renal function have been reported but, at a clinically significant level, these are rare.[32]

Exactly how long a drowning or near-drowning victim has been submerged is hardly ever known. The degree of arterial hypoxemia and, therefore, the potential for brain damage and cardiac arrest, are directly proportional to the duration of time from the onset of submersion to the administration of effective resuscitative measures. Since ventilation usually stops before circulation, it is prudent to begin mouth-to-mouth ventilation as soon as possible, preferably in the water, if the rescuer is able to perform mouth-to-mouth ventilation without putting himself or herself at risk. If effective mouth-to-mouth ventilation is performed and the victim's heart is still beating, there will be improved oxygenation of the myocardium followed by an increase in cardiac output. If the victim has not aspirated water, a prompt, full recovery may be expected. If the victim has aspirated water, alteration of pulmonary function will undoubtedly occur and further therapy will be necessary. If the rescuer cannot feel a pulse, closed-chest cardiac massage, in addition to mouth-to-mouth ventilation, is imperative.

While some have advocated the use of the abdominal thrust, or Heimlich Maneuver, in the treatment of near-drowned victims,[13] I agree with the American Heart Association,[33] the American Red Cross, and the Institute of Medicine's[34] findings, namely, that basic cardiopulmonary resuscitation is the preferred therapy. I further believe that the use of the Heimlich Maneuver may increase the interval before administration of effective CPR, thereby potentially increasing the duration of cerebral hypoxia. Furthermore, with an abdominal thrust maneuver, it is unlikely that a significant quantity of water will be expelled from the lungs. This is particularly true in freshwater near-drowning where the water is absorbed very rapidly from the lungs into the circulation. If water is expelled, it is more likely swallowed water from the stomach. Should the victim take a breath during the time the water is being expelled, he or she may aspirate this material, thus compounding pulmonary injury and complicating the aspiration of water with the aspiration of stomach contents, which, in general, produces a more severe lesion.[35]

Since the poolside observer frequently does not know whether or not aspiration has occurred, it is prudent that all near-drowning victims be transported by appropriate rescue vehicle to an emergency room facility, where a physician can examine the patient and perform laboratory tests, as needed, to evaluate the severity of the injury and the treatment indicated.

When emergency medical technicians arrive, it is important that they evaluate the patient to determine what type of further emergency therapy is necessary. I believe that all near-drowning victims should be given supplemental oxygen en route to the hospital since it is not possible for the initial responders to know with certainty the adequacy of the patient's arterial oxygenation. If the patient is awake and talking, that is a very positive sign; however, one does not know how close the patient may be to losing consciousness due to a slight further drop in arterial oxygen tension. If the patient is not able to maintain an airway, then that airway must be supported manually by the emergency medical technician; the need for an oropharyngeal airway or even endotracheal intubation should be evaluated. It should be remembered, however, that if the patient has active oropharyngeal reflexes, inserting an oropharyngeal airway may lead to laryngospasm or to vomiting with subsequent aspiration of stomach contents. Endotracheal intubation should be attempted only by those who are skilled in the technique and then the patient should be thoroughly evaluated to ensure that the endotracheal tube is properly placed in the trachea rather than in the esophagus or one of the mainstem bronchi. Demonstrating carbon dioxide on exhalation is highly desirable as a method of confirming tracheal placement of the tube. At a minimum, however, the laryngoscopist must listen over both sides of the patient's chest and the epigastrium to check for proper placement of the endotracheal tube.

Transmitting the patient's electrocardiogram via telemetry to the hospital is useful in helping the emergency medical technician to determine whether significant cardiac arrhythmias are present. Obviously, blood pressure should be measured and inotropic support administered, if indicated. In my experience, however, support of the circulation of the near-drowning victim with inotropic agents is usually not necessary if adequate oxygenation is achieved. An intravenous line should be started so that the emergency medical technician has access to the circulation should the administration of intravenous drugs be necessary. The patient should be monitored with pulse oximetry if the appropriate equipment is available in the rescue vehicle. For patients who are not adequately oxygenated as evidenced by pulse oximetry, the application of positive airway pressure may be used if the appropriate equipment is available and the emergency medical technician is familiar with its use and potential complications.

Once the patient arrives at the hospital, arterial blood gas tensions and pH should be measured in order to ensure that there is adequate arterial oxygenation and carbon dioxide removal. The pH of the blood will indicate whether there remains a metabolic acidosis secondary to a significant period of hypoxia. Respiratory acidosis, if it exists, also will become evident. A metabolic acidosis resulting in a pH of less than 7.2 should be treated with sodium bicarbonate; however, a pH above 7.2 is probably best left to correct itself, provided the patient has adequate circulation and respiration either spontaneously or artificially.

Any question regarding the adequacy of the patient's effective circulating blood volume can be evaluated by a central venous catheter or preferably a pulmonary artery catheter, which will give the clinician the opportunity to evaluate pulmonary artery occlusion pressure and, thus, guide further fluid therapy. An echocardiogram may be useful for this purpose as well. Initial laboratory evaluation should consist of arterial blood gas measurements, a hemoglobin or hematocrit, plasma hemoglobin concentration, and serum electrolyte concentrations; urinalysis should also be performed. It is unlikely that a significant abnormality in any of the above tests, other than the blood gas results, will be seen unless the victim has aspirated a substantial quantity of water. This occurs in less than 15% of the population.[19] The magnitude of intensive respiratory support, cardiovascular support, and fluid administration required will depend on the individual patient and must be left to the judgment of the intensivist physician responsible for the patient's hospital care.

It is important to realize that there is no single clinical observation or laboratory test available at the scene of the accident that permits one to predict with certainty the outcome of the patient.[36] This becomes particularly difficult in the comatose patient because one does not want to withhold therapy from any patient who has a chance of normal survival. On the other hand, prolonged intensive therapy administered to the patient who has irreversible brain damage takes a significant toll on friends and relatives, in addition to being extremely costly. Perhaps the most reliable single indicator of whether the victim can regain normal brain function is appropriate response to evoked potential monitoring.[37] This technique, however, requires special equipment within the hospital and is not available either at the scene or in transit to the hospital. Knowing there is no single clinical observation or test that will accurately and uniformly predict survival or brain death,[36] near-drowned patients who are awake and alert when they arrive in the emergency room have been reported in two studies to have a 100% normal survival rate.[38–39] Occasionally, however, such an individual will die, usually from progressive pulmonary complications. Patients who have a blunted level of consciousness upon arrival at the emergency room have a survival rate of approximately 90%.[38] It is patients who are comatose upon arrival at the emergency room who are most likely to subsequently die or live with significant incapacitating brain damage. In this particular group of patients, the normal survival rate was in the 40–50% range, unless they were flaccid upon admission to the emergency room, or were still in a state of cardiac arrest, in which case the prognosis is very grim, with a survival rate of 7% at best.[38–39]

Although it is not the purpose of this chapter to discuss pool safety, I feel very strongly that pools should have a protective enclosure that minimizes the risk of someone inadvertently entering the water. I also firmly believe that young children should be taught to swim so that they can remove themselves from the water should they accidently fall in.

When someone in a pool is submerged, all too frequently bystanders and even some professional lifeguards assume the victim is not in distress but rather "horsing around." Whenever someone is submerged and not making purposeful movements it should be assumed that he or she is in serious trouble and that person should be removed from the water immediately.

Finally, I would like to condemn the teaching of hyperventilation prior to underwater swimming as a method by which one can prolong breath-holding, and thus increase time under water. This potentially lethal exercise should be avoided by prudent people.

REFERENCES

1. Herholdt, J. D. and Rafn, C. G., *An attempt at a historical survey of life-saving measures for drowning persons and information of the best means by which they can again be brought back to life*, H. Tikiob's Bookseller, Copenhagen, 1796.
2. Kouwenhoven, W. B., Jude, J. R., and Knickerbocker, G. G., "Closed-chest cardiac massage," *JAMA* 173:1064, 1960.
3. Lowson, J. A., "Sensations in drowning," *Edinburgh Med. J.* 13:41–45, 1903.
4. Karpovich, P. V., "Water in the lungs of drowned animals," *Arch. Path.* 15:828–833, 1933.
5. Craig, A. B., Jr., "Underwater swimming and loss of consciousness," *JAMA* 176:255–258, 1961.
6. Craig, A. B., Jr., "Causes of loss of consciousness during underwater swimming," *J. Appl. Physiol.* 16:583–586, 1961.
7. Dumitru, A. P. and Hamilton, F. G., "A mechanism of drowning," *Anesth. Analg.* 42:170–176, 1963.
8. Modell, J. H., "Resuscitation after aspiration of chlorinated fresh water," *JAMA* 185:651–655, 1963.
9. Modell, J. H., *Pathophysiology and treatment of drowning and near-drowning*, Thomas, Springfield, 1971, pp. 74–82.
10. Modell, J. H., *Pathophysiology and treatment of drowning and near-drowning*, Thomas, Springfield, 1971, pp. 8–12.
11. Modell, J. H., "Drown vs. near-drown: a discussion of definitions," *Crit. Care. Med.* 9:351–352, 1981.
12. Cot, C., *Les asphyxies accidentelles (submersion, électrocution, intoxication oxycarbonique). Étude clinique, thérapeutique et préventive*, Éditions Medicales N. Maloinc, Paris, 1931.
13. Heimlich, H. J., "Subdiaphragmatic pressure to expel water from lungs of drowning persons," *Ann. Emerg. Med.* 10:476–480, 1981.
14. Swann, H. G. and Brucer, M., "The cardiorespiratory and biochemical events during rapid anoxic death. VI. Fresh water and sea water drowning," *Tex. Rep. Biol. Med.* 7:604–618, 1949.

15. Swann, H. G., Brucer M., Moore, C., and Vezien, B. L., "Fresh water and sea water drowning: a study of the terminal cardiac and biochemical events," *Tex. Rep. Biol. Med.* 5:423–437, 1947.

16. Modell, J. H., Graves, S. A., and Ketover, A, "Clinical course of 91 consecutive near-drowning victims," *Chest* 70:231–238, 1976.

17. Modell, J. H., Moya F., Newby, E. J., Ruiz, B. C., and Showers, A. V., "The effects of fluid volume in seawater drowning," *Ann. Intern. Med.* 67:68–80, 1967.

18. Modell, J. H. and Moya F., "Effects of volume of aspirated fluid during chlorinated fresh water drowning," *Anesthesiology* 27:662–672, 1966.

19. Modell, J. H. and Davis, J. H., "Electrolyte changes in human drowning victims," *Anesthesiology* 30:414–420, 1969.

20. Modell, J. H., Kuck, E. J., Ruiz, B. C., and Heinitsh, H., "Effect of intravenous vs. aspirated distilled water on serum electrolytes and blood gas tensions," *J. Appl. Physiol.* 23:579–584, 1972.

21. Modell, J. H., "Drowning," *N. Engl. J. Med.* 328:253–256, 1993.

22. Biggart, M. J. and Bohn, D. J., "Effect of hypothermia and cardiac arrest on outcome of near-drowning accidents in children," *J. Pediatr.* 117:179–183, 1990.

23. Giammona, S. T. and Modell, J. H., "Drowning by total immersion. Effects on pulmonary surfactant of distilled water, isotonic saline and sea water," *Am. J. Dis. Child* 114:612–616, 1967.

24. Modell, J. H., Calderwood, H. W., Ruiz, B. C., Downs, J. B., and Chapman, R., Jr., "Effects of ventilatory patterns on arterial oxygenation after near-drowning in sea water," *Anesthesiology* 40:376–384, 1974.

25. Modell, J. H., Moya, F., Williams, H. D., and Weibley, T. C., "Changes in blood gases and A-aDO$_2$ during near-drowning," *Anesthesiology* 29:456–465, 1968.

26. Ruiz, B. C., Calderwood, H. W., Modell, J. H., and Brogdon, J. E., "Effect of ventilatory patterns on arterial oxygenation after near-drowning with fresh water: comparative study in dogs," *Anesth. Analg.* 52:570–576, 1973.

27. Berquist, R. E., Vogelhut, M. M., Modell, J. H., Sloan, S. J., and Ruiz, B. C., "Comparison of ventilatory patterns in treatment of fresh water near drowning in dogs," *Anesthesiology* 52:142–148, 1980.

28. Tabeling, B. B. and Modell, J. H., "Fluid administration increases oxygen delivery during continuous positive pressure ventilation after fresh water near drowning," *Crit. Care Med.* 11:693–696, 1983.

29. Modell, J. H., Davis, J. H., Giammona, S. T., Moya, F., and Mann, J. B., "Blood gas and electrolyte changes in human near-drowning victims," *JAMA* 203:337–343, 1968.

30. Calderwood, H. W., Modell, J. H., and Ruiz, B. C., "Ineffectiveness of steroid therapy for treatment of fresh-water near drowning," *Anesthesiology* 43:642–650, 1975.

31. Wynne, J. W., Reynolds, J. C., Hood, I., Auerbach, D., and Ondrasick, J., "Steroid therapy for pneumonitis induced in rabbits by aspiration of foodstuff," *Anesthesiology* 51:11–19, 1979.

32. Munroe, W. D., "Hemoglobinuria from near-drowning," *J. Pediatr.* 64:57–62, 1964.

33. American Heart Association, "Standards and guidelines for cardiopulmonary resuscitation (CPR) and emergency cardiac care (ECC): Special resuscitation situations," *JAMA* 26:2242–2250, 1992.

34. Rozen, P., Stoto, M., and Harley, J., Eds., *The use of the Heimlich maneuver in near-drowning.* Committee on the treatment of near-drowning victims, Division of Health Promotion and Disease Prevention. Institute of Medicine, Washington, DC, August 1994.

35. Modell, J. H., "Is the Heimlich maneuver appropriate as first treatment for drowning," editorial, *Emerg. Med. Serv.* 10:63–64, 66, 1981.
36. Modell, J. H., "Drowning: to treat or not to treat? — an unanswerable question," editorial, *Crit. Care Med.* 21:313–315, 1993.
37. Goodwin, S. R., Friedman, W. A., and Bellefleur, M., "Is it time to use evoked potentials to predict outcome in comatose children and adults?" *Crit. Care Med.* 19:518–524, 1991.
38. Modell, J. H., Graves, S. A., and Kuck, E. J., "Near-drowning — correlation of level of consciousness and survival," *Can. Anaesth. Soc. J.* 27:211–215, 1980.
39. Conn, A. W., Montes, J. E., Barker, G. A., and Edmonds, J. F., "Cerebral salvage in near-drowning following neurological classification by triage," *Can. Anaesth. Soc. J.* 27:201–210, 1980.

3 What is Happening with Drowning Rates in the United States?

Christine M. Branche

Between 1988 and 1992, U.S. drowning rates declined steadily. In 1993, however, they suddenly rose by 4.8%, claiming the lives of 4,390 persons. Why did the rates decline during those five years and then increase sharply? Was 1993 a statistical outlier, or did certain circumstances or interventions play a role in this sharp increase? Are changes in drowning rates uniform across all groups of individuals? Are drowning rates the same in all recreational waters?

Before we can answer these questions, we must examine the major risk factors for drowning — age, sex, race, and setting — and a number of behavioral risk factors. Only then can we begin to understand the complexities of recent drowning trends and develop appropriate interventions. First, let us review some important background information.

BACKGROUND

Drowning is the fourth leading cause of unintentional injury death in the United States after motor vehicle crashes, falls, and fires. In addition to claiming thousands of lives each year, drowning contributes to enormous healthcare costs. Rescue, hospitalization, and rehabilitation costs associated with drownings and near-drownings totaled $2.5 billion dollars in 1985 alone (Rice et al. 1989).

To provide a better indication of the impact of the costs, let us examine data from one state. Recent data from a California Department of Health study (1992 drowning rate was 1.6 per 100,000 population) showed that total charges for initial hospitalization, excluding physician's fees, were $11.4 million (Ellis and Trent 1995).

Until 1993, drowning rates* (per 100,000 population) have been declining since 1986 (Figure 1) from a high of 2.38 (5,700 drownings) in 1986 to 1.65 (4,186 drownings) in 1992. Preliminary data indicates that 1993 was an unusual year for

---

* Age-adjusted rates exclude data on persons of unknown age. The standard population is based on the U.S. population in 1940, all races and both sexes. Data sources: National Center for Health Statistics mortality data tapes for number of deaths; U.S. Bureau of the Census populations estimates (intercensual data are used for 1984–1989, and decennial census data are used for 1990). Demo-detail postcensual population estimates are used for 1991–1992.

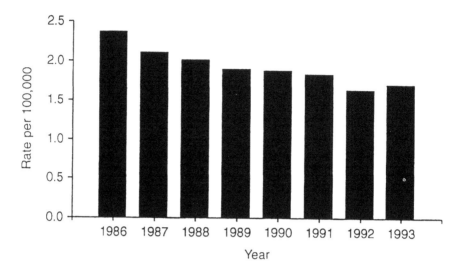

FIGURE 1   U.S. drowning rates 1986–1993.

drownings. There were 4,390 drownings (1.72 per 100,000 population), reflecting a 96% increase over 1992 and a reversal of previous trends.

RISK FACTORS

When we take a closer look at recent drowning rates, we see that trends vary in different populations. As we examine these trends, we can begin to understand why differences occur. Let us focus on the four main covariates, or risk factors, for drowning rates: age, sex, race, and setting.

AGE

From 1986 through 1993, drowning rates for each age group have followed the same general trend: drowning rates fell over time; mortality data from selected years confirm this trend (Figure 2). Drowning rates are highest mainly for two age groups: children under 5 years of age, and persons 15–24 years of age (Branche-Dorsey et al. 1994; Brenner et al. 1994; Gulaid and Sattin 1988). Persons aged 85 or older generally have the next highest drowning rates, but the numbers of death are usually small, with an average of 70 deaths for 1986–1993. This trend has remained virtually unchanged for many years. High drowning rates among small children, adolescents, and young adults result from many different factors. Risk factors for drowning differ by age. Drownings among young children usually occur in water sources around the household, including bathtubs, buckets, toilets, large puddles, and swimming pools (Robertson et al. 1992); this is true in both rural and urban settings. Small children can drown in as little as one inch of liquid, and in only 30 seconds (American Red Cross 1995). As is true for other types of unintentional injury and death, lapses in adult supervision caused by chores, socializing, or phone calls, for example, are

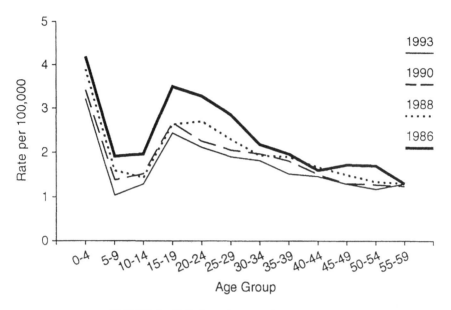

FIGURE 2   U.S. drowning rates by age group.

implicated in most drowning incidents among children under five years of age (Robertson et al. 1992). The danger of drowning also increases with the number of young children present because of the difficulty of supervising several children at once. In one study of bathtub drownings involving young children, all of the drownings occurred while the victim was bathing with a younger sibling (Jensen et al. 1992). A lapse in adult supervision, furthermore, does not have to be long — young victims were out of sight for five or fewer minutes in one study of pool drownings (Present 1987).

Among adolescents and adults, drowning occurs during swimming, wading, and boating in natural bodies of water, particularly when alcohol is involved (Patetta and Biddinger 1988; Wintemute et al. 1988). An estimated 40–45% of drownings in these age groups occur during swimming (Dietz and Baker 1974; CDC 1986), whereas 12–29% are associated with boating (Dietz and Baker 1974; Gulaid and Sattin 1988). The risk factors that contribute to the role of age in drowning have been consistent over time. Such risk factors include drinking alcohol, swimming alone, and not wearing a personal flotation device while engaged in water sports or recreation.

Sex

Drowning rates have fallen in general for both sexes, but with more dramatic decreases for males than for females (Figure 3). Drowning rates, however, were almost five times greater for males than for females during the years 1987–1993, whereas in previous years, they were only four times greater (Gulaid and Sattin 1988). This male–female difference is evident in every year from childhood through older age (Wintemute et al. 1988).

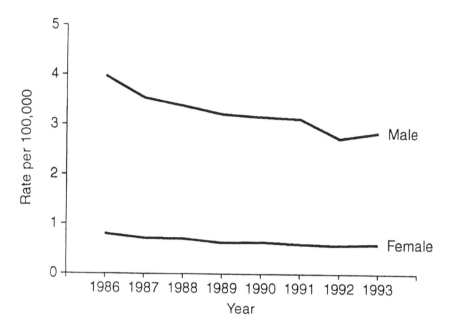

FIGURE 3   U.S. drowning rates by sex.

The increased risk for males is primarily related to alcohol consumption. Alcohol use is a well-documented risk factor in drowning and other fatalities occurring during water recreation (CDC 1987; Howland et al. 1990). A summary of studies showed that 25–50% of adult drowning victims were exposed to alcohol at the time of death (Howland and Hingson 1988; Hingson and Howland 1993). In one study of drowning, as many as 47% of adult victims were positive for alcohol at autopsy (Hingson and Howland 1993). In a national survey on the use of alcohol during aquatic activity, men reported consuming more alcoholic beverages than women, with a mean of 4.5 alcoholic beverages compared with 2.9 for women on their last reported day on or near the water (CDC 1993). Alcohol can reduce body temperature and, through its effect on the central nervous system, can impair swimming ability (CDC 1990). Because alcohol use affects vision, balance, and movement, it is a risk factor for injury and death for swimmers, boat operators, and passengers, who can fall overboard while intoxicated (Howland and Hingson 1988; Howland et al. 1993).

RACE

Race is a demographic curiosity in the overall assessment of drowning rates in the United States (Figure 4). During 1986–1992, drowning rates fell, and this trend was true generally for all racial groups, except African-American (*Black*) males (Figure 5), *Other* males, and *Other* females.* These three groups experienced erratic

---

* The National Center for Health Statistics uses *White, Black,* and *Other* (Asian, Pacific Islander, American Indian, Alaska Native) as broad racial categories.

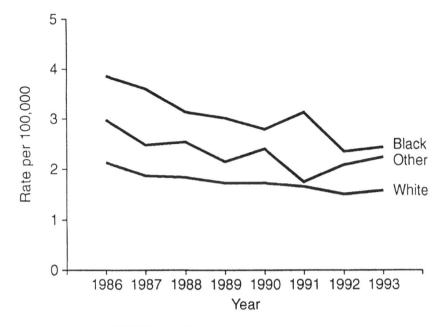

FIGURE 4   U.S. drowning rates by racial group.

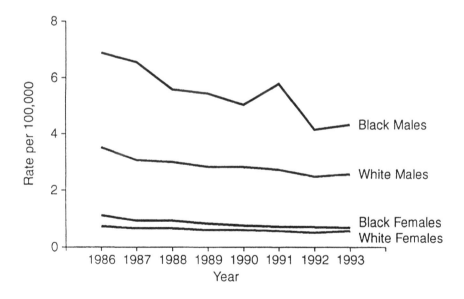

FIGURE 5   U.S. drowning rates by sex and racial group.

rises and falls in rates throughout the eight-year period, and this pattern was most pronounced among African-American males.

Drowning rates among African-Americans are twice those among white Americans (Wintemute et al. 1987; Gulaid and Sattin 1988) (Figure 4); however, this is not true for all age groups. For example, white American children aged 1–4 years have twice the drowning rate as do African-American children of these ages, largely because of drownings in residential swimming pools, which are not typically available to minority children in the United States. But for children aged 5–19 years, African-Americans drown two to four times more often than white Americans (Rodriguez and Brown 1990). In one study of drowning among African-American and Hispanic children 0–19 years of age, drownings among Hispanic children exceeded drownings among white American children by as much as 19% (Warneke and Cooper 1994).

Among American Indians and Alaskan Natives, drowning rates fell from 7.2 in 1987 to 5.7 in 1992, but they remained higher than rates for African-Americans. Data from U.S. Indian Health Service Areas shows that drowning rates for most areas were similar, except in the Alaska area, where rates were four times higher than the Indian Health Service area with the next highest rate. Drowning rates were high among young American Indian and Alaskan native children, and those aged 15–34 years. Males experience the highest rates, seven times higher than rates for American Indian and Alaskan native females and two times higher than for African-Americans. American Indians and Alaskan natives have such high drowning rates for several reasons, including common use of natural waterways for daily activities, alcohol use, and limited access to emergency rescue and trauma care services.

But is it race or ethnicity alone that is a risk factor for drowning? Research indicates that race may determine buoyancy or other physiological differences but not ability to learn to swim (Mael 1995). Learning to swim requires access to water on a regular basis, and such access has not always been available to everyone equally. Also, valuing learning to swim and choosing water recreation during leisure time would have a direct effect on drowning prevention strategies. Cultural differences may have an effect on desires to learn to swim and selecting water recreation during leisure time, and these cultural differences may explain, in part, differences in drowning rates by race.

SETTING

Differences in drowning rates in the United States reflect several factors that include climate; availability of beaches, lakes, and other natural and artificial water sources; and parks and water recreational equipment and products (e.g., personal watercraft). Overall, between one half and three quarters of drownings occur in lakes, ponds, rivers, and the ocean (Dietz and Baker 1974; CDC 1986).

Region

Drowning rates differ by region of the country. Coastal areas and regions adjacent to the southern Mississippi River have high drowning rates (Devine et al. 1990). Rates for drownings that do not involve boats are generally highest in southern and mountain states. The 1993 floods that occurred in the Mississippi River valley may have affected drowning rates for states that line the river, but evidence suggests that it was only minimal.

Alaska, Louisiana, Idaho, Arkansas, Hawaii, and South Carolina were among the states with the highest drowning rates in 1993. Alaska has the highest rate (7.67 per 100,000 population), which exceeds the rate for motor vehicle-related deaths in Alaska and is more than twice the drowning rate in the state with the next highest rate, Louisiana, with a rate of 3.70 per 100,000 population. A major factor in the extremely high rate in Alaska is the very low water temperature, which reduces a person's chance of survival after falling into the water.

Recreational Boating Sites

More than 75 million people engage in recreational (noncommercial) boating annually in the United States (U.S. Coast Guard 1995). Among enthusiasts, a variety of boating-related injuries can ensue, ranging from drownings to falls, burns, and trauma, which can precede drowning. We can expect drownings and falls overboard to be frequent outcomes (CDC 1987). In one study, lacerations were the most frequently reported boat-related injury (26.9%) (Branche-Dorsey et al. in press). Personal watercraft use is growing, and with lighter, more manageable, and less expensive models entering the market each year, many more people are using personal watercraft on all forms of natural waters. Personal watercraft use is associated with a growing number of injuries (Branche-Dorsey et al. in press) and less so with drowning; nevertheless, we must monitor the number of drownings associated with personal watercraft use, as these watercraft become more popular. We have limited data on African-Americans, their boating habits, and their drowning risks while boating, but the data available indicates that more white Americans than African-Americans drown in boating-related incidents.

Swimming Pools

Swimming pools greatly influence drowning rates in warmer climates (Baker et al. 1992). Young children account for the largest proportion of drownings in residential swimming pools (Ellis and Trent 1995). Adults often expect small children to splash and show obvious signs of distress when they are having trouble in the water, yet drowning children rarely display such signs of distress or call for help.

Water Parks

Water parks provide water recreation in large urban and remote rural areas. Water parks allow a greater opportunity for water recreation among persons who would not usually partake of water sports and recreation, and they provide water recreation facilities to millions of visitors annually. Many water park visitors classify themselves as nonswimmers (Ellis and Trent 1995). In fact, in one survey of persons rescued at water parks, 39% said they never intended to go swimming. This finding may be because many water parks are juxtaposed or contained within other large amusement parks, and many patrons go to the water park simply for relief from the summer heat when visiting other amusement parks.

Many of the persons who frequent water parks would not customarily participate in water recreation at conventional swimming pools or natural bodies of water (Ellis and Trent 1995). The simulation of surf waves without the danger of real tidal activity, as well as the flumes, slides, and other attractions, lure patrons in large numbers — up to 900,000 visitors annually in some locations (Ellis and Trent 1995). Drownings are rare at these facilities, probably because of the large number of lifeguards on staff. Where water hazards are evident (e.g., slide flumes that drop patrons into deep water), multiple guards scan the area.

PREVENTIVE STRATEGIES

Declines in drowning rates in the United States can be attributed, in part, to successful interventions and other preventive strategies. The nature of these strategies can be environmental or engineering (changing the area where water recreation occurs), educational (training water enthusiasts about dangers associated with water recreational activities), behavioral (adopting water safety practices), or legislative (adopting and enforcing policies that protect the public from unacceptable risks).

SUPERVISING YOUNG CHILDREN

Parents need to constantly supervise their young children around all household and outdoor water sources to prevent drownings. During well-baby and well-child visits, physicians can warn parents of how quickly and under what circumstances their children can drown.

ISOLATION POOL FENCING

Isolation pool fencing, which separates the residential swimming pool from the house and remaining yard, has been widely regarded as an effective barrier method of prohibiting access to the swimming pool by unsupervised children (Pitt and Balanda 1991). Not to be confused with property-line fencing, which separates properties with residential pools from neighboring yards and properties, isolation pool fencing has been recommended by the American Medical Association. Isolation pool fencing, however, has met with criticism, particularly in jurisdictions with ordinances requiring it. For homes equipped with swimming pools where small children do not reside or rarely visit, such a requirement can be perceived as intrusive. Critics have recommended that pool covers, pool alarms, door alarms, and child alarms provide equally satisfactory protection for children. Additional research is needed to determine the degree of protection these alternative methods provide to children.

PERSONAL FLOTATION DEVICES

Personal flotation devices (PFDs) or life jackets are not substitutes for knowing how to swim, but they do offer a degree of protection for swimmers in rough or uncertain waters and for individuals who cannot swim or who swim poorly (Bever 1996). Personal flotation devices are recommended for all boat operators and passengers on all boating vessels on all waterways. A personal flotation device is required to be on board for each person on the vessel if the vessel is under 16 ft.

CARDIOPULMONARY RESUSCITATION (CPR)

With improved emergency rescue services, improved emergency treatment modalities and the recommendation that parents, swimming pool owners, and recreational boat users learn CPR, effective conversion of near-drowning victims appears to be possible more often (Kyriacou et al. 1994). The outcome in the emergency department appears to be improved for near-drowning victims only if they have nearly drowned in ice water (Fields 1992). The study from which this conclusion was drawn was conducted only on children. CPR requirements for pool owners and other legislation seem to be likely preventive strategies (Liller et al. 1993).

LEGISLATION REGARDING ALCOHOL

Over the past decade, more communities have adopted laws that prohibit people from buying, selling, possessing, and using alcoholic beverages at water recreation facilities. Laws that govern the consumption and sale of alcoholic beverages at water recreation facilities have been slowly changing. Legislation that prohibits alcohol use during boating is on the rise. Such legislation may have contributed to the decline in drownings, especially during the last few years.

RESEARCH AND SURVEILLANCE

We have a limited understanding of several risk factors for drowning. Recently, federal health agencies have called for more research in drownings among adolescent and adult African-Americans and other minority populations (Robertson et al. 1992), especially studies of the circumstances of such drownings. Several questions need to be answered: Are persons who drown less likely to know how to swim? If so, are the waters in which they drown appropriate for swimming only or for boating and other activities only? Also, what is the clear relationship between alcohol use and water recreation injuries, including drownings?

We would have an easier time answering these questions and gaining a better understanding of recent drowning trends if we had a faster, more efficient system for collecting data on confirmed drowning cases. Current national data on drowning is drawn from reliable data provided by the National Center for Health Statistics. Surveillance systems would be ideal, but such systems for injury conditions, including drownings, are very limited. Few states and municipalities have invested the resources to support surveillance activities, that is, the ongoing systematic collection, analysis, and interpretation of health event data for use in public health practice (Thacker 1994). The few drowning surveillance activities that are in place do not focus on all conditions and settings. For example, the Arizona Department of Health Services, in cooperation with Maricopa County and Phoenix health and safety officials, has developed a drowning surveillance system that collects data important to our understanding of all components of drowning, both environmental and behavioral (CDC 1990). The system, however, focuses mainly on drownings among small children in swimming pools. Most of the collected information would be relevant to any drowning surveillance system, but it would have to be expanded to include settings other than pools. As another example, the Water Safety Division, Department of Parks and Recreation Department of the City and County of Honolulu, Hawaii, maintains a data collection system for use by water safety officers located at selected beaches on the island of Oahu. Data collection is comprehensive for beach locations where water safety officers are stationed, but it is not available for beaches where lifeguards are not assigned. Drownings in inland waters, swimming pools, and household water sources are not included, as is the case with most drowning surveillance systems.

Surveillance of the circumstances and locations of drownings is essential for targeting specific interventions to specific circumstances (Robertson et al. 1992). Ideally, each state would institute surveillance systems for drowning and other injury conditions. Such surveillance activities would need to be coordinated nationally to standardize definitions and monitor trends. National surveillance efforts would allow us to monitor the effectiveness of innovative intervention strategies, technology, and education, as well as to track the number of drownings and near-drownings.

The type of information to be captured by surveillance systems includes demographic data (e.g., age and sex), the circumstances surrounding the submersion, how the event occurred, the type and condition of any existing barriers, the type and use of resuscitation (e.g., CPR) administered, the type of medical care administered, and the outcome of the incident.

SUMMARY

Are drowning rates rising or falling? After examining the data by key demographic parameters and by major risk factors, drowning rates appear to be declining over time, and 1993 may simply have been a statistical outlier. We will not know for certain whether 1993 was an unusual year until we see data for 1994 and subsequent years. Drowning remains an important public health problem, regardless of trends in drowning rates. We need to continue our drowning prevention efforts for all persons and on all bodies of water. More data is needed on specific risk factors to fully understand their role in drownings among African-Americans, persons of Hispanic ethnicity, and other minorities. Furthermore, more research is needed to determine the effectiveness of several newer interventions.

REFERENCES

American Red Cross, 1995, *Lifeguarding Today*, Mosby-Year Book, St. Louis, MO.

Baker, S. P., O'Neill, B., Ginsburg, M. J., and Li, G., 1992, *The Injury Fact Book*, 2nd edition, Oxford University Press, New York.

Bever, D. L., 1996, *Safety: A Person Focus*, 4th edition, Mosby-Year Book, St. Louis, MO.

Branche-Dorsey, C. M., Russell, J. C., Greenspan, A. I., and Chorba, T. C., 1994, "Unintentional injuries: the problems and some preventive strategies," in *Handbook of Black American Health: The Mosaic Of Conditions, Issues, Policies and Prospects*, Livingston, I. L., Ed. Greenwood Publishing Group, Westport, CT.

Brenner, R. A., Smith, G. S., and Overpeck, M. D., 1994, "Divergent trends in childhood drowning rates, 1971 through 1988," *JAMA* 271:1606–08.

Centers for Disease Control, 1986, "North Carolina drownings," 1980–1984, *Morbidity and Mortality Weekly Report* 35:635–38.

Centers for Disease Control, 1987, "Recreational boating fatalities — Ohio, 1983–1986," *Morbidity and Mortality Weekly Report* 36:321–24.

Devine, O. J., Annest, J. L., Kirk, M. L., Holmgreen, P., and Emrich, S. S., 1990, *Injury Mortality Atlas of the United States, 1979–1987*, National Center for Injury Prevention and Control, Centers for Disease Control and Prevention, Atlanta, GA.

Dietz, P. and Baker, S., 1974, "Drowning: epidemiology and prevention," *Am. J. Pub. Hlth.* 64:303–12.

Ellis, A. A. and Trent, R. B., 1995, "Hospitalizations for near-drowning in California: Incidence and costs," *Am. J. Pub. Hlth.* 85:1115–18.

Fields, A. I., 1992, "Near-drowning in the pediatric population," *Critical Care Clinics* 8:113–29.

Gulaid, J. A. and Sattin, R. W., 1988, "Drowning in the United States, 1978–1984," *Morbidity and Mortality Weekly Report* 37:27–33.

Hingson, R. and Howland, J., 1993, "Alcohol and non-traffic unintended injuries," *Addiction* 88:877–83.

Howland, J. and Hingson, R., 1988, "Alcohol as a risk factor for drownings: a review of the literature (1950–1985)," *Accident Analysis and Prevention* 20:19B25.

Howland, J., Mangione, T., Hingson, R., Levenson, S., Winter, M., and Altwicker, A., 1990, "A pilot survey of aquatic activities and related consumption of alcohol, with implications for drowning," *Public Health Reports* 105:415–19.

Howland, J., Smith, G. S., Mangione, T., Hingson, R., DeJong, W., and Bell, N., 1993, "Missing the boat on drinking and boating," commentary, *JAMA* 270:91–92.

Jeff Ellis & Associates, 1995, *Rescue statistics summary*, Jeff Ellis & Associates, Kingwood, TX.

Jensen, L. R., Williams, S. D., Thurman, D. J., and Keller, P. A., 1992, "Submersion injuries in children younger than 5 years in urban Utah," *West. J. Med.* 157:641–44.

Kyriacou, D. N., Arcinue, E. L., Peek, C., and Kraus, J. F., 1994, "Effect of immediate resuscitation on children with submersion injury," *Pediatrics* 94:137–42.

Liller, K. D., Kent, E. B., Arcari, C., and McDermott, R. J., 1993, "Risk factors for drowning and near-drowning among children in Hillsborough County, Florida," *Public Health Reports* 108:346–53.

Mael, F. A., 1995, "Staying afloat: Within-group swimming proficiency for whites and blacks," *J. App. Psych.* 80:479–90.

National Committee for Injury Prevention and Control, 1989, *Injury prevention: Meeting the Challenge*, Oxford University Press, New York.

Patetta, M. J. and Biddinger, P. W., 1988, "Characteristics of drowning deaths in North Carolina," *Public Health Reports* 103:406–11.

Pitt, W. R. and Balanda, K. P., 1991, "Childhood drownings and near-drownings in Brisbane: the contribution of domestic pools," *Med. J. As.* 154:661–65.

Present, P., 1987, *Child Drowning Study: A Report on the Epidemiology of Drownings in Residential Pools to Children Under Age Five*, U.S. Consumer Product Safety Commission, Directorate for Epidemiology, Washington, DC.

Rice, D. P., MacKenzie, E. J., Jones, A. S., et al., 1989, *Cost of Injury in the United States: a Report to Congress*, The Johns Hopkins University and Injury Prevention Center, University of California, Institute for Health and Aging, San Francisco.

Robertson, L., Stallions, L., Branche-Dorsey, C. M., et al., 1992, "Home and leisure injury prevention," in *Position Papers from the Third National Injury Control Conference: Setting the National Agenda for Injury Control in the 1990s*, Centers for Disease Control, Atlanta, GA.

Rodriguez, J. G. and Brown, S. T., 1990, "Childhood injuries in the United States," *Am. J. Diseases Child.* 144:627–46.

Thacker, S. B., 1994, "Historical development," in *Principles and Practice of Public Health Surveillance*, Deutsche, S. M. and Churchill, R. E., Eds., Oxford University Press, New York.

U.S. Coast Guard, 1995, *Boating Statistics 1994*, Publication No. COMDTPUB P16754.8, U.S. Department of Transportation, Washington, DC.

Warneke, C. L. and Cooper, S. P., 1994, "Child and adolescent drownings in Harris County, Texas, 1983 through 1990," *Am. J. Pub. Hlth.* 84:593–98.

Wintemute, G. J., Kraus, J. F., Turret, S. P., and Wright, M. A., 1987, "Drowning in childhood and adolescence: A population-based study," *Am. J. Pub. Hlth.* 77:830–32.

Wintemute, G. J., Kraus, J. F., Turret, S. P., and Wright, M. A., 1988, "The epidemiology of drownings in adulthood: Implications for prevention, *Am. J. Prove. Med.* 4:343–48.

4 Racial Variations in Drowning: Cultural or Biological?

Fred A. Mael

The views expressed in this paper are those of the author and do not necessarily reflect the views of the U.S. Army Research Institute, the U.S. Military Academy, or the Department of the Army.

As a form of strenuous exercise which can be performed outdoors in pleasant weather or indoors in all climates, as an enjoyable activity which is associated with beach trips and splash parties, or as a competitive sport, swimming serves many purposes. For most, however, swimming would or should be viewed, perhaps primarily, as a survival skill. The inability to swim not only deprives people of the health benefits and pleasures of swimming, but may even jeopardize their lives. Drowning is a potential problem not only for those engaged in recreational swimming, but also as a result of flash floods, hurricanes, swimming, and auto, boating, and fishing mishaps (Campbell, 1991). According to the Centers for Disease Control and the National Safety Council, 4,600 drownings occurred in the U.S. in 1989. Although this figure is down from 1986 (5,596) and 1980 (7,257), the number is not trivial. The estimated cost of drownings and near-drownings, including rescue, hospitalization, and rehabilitation costs, is $2.5 billion dollars (NCIPC, 1989). Drowning is the third most common cause of unintentional injury death for all ages, and ranks second for ages 5–44 (Baker, O'Neill, Ginsburg, and Li, 1992). About 40–45% of drowning deaths occur during swimming, with 12–30% occurring during boating (Dietz and Baker, 1974). In the U.S. Army, water-related fatalities accounted for 50% of all recent recreational deaths, 75% of which were swimming related (Green, 1992). Because they overestimate their skills, beginners are often at greater risk than nonswimmers (Allinder, 1989).

Differences in drowning rates between the races is paralleled by differences in swimming ability. At every level of swimming, from minimal competency to representation in world-class competition, there are stark differences in the performance or participation of African-Americans relative to American whites (Allinder, 1989; Hoose, 1990; Teplitzky, 1992). This discrepancy has a range of negative implications for African-Americans, ranging from increased drowning risk to underrepresentation in occupations and sports requiring swimming skill. It should be obvious that there are many causes of drowning other than inability to swim. These include alcohol and drug consumption; hazards caused by weather, such as flash floods and hurricanes; variations in tides and currents; boating and automobile mishaps; and other factors. It would seem farfetched to attribute racial differences in drownings caused by these other factors to either cultural or genetic differences. What *can* be done is to try to understand differences in swimming ability between the races. For cases in which lack of swimming ability leads to drowning, this will be directly relevant. In other cases, the connection may be more indirect. For example, a drunk person who falls off a pier may or may not have the faculties to save himself or herself; perhaps the person's swimming ability (or reduced panic in the water) could mean the difference between life and death, but so would the degree of inebriation. In every natural disaster, be it riptide, flood, or storm at sea, swimming ability may or may not make a difference in whether one could survive.

In this chapter I focus on the controllable aspect of drowning that has known racial differences. The title — *Racial Variations in Drowning: Cultural or Biological?* — may be somewhat misleading, in that it appears to preclude some degree of interaction between the two factors. I summarize my earlier research (Mael, 1995) on possible reasons for African-American–white swimming differences, and more importantly, on reasons for within-group differences among African-Americans. I also describe a more recent replication and extension of that work with a much larger sample of military personnel that is more heterogeneous in terms of race, academic accomplishment, physical ability, and socioeconomic status (SES) than was the original sample (Mael, 1996). I begin by reviewing evidence of African-American–white differences in swimming.

GROUP DIFFERENCES IN SWIMMING
AND WATER SAFETY PROFICIENCY

The rate of drowning among U.S. African-Americans is two to three times as high as the white rate (Baker et al., 1992; Gulaid and Sattin, 1988; Kizer, 1983; Wintemute, Kraus, Teret, and Wright, 1988). For example, drowning rates for African-Americans in Maryland were 2.6 times as high (5.8 deaths per 100,000) as those of whites (2.3 per 100,000) (Dietz and Baker, 1974). During 1984–1988, 80% of the drowning fatalities in Florida were minorities, while African-Americans accounted for 44% of the drownings in Georgia during that period (Campbell, 1991; cf., Fife and Goldoft, 1994). In a study of Navy fatalities, the percentage of African-American fatalities by drowning (23% of all deaths) was more than twice that of whites (10%) (Palinkas, 1985). Of the 1,107 drowning fatalities that occurred on U.S. Army Corps of Engineers projects during 1986–1990, 35% involved minorities. It is currently unknown to what degree higher rates of drowning among African-Americans are directly the result of inability to swim, compared to other possible reasons related to use of alcohol, use of unsafe areas for water recreation, or other factors (Branche-Dorsey, Russell, Greenspan, and Chorba, 1994).

Differences in terms of water safety awareness are also evidenced from an unpublished 1991 study of lifeguard rescues, conducted by Ellis & Associates, a national aquatic safety consulting firm. Out of 16,333 rescues at 150 water parks servicing almost 24 million guests, 33% were of African-Americans, compared to

43% white, even though the water parks were not concentrated in urban or predominantly African-American areas.

In terms of minimal swimming proficiency, there are also significant differences. Allinder (1989) found attrition from Navy training due to failure of swimming requirements much higher for African-Americans (6.46%) than whites (0.62%) at all three Navy Recruit Training Centers. At one center, African-Americans accounted for 75% of all swim failures in 1987 and for 78% in 1989, though they comprised only 15% of trainees. The same problem was found at the Navy's Aviation Officer Candidate School (AOCS), where African-Americans attrited disproportionately from the TADPOLE preparatory swim program or from AOCS (Chief of Naval Operations, 1988). Palinkas (1985) suggests that even those African-American males who pass the Navy swim test may be less safety-aware and comfortable in the water, leading to their higher drowning rate. Similar discrepancies were found with regard to the 50-yd swimming test requirement of the U.S. Army's Special Forces Assessment and Selection (SFAS) course. During FY 1991, 15.4% of African-Americans (24/156) failed the pre-SFAS swim test, as opposed to 2.8% (74/2597) of whites and 4.6% (8/166) of other minorities (cf. Teplitzky, 1992). As swimming ability is required to be a member of the Special Forces, the Army Rangers, and the Marines, as well as other elite military units, the inability to swim could thus limit the nonswimmer's chances for employment and promotions in military careers. Inability to swim could also adversely affect participation in a wide range of civilian careers such as maritime commerce and engineering, fishing, marine research, lifeguarding, and offshore oil exploration and drilling. Even a career such as a flight attendant often has swimming or water safety requirements. Finally, there are African-American–white differences in competitive swimming. African-Americans are underrepresented in elite competitive swimming, and no African-American swimmer has ever been on a U.S. Olympic team (Hoose, 1989, 1990).

REASONS ADVANCED FOR GROUP AND INDIVIDUAL DIFFERENCES

A number of reasons have been advanced for African-American–white differences in swimming. One school of thought focuses on physiological differences (Arnot and Gaines, 1986; Burfoot, 1992). For example, African-Americans as a group have less subcutaneous fat and are less buoyant than whites (Baker and Newman, 1957; Burdeshaw, 1968; Campbell, 1991; Lane and Mitchum, 1964; Malina, 1972; Patterson, 1972). African-Americans as a group have denser bones, resulting in denser lean body mass (Malina, 1972; Schutte et al., 1984). These differences could have both direct and indirect influences on the ability to float, the ability to relax and maintain body heat in cold water, and thus the motivation to persevere at learning to swim (Burdeshaw, 1968; Campbell, 1991; Costill, Maglischo, and Richardson, 1992; Page, 1975; Ryan, 1974). However, most researchers doubt that physiological differences play a primary role in minimal swimming competency (Mullen, 1993), and there is no evidence that the discrepancies in swimming ability found in the U.S are true of other countries and cultures. Similarly, "previous studies suggest that swimming success is dependent more on the swimmer's skill than on muscular strength and endurance"

(Costill, Maglischo, and Richardson, 1992, p. 26). As described below, Mael's (1995) findings at the United States Military Academy (USMA) demonstrated that even when there are no body-fat differences between whites and African-Americans in a given sample, there are still stark differences in performance.

SOCIAL DIFFERENCES

Sociocultural factors have generally been viewed as more important reasons for poor African-American swimming (Allinder, 1989; Campbell, 1974, 1991; Hoose, 1989). Observers such as former Mayor Andrew Young of Atlanta (cited in Hoose, 1989) claim that racism has traditionally been most strident regarding common use of swimming facilities. The mingling of African-Americans and whites in the minimally-dressed, close contact milieu of the swimming pool was especially abhorred by segregationist whites. Some pool proprietors, if unable to mandate separate facilities for African-Americans, would change the pool water after each use by African-Americans (Hoose, 1989, 1990).

Campbell (1991) and Hoose (1989) also describe the lack of quality swimming facilities for inner-city youth. Like golf and tennis, in which African-Americans are underrepresented (Potter, 1992), swimming can require facilities which may be too expensive for or inaccessible to many African-Americans. The time and financial demands that organized and competitive swimming makes on parents are even more daunting for single mothers, who are overrepresented in the inner-city, African-American community. Anecdotal evidence (Hoose, 1989) suggests that many African-Americans also develop negative attitudes and presumptions of failure towards swimming.

Unfortunately, much of what is written from this perspective tends to treat race and lower socioeconomic (SES) status as synonymous, with the concomitant, untested assumption that rates of swimming among middle-class African-Americans are similar to those of whites. As described below, although there are swimming differences *between* African-Americans that are correlated with SES, African-American–white differences in swimming exist even when correlations have been statistically controlled for SES.

THE INITIAL STUDY

Using a sample of over 2,500 cadets (6% African-American) from the U.S. Military Academy classes of 1994 and 1995, I simultaneously evaluated physiological, demographic, and biodata factors as predictors of swimming proficiency (Mael, 1995). The criterion used to assess swimming ability was a swimming test that is regularly administered to all cadets shortly after arrival at USMA. Each cadet was categorized as a (1) nonswimmer (unable to swim 50 yds), (2) beginner (can swim 51–160 yds), (3) low intermediate (can swim 161–200 yds within five minutes), (5) high intermediate (201–260 yds within five minutes, or (6) advanced (261+ yds within five minutes).

Among the cadets, 2.5% of whites were classified as nonswimmers. In contrast, 29% of African-Americans were nonswimmers, and another 44.3% were categorized as beginners. At the other extreme, 12% of whites were coded as advanced swimmers, compared to under 2% of African-American cadets. Thus, African-Americans, who made up 6.2% of these classes, accounted for 37.4% of the nonswimmers, and only 1.9% of advanced swimmers. The African-American–white differences were statistically significant ($X^2(5) = 336$, $p < .001$). Noteworthy is that, unlike previous research, albeit with less select samples, African-Americans' and whites' scores on the Body Mass Index (BMI) were not different (23.51 and 23.59, respectively). In addition, BMI scores were unrelated to either swimming ability or learning to swim earlier for either African-American or white cadets.

That study's analyses indicated that the age at which a cadet had learned to swim (if at all) was the single best predictor of subsequent swimming ability. Excluding those who had never learned to swim, age of learning had a correlation with swimming ability of .43 for African-Americans and .32 for whites. Moreover, African-Americans and whites showed stark differences in the age at which they learned to swim: Over 90% of whites learned to swim by age 9, compared to 58% of African-Americans. Conversely, while only 1% of whites had never learned to swim, 16% of African-Americans had not. Moreover, African-Americans were also less proficient swimmers than whites who learned to swim at the same age. For example, 64% of African-Americans who learned to swim by age 5 were coded as low intermediates or higher. For those who learned between 6 and 9, that number dropped to 30%. Less than 7% of those learning after age 9 were low intermediates or higher. By contrast, among whites, the equivalent rates of proficiency were 90% (by 5), 70% (between 6–9), and 35% (over 10), respectively.

In addition to finding African-American–white differences in ability and age having learned to swim, Mael found a number of background and behavioral variables that explained differences in swimming ability within the subsample of African-Americans. The background differences fell into the following categories.

PHYSICAL CONDITION AND EXERCISE

Hours of exercise per week and scores on USMA's Physical Aptitude Exam were significant correlates of swimming proficiency and/or earlier swimming for African-Americans. Also, those who preferred individual-oriented sports and who were involved in rugged, outdoor activities were more capable swimmers, with significant correlations for whites and correlations of equivalent magnitude for African-Americans.

PHYSIOLOGICAL DIFFERENCES

Although BMI scores were unrelated to either criterion for this sample, heavier cadets were both better swimmers and earlier learners, with significant correlations for whites and equivalent correlations for African-Americans.

SWIMMING AND SOCIOCULTURAL OPPORTUNITY

Three items were significant indicators for African-Americans only. Those cadets who watched less television than others and those who favored social studies over other core high school courses were better swimmers. Those cadets were also more likely to have learned to swim earlier, as were those who had been Boy or Girl

Scouts. Conversely, music lessons were a significant correlate of learning to swim earlier among whites. These variables have implications for socioeconomic differences in childrearing and lifestyle (Elkin and Handel, 1989; Farber, 1964), and were particularly salient as within-group predictors of swimming ability.

TENDENCIES TO AVOID SWIMMING

Among both African-Americans and whites, those who were more studious or were top academic performers were poorer swimmers. Among whites, cadets with more extroverted styles, as expressed in a preference for socializing in larger groups, tended to be better and earlier swimmers. Both African-Americans and whites who had earlier part-time work experiences were better swimmers. Finally, birth order was a significant swimming correlate for African-Americans: oldest and only children learned to swim later, and swam more poorly, than later-born siblings. It is possible that these relationships are indicative of the role of dispositional tendencies, such as risk-aversiveness and introversion, in the tendency to learn how to swim proficiently (Behrman, 1967; Nisbett, 1968; Yiannakis, 1976; Whiting and Stembridge, 1965).

GENDER

This variable alone had statistically significant correlations in opposite directions for African-Americans vs. whites. African-American males were significantly more likely than African-American females to have learned to swim at an earlier age, while among whites, the reverse was true. Possible reasons are discussed in Mael (1995).

THE REPLICATION STUDY RESEARCH

For the replication study, data was obtained from a larger, more heterogeneous sample, although that sample also was limited to military personnel. Although I was afforded only limited input into the survey instrument used, better measurement of various dimensions of swimming was possible, as well as replication of previously found relationships. The sample for this study was the randomly chosen U.S. Army personnel who participated in the Fall 1994 Sample Survey of Military Personnel, which is a regularly administered, large-scale survey of United States Army officers (n = 4,241) and enlisted personnel (n = 4,788). In the officer sample, 88% of the officers were male, 84% were white, 9% African-American, 4% Hispanic, and 3% belonged to other groupings. In the enlisted sample, 87% of the officers were male, 60% were white, 27% African-American, 8% Hispanic, and 5% belonged to other groupings. Thus, the total African-American sample was over five times as large as the original USMA African-American sample. The larger sample could be expected to be more representative and stable than the that obtained at USMA. While I describe portions of the results regarding white, African-American, and Hispanic swimming proficiency, I again limit description of the correlational analyses to testing African-American–white and within African-American hypotheses. For descriptive analyses, the officers and enlisted personnel are described separately; however, for correlational analyses, the groups were combined, and officer/enlisted status was treated simply as an additional predictor variable.

SWIMMING ITEMS

The following swimming items were added to the Fall 1994 iteration of the survey. The first was "About how old were you when you first learned to swim?" This variable was computed in two ways. The first computation included those who said that they had never learned to swim at all. The second excluded nonlearners, and so essentially measured the age at which someone who eventually learned to swim *had* learned to swim. The second item was "Which of the following comes closest to the longest distance you have ever been able to swim *without* stopping?" The next four items stated: "How would you rate your ability to swim using the following swimming strokes?" The four listed strokes were backstroke, breaststroke, crawl, and sidestroke. All survey items were self-report items. The relative weakness of the replication study data was the lack of an objective measure of swimming proficiency, whereas its advantage was the greater detail provided in terms of aspects of swimming ability, and the greater sample stability and heterogeneity.

ADDITIONAL ITEMS

Although the majority of the survey was not focused on swimming issues, other items provided a way to test other hypotheses or replicate the previous research at USMA. These include the participant's current age, which could be indicative of current fitness level, but is more importantly a measure of the person's age cohort and the likeliness of available swimming instruction during the person's formative years. I hypothesized that younger persons would have learned to swim at an earlier age, on the assumption that availability of swimming instruction and facilities is typically on the rise in most, though surely not all, communities. Also included as a variable was race, with the hypothesis that whites would have learned to swim earlier and more than Hispanics, who in turn would have achieved greater proficiency than African-Americans. However, as mentioned above, race was used primarily to study within-group variations in swimming proficiency.

Gender was included in the study as well. Based on the USMA research, it was hypothesized that white females would learn earlier than males, and that African-American females would learn later than their male counterparts. Also measured was the person's highest achieved educational degree, which may be a measure of both intellectual capability and socioeconomic status. Similarly, status as either officer or enlisted person was viewed as a partial surrogate for socioeconomic status, as described below. Finally, two questions measured the person's self-reported frequency of exercise (times per week) in two categories: muscle strength (such as push-ups, sit-ups, and weightlifting, and aerobic (such as biking, running, and swimming). Based on the USMA and Special Forces research described earlier, I hypothesized that both forms of exercise would be associated with more proficient swimming.

RESULTS: DESCRIPTIVE STATISTICS

SWIMMING ABILITY

As a group, most of these Army personnel knew how to swim: only 5% of officers and 20% of enlisted personnel stated that they were unable to swim. However, 25%

of African-American officers and 42% of African-American enlisted personnel were unable to swim, compared to 3% and 9% of white officers and enlisted personnel, respectively. In other words, the rate of nonswimming among African-Americans was 4–5 times as high as among whites. Rates of nonswimming among Hispanics were 10% and 24%, respectively, indicating some degree of nonswimming among Hispanics, though nowhere near the magnitude of African-Americans. These numbers are also consistent with the findings at the Special Forces SFAS course described above, in which Hispanics occupied a middle ground between whites and African-Americans.

Age Learned to Swim

In this survey, as in USMA, African-American–white differences on this variable were found again. Among officers, 84% of whites had learned to swim by age 10, as opposed to only 33% of African-Americans (and 63% of Hispanics). Among enlisted soldiers, the rates were 79%, 28%, and 55%, respectively.

In the previous USMA research, the same variable (age of learning to swim) was used, and was compared to objective swimming tests taken upon entry at USMA. It was evident that not everyone who said that they learned to swim at a certain age was now a competent swimmer, and a number who claimed to have learned to swim were categorized as nonswimmers or beginners. Thus, the item has to be understood generally as when one was first able to do some rudimentary swimming, although the skill may later have been lost, or was never properly mastered.

Quality of Swimming Ability

Assessment of swimming ability (in terms of distance and stroke proficiency) is limited to those who said that they had learned to swim, and provide a picture of quality of swimming ability even among those who claim they can swim. Among those claiming that they had learned to swim at some age, we find that 61% of African-American officers could only swim 100 yds or less, compared to 23% of whites and 17% of Hispanics. (This was a rare case where Hispanic swimming skill surpassed that of whites). For enlisted personnel, the rates were 70%, 26%, and 43%, respectively. Naturally, if those who said they had never learned to swim were included, the percentage for each race of those who could not swim 100 yds would be higher, as would be true for the percentages claiming proficiency in various strokes.

No "Different Strokes for Different Folks"

In general, there were few differences within each group in ability to perform the four basic swimming strokes included in the survey. Among the enlisted respondents, there were virtually no differences in self-rated ability to do the various strokes, at least at the level of minimal ability. Among officers, slightly fewer rated themselves as "can't swim" or "poor" on the crawl (13.5%) or sidestroke (12.7%) than they did on the backstroke (17.8%) or breaststroke (20%). Whether a self-evaluative halo effect was operating, or whether there were really no differences in proficiency, cannot be sufficiently determined from this data. It is likely that actual tests of proficiency in the different strokes would show greater variance (cf., Campbell, 1974).

In terms of racial differences in specific stroke competencies, the percentage of white officers who said they could perform each stroke at either the "good," "very good," or "excellent" level ranged from 25–31% higher than the equivalent percentage of African-American officers. Among enlisted personnel, the white–African-American differences in percentages for the four strokes ranged from 18–23%. Once again, Hispanics generally occupied a middle level of proficiency.

MALE–FEMALE DIFFERENCES

In the current sample, male officers were less likely to be nonswimmers (4%) than female officers (13%), and the same was true among enlisted personnel (men, 17% nonswimmers; women, 35%). Similarly, a greater percentage of male officers learned to swim by age 10 (80%) than did female officers (70%). An even larger disparity was seen among enlisted personnel (men, 65% learned by age 10; women, 49%). Even among those who learned to swim, there were significant differences in the minimal competency of men and women. Among officers, 34% of women could only swim 100 yds or less, vs. 19% of males. Among enlisted soldiers, the rates were 57% and 21%, respectively. However, gender differences in ability to do the four strokes well were minimal.

GENDER–RACE INTERACTIONS

Previous research indicated that gender differences in age of learning to swim may primarily be a function of racial differences, in that African-American females may have swimming constraints compared to men, whereas, at least at USMA, white women tended to learn earlier than white males. The findings for African-Americans were confirmed with this larger sample, whereas findings for whites were more equivocal.

Among African-American officers, males were much more likely to have ever learned to swim than females (80% vs. 55%). Of those who learned to swim, males were most likely to learn during ages 5–9, whereas females were more likely to learn from ages 10–14. Among enlisted personnel, 61% of African-American males learned to swim, vs. only 42% of females. Thus, enlisted African-American females are the only group in the sample in which over 50% of the members never learned to swim. However, there were no differences in age of learning for those who did learn. Among Hispanics, males were also more likely to have learned to swim; in addition, enlisted Hispanic male officers were about three times as likely as their female counterparts to have learned to swim before the age of 5. Strangely, however, enlisted Hispanic females were about three times as likely to have learned to swim before the age of 5 as their officer peers. Among whites, the reverse is true: More females learned to swim in the under-5 period, whereas more males learned between ages 5–9. About twice as many females never learned to swim, although the numbers were small for both genders. Among white enlisted personnel, there were no male–female differences. This may suggest an interaction between gender and SES among whites; the officers would be more comparable to the USMA cadets, who are future officers, than they would be to the enlisted sample.

In terms of swimming distances, both white and African-American females were more likely to be unable to swim 25 yds or less, or 100 yds or less. Evidently, among white females, earlier learning does not translate into greater proficiency or endurance in swimming. On the subject of self-rated proficiency in various swimming skills, with few exceptions males of all races were more likely to rate themselves as "very good" or "excellent" at each of the four strokes than females.

IMPLICATIONS OF ENLISTED–OFFICER DIFFERENCES

A higher percentage of officers learned to swim than did enlisted personnel (95% vs. 81%). Similarly, of those who learned to swim, more officers could swim 100 yds or more without stopping (79%) than could enlisted personnel (64%). Differences in rated ability to do each of the four strokes were not great. The enlisted-officer differences may be indicative of typical socioeconomic differences between these two groups, and may also reflect the greater racial diversity of the enlisted ranks. In order to clarify many of these issues, correlational and regression analyses are needed to sort out the unique impact of many of the relationships.

CORRELATES OF SWIMMING ABILITY

All measures of swimming proficiency were consistently related, although they were admittedly subject to inflation, as self-report surveys without external criterion measure are prone to common method variance. Because of the lack of distinction and high intercorrelations of the four independent items regarding stroke proficiency, the items were combined into a single-stroke proficiency scale for subsequent analyses. In addition to the evidence of racial differences, the other correlates of swimming ability included in this survey also supported hypothesized and previously found relationships. Tables showing the intercorrelations between all variables and the multiple regression analyses appear in Mael (1996).

AGE

Younger personnel had learned to swim earlier. Though they could not swim farther, younger personnel consistently rated themselves as more proficient at the various strokes. The consistent relationship to age having learned to swim would appear to support the contention that more recent cohorts have had greater access to swimming instruction at earlier ages.

GENDER

Across the total sample, males learned to swim earlier, could swim farther, and were minimally more proficient on some strokes. Unlike the USMA sample, even white females learned to swim somewhat later than white males. However, the gender gap in age of learning was more pronounced among African-Americans than whites, so that African-American–white differences were still in evidence. Possible reasons for male–female differences among African-Americans (Wessel, 1994; Woodham, 1994) include the difficulties with hair care that African-American women face following engaging in swimming.

EDUCATION

More educated members of the sample learned earlier, swam farther, and were minimally more proficient in some strokes. One anomaly, however, is that when limited to those who had learned to swim at some point, more educated soldiers were more likely to learn to swim later. One possible conjecture is that to the extent that education is a function of SES, those with poor educational backgrounds were more likely not to have learned to swim at all. However, when limiting the sample to those who were exposed to swim training, it is possible that the most highly educated subjects were slower learners. This would be consistent with findings in the USMA sample that those who were in the top 10% of their high school classes were later learners. If this is correct, it would lend support to previous indications that highly studious and somewhat introverted persons are less likely to master swimming early. Also revealing were the African-American–white differences in beta weights in the regression analysis. Among whites, more educated soldiers had swum farther, although they were no more proficient in various strokes, whereas among African-Americans, more educated personnel had not swum farther and were somewhat less proficient in swimming strokes.

OFFICER–ENLISTED

Personnel who were officers consistently learned to swim earlier and were more proficient swimmers. As there are clear SES differences between the two groups, these data may support the findings of Mael (1995) that SES differences explain significant differences in swimming ability, a finding that is intuitive, given that some level of financial resources is usually needed to learn how to swim (Campbell, 1991; Hoose, 1989).

CURRENT PHYSICAL FITNESS

Both those who spent more time on strength-building exercise and those who spent more time on aerobic exercise had learned to swim earlier, could swim farther, and rated themselves more proficient in each of the strokes. Whereas both indices of exercise were considerably related to each other, there were some small distinctions between those emphasizing one or the other mode. It should also be noted that contrary to other research, albeit with civilian populations (Kelley and Kelley, 1994), showing that African-Americans are less involved in physical activity as a group, there were no differences between the races on amount of physical activity.

THE ROLE OF RACE

African-American–white differences in swimming remained even after controlling for the effects of all the other variables. This was most noticeable in the prediction of age of learning to swim, though race also contributed unique variance to the skill criteria. Once again, lack of access to early training appears to be the strongest predictor of swimming proficiency, for whites as well as African-Americans.

Nevertheless, there is no basis to conclude that genetics or physiology account for these race differences. Even though some gross measures of SES were included, more specific aspects of access to swimming resources were not, nor were measures of parental swimming ability. Additional predictors that should appear in future research are discussed below.

NEEDED FUTURE RESEARCH DIRECTIONS

LIMITATIONS OF THE CURRENT STUDIES

Although the research at USMA and with the Army would appear to aid in our understanding of these phenomena, both have serious limitations, most of which are attributable to the fact that they were part of research instruments that were designed for other purposes, and that direct interaction with the participants was not possible. In addition, the USMA research used a relatively small sample of African-Americans and a rather select group of participants. The Army survey research compensated with a much larger sample, and primarily replicated previous findings, although the study is marred by the use of a self-report criterion in place of actual tests of swimming ability. In addition, the Army survey did not have any measures of subjects' physiological characteristics. Both studies were limited in their lack of direct assessment of possible individual impediments to learning how to swim.

THE NEED FOR COLLABORATIVE RESEARCH

It could be argued that it is time to move beyond surveys of this nature. Optimal research in this field of endeavor would require multidisciplinary, collaborative effort that would bring together researchers and practitioners with various skills. In this final section, I try to set forth a rough idea of what a more complete effort would include.

(a) *Complete definition and measurement of the criterion domain.* What is the criterion of concern? Drowning statistics are "hard" criteria, meaning that they are not tinged by the subjectivity of ratings. However, they suffer from so-called "criterion contamination" and "criterion deficiency" in the parlance of industrial/organizational psychology (Blum and Naylor, 1968; Brogden and Taylor, 1950). There is lack of consensus as to what is considered a rescue, a drowning, or a near-drowning. In addition, a myriad of factors, whether use of alcohol or other self-destructive behavior, injury, or an unrelated sudden illness such as stroke or heart attack, could precede a drowning episode, such that the drowning or near-drowning could not be clearly attributed solely to a lack of swimming skill. Thus, caution must be used in interpreting drowning statistics as direct criterion measures of swimming ability.

(b) *Better physiological measurement.* Sports psychologists and physiologists should be participants in the determination of the most sophisticated, economical, and accurate ways to measure buoyancy, body fat levels, muscle density, fast-twitch and slow-twitch muscle fibers, and other relevant indices.

Better measurement of how alcohol and drug use directly affects the ability to swim, to float, and to navigate toward safety would be helpful, as would determining if there are racial or ethnic differences in this realm. Other less obvious physiological issues to explore would be allergic reactions to chlorine, otherwise sensitive skin, effects of swimming on hair care and maintenance, and tolerance for cold water. On a practical level, different ways of addressing the hair care issues of African-American woman who are interested in swimming (Wessel, 1994; Woodham, 1994) must be considered.

(c) *Better background measurement.* Greater focus on specific aspects of background that may have affected learning to swim or subsequent practice is needed. This would include parental attitudes toward swimming and ability; peer swimming ability and interest; experience with siblings or friends involving life-threatening water rescues or drownings; geographical location of home and access to pools, all-season indoor pools, and instructors; makeup of family, including access to a same-sex parent; and whether local instructional opportunities are gender-integrated or separate-sex.

(d) *Better measures of dispositional factors.* More complete measurement would have to include measures of anxiety and risk-taking, as well as a number of other temperament constructs. The processes by which persons panic in potentially dangerous situation involving water, and the ways in which different personality types could be trained to resist such panic reactions, could be better documented.

(e) *Measuring the same sample on all predictors and criteria.* This would include developing a sample that is balanced by race, gender, and age. It is almost certain that a consortium made up of researchers and professionals from different milieus would be in a better position to achieve this goal than would be any single researcher at a given campus or swimclub setting. It would also be highly desirable for "hands-on" researchers to include team researchers who are comfortable with multivariate statistics such as multiple regression, factor analysis, and structural equation analysis.

CONCLUSION

Although there are stark differences in African-American–white swimming and drowning rates, there are ample signs of improvements in African-American swimming (Mullen, 1993). New urban pools and swim clubs are introducing more young African-Americans to aquatics and successful competitive swimming (Hoose, 1989, 1990). A recent national swim meet, showcasing over 600 primarily African-American members of urban swim teams, underscores this trend (Backover, 1993). The consensus is that given sufficient opportunity, the rate of African-American swimming will increase and the African-American–white gap will be narrowed. However, drowning continues to be a concern. African-Americans remain disproportionately vulnerable to both drownings and near-drownings, which underscores the desirability and urgency of continued investigation, especially collaborative, multidisciplinary research.

REFERENCES

Allinder, G. E., 1989, *Swim and survival at sea training: Does it meet the Navy's needs?* Masters thesis, DTIC # AD-A215 114, Naval Postgraduate School, Monterey, CA.

Arnot, R. B. and Gaines, C., 1986, *SportsTalent*. Penguin, New York.

Backover, A., Feb. 13, 1993, "600-plus here in showcase of black talent," *Washington Post*, p. D8.

Baker, P. T. and Newman, R. W., 1957, "The use of bone weight for human identification," *Am. J. Anthro.*, 15, 601–618.

Baker, S. P., O'Neill, B., Ginsburg, M. J., and Li, G., 1992, *The injury fact book*. 3rd edition, Oxford University Press, New York.

Behrman, R. M., 1967, "Personality differences between nonswimmers and swimmers," *Research Quarterly*, 38, 163–171.

Blum, M. L. and Naylor, J. C., 1968, *Industrial psychology, its theoretical and social foundations*. Harper & Row, New York.

Branche-Dorsey, C. M., Russell, J. C., Greenspan, A. I., and Chorba, T. L., 1994, "Unintentional injuries: the problems and some preventive strategies," in Livingston, I. L., Ed., *Handbook of Black American health: The mosaic of conditions, policies, and prospects*, pp. 190–204, Greenwood Press, Westport, CT.

Brogden, H. E. and Taylor, E. K., 1950, "The theory and classification of criterion bias," *Educational and Psychological Measurement*, 10, 159-186.

Burdeshaw, D., 1968, "Acquisition of elementary swimming skills by Negro and white college women," *Research Quarterly*, 39, 872-879.

Burfoot, A., August 1992, "White men can't run," *Runner's World*, 27(8), 89–95.

Campbell, W. A., Jr., 1974, *The self-concept of the black competitive swimmer: A psychocultural analysis*. Unpublished doctoral dissertation, Springfield College, Springfield, MA.

Campbell, W. A., Jr., 1991, *Aquatics: shades of black and white*. Kendall-Hunt, Dubuque, IA.

Costill, D. L., Maglischo, E. W., and Richardson, A. B., 1992, *Swimming*. Blackwell Scientific Publications, Oxford, U.K.

Dietz, P. E. and Baker, S. P., 1974, "Drowning: Epidemiology and prevention," *Am. J. Pub. Hlth.*, 64, 303–312.

Elkin, F. and Handel, G., 1989, *The child and society*. 5th edition, Random House, New York.

Ellis & Associates, 1991, *Aquatic safety consultants' 1991 rescue statistics*, Unpublished manuscript.

Farber, B., 1964, *Family: Organization and interaction*. Chandler, San Francisco.

Fife, D. and Goldoft, M., 1994, "Swimming capabilities and swimming exposure of New Jersey children," *J. Safety Res.*, 25, 159–165.

Green, W., April 1992, "Water sports top list of fatality producers," *Countermeasure: Army Ground Accident Report*, 13, 3.

Gulaid, J. A. and Sattin, R. W., 1988, "Drowning in the United States, 1978–1984," *Morbidity and Mortality Weekly Report*, 37, 27-33.

Hamilton, E. M., Whitney, E. N., and Sizer, F. S., 1988, *Nutrition: Concepts and controversies*. West Publishing, St. Paul, MN.

Heyward, V., 1991, *Advanced fitness assessment and exercise prescription*. Human Kinetics, Champaign, IL.

Hoose, P., 1989, *Necessities*. Random House, New York.

Hoose, P., April 29, 1990, "A new pool of talent," *New York Times Magazine*, 48–61.

Kelley, G. A. and Kelley, K. S., 1994, "Physical activity habits of African-American college students," *Research Quarterly for Exercise and Sport*, 65, 207–212.

Kizer, K. W., 1983, "Resuscitation of submersion casualties," *Emergency Medicine Clinician of North America*, 1, 643-652.

Lane, E. C. and Mitchum, J. C., 1964, "Buoyancy as predicted by certain anthropometric dimensions," *Research Quarterly*, 35, 21–28.

Mael, F. A., 1995, "Staying afloat: Within-group swimming proficiency for whites and blacks," *J. App. Psych.*, 80, 479–490.

Mael, F. A., 1996, "Differences in swimming proficiency within and between racial groups: Replication and future directions," *Int. J. Aquatic Res. Edu.*, 1, 9–19.

Malina, R. M., 1972, "Anthropology, growth and physical education: Specific applications to physical education," in Singer, R. N., Lamb, D. R., Loy, J. W., Jr., Malina, R. M., and Kleinman, S., Eds., *Physical Education: An interdisciplinary approach*, pp. 276–309. Macmillan, New York.

Mullen, P. H., April 1993, "No limits," *Swimming World and Junior Swimmer*, 30–35.

National Committee for Injury Prevention and Control (NCIPC), 1989, *Injury prevention: Meeting the Challenge*. Oxford University Press, New York.

Nisbett, R. E., 1968, "Birth order and participation in dangerous sports," *J. Personality Soc. Psych.*, 8, 351–353.

Page, R. L., 1975, "The role of physical buoyancy in swimming," *J. Hum. Move. Stud.*, 1, 190–198

Palinkas, L. A., 1985, "Racial differences in accidental and violent deaths among U.S. Navy personnel," *Military Medicine*, 150, 587–592.

Patterson, G. T., 1972, *A comparative study of the performance of black students in beginning swimming using the Red Cross method and the Silva method*, Unpublished masters thesis, North Carolina Central University.

Potter, J., Oct. 21, 1992, "Minorities try to forge link with golf," *U.S.A. Today*, 1C–2C.

Ryan, A. J., August 1974, "A need to know: Can blacks float?" *The Physician and Sports Medicine*, 11.

Schutte, J. E., Townsend, E. J., Hugg, J., Shoup, R. F., Malina, R. M., and Blomqvist, C. G., 1984, "Density of lean body mass is greater in blacks than in whites," *J. App. Physiol.*, 56, 1647–1649.

Teplitzky, M. L., 1992, *Minority representation in the enlisted Special Forces*, Research Report 1629, U.S. Army Research Institute for the Behavioral and Social Sciences, Alexandria, VA.

Wessel, H., June 27, 1994, "Black kids get into swim: New efforts focus on a long-neglected group," *Orlando Sentinel*, E1–2.

Wintemute, G. J., Kraus, J. F., Teret, S. P., and Wright, M. A., 1987, "Drowning in childhood and adolescence: A population-based study," *Am. J. Pub. Hlth.*, 77, 830–832.

Woodham, M., July 21, 1994, "Turning the tide," *Atlanta Constitution*, G1, G4.

Whiting, H. T. A. and Stembridge, D. E., 1965, "Personality and the persistent non-swimmer," *Research Quarterly*, 36, 348–356.

Yiannakis, A., 1976, "Birth order and preference for dangerous sports among males," *Research Quarterly*, 47, 62–67.

5 Drowning in a Hypothermic Environment

Desmond Bohn

INTRODUCTION

Drowning and near-drowning accidents associated with hypothermia are generally confined to the higher geographic latitudes and represent a small proportion of the total number seen each year. They are of particular interest and importance because of the well-documented cases of prolonged submersion, usually in children, where cardiac arrest has been associated with intact neurological survival. This is in contrast to submersion accidents in warm water environments where victims who arrive in hospital with no vital signs have a universally poor outcome. It is now quite evident that submersion in hypothermic conditions can lead to rapid core cooling which allows the brain some protection against the effects of cerebral hypoxia. In addition, we need to consider the physiological changes that occur during immersion accidents where the victim is not submerged but maintains flotation. Many of these victims will subsequently drown due to the effects of hypothermia.

PATHOPHYSIOLOGICAL CHANGES FOLLOWING SUBMERSION

The sequence of events that occurs immediately after a submersion accident has been the subject of considerable speculation in the medical literature. Much of this speculation has centered on the importance of the "diving reflex," the amount of fluid aspiration during submersion and the concept of "dry drowning," and whether there are important physiological differences between salt and fresh water drowning. Many of the conclusions have been based on either experiments in anesthetized animals with direct flooding of the lungs with water or deductions from postmortem studies in humans. The reality is that pathophysiological changes that occur during and immediately after a near-drowning accident vary according to the circumstances in which the submersion occurs. The enthusiasm for the use of cerebral protection regimes in the 1970s and 1980s has tended to obscure the fact that near-drowning is more than just a problem of cerebral hypoxia. It is, in reality, a global hypoxic insult, which frequently results in multiple organ damage, with the brunt of the damage taken by the central nervous system and the lungs. The pathophysiological changes in near-drowning should therefore be considered as a global hypoxic insult, which may be complicated by hypothermia, and the pathophysiological changes considered according to the effect on the principal systems involved.

THE CARDIORESPIRATORY EFFECTS OF SUBMERSION

The cardiorespiratory changes seen in near-drowning depend on whether the accident results in immediate submersion or whether there is immersion (maintenance of flotation). In the former, the most common scenario in infant and toddler accidents in swimming pools and bathtubs, the onset of hypoxia is immediate. Immersion followed by drowning is exclusive to older children and adults, is seen in boating and swimming accidents, and frequently involves salt water.

Immediately following immersion or submersion there is frequently a reflex bradycardia, which is commonly seen with facial immersion in cold water. This, together with prolonged breath holding and shunting of blood flow from the periphery to the core, are part of the so-called "diving reflex" by which diving mammals maintain cerebral oxygenation and survive prolonged periods in an hypoxic environment (Elsner et al., 1966). This mechanism is frequently invoked to explain some of the dramatic survivals seen in children with prolonged submersions in hypothermic conditions. However, studies on breath-holding in humans performed by Hayward suggest that this mechanism is unlikely. They show that the maximum breath hold in children under experimental conditions is less than 20 seconds and that this is reduced in cold water (Hayward et al., 1984). These same studies show that the magnitude of the reflex bradycardia is the same in adults and children (Ramey, Hayward, and Hayward, 1987). In fact, both facial immersion in water and breath-holding result in similar degrees of bradycardia (Paulev et al., 1990). A much more likely explanation for this preservation of brain function is rapid core cooling due to aspiration of cold water into the lung (Conn et al., 1995).

Following submersion it is likely that spontaneous respiratory efforts will continue for around 60 seconds. This conclusion is based on an animal study performed in 1951 on resuscitation in unanesthetized drowned dogs (Fainer, Martin, and Ivy, 1951), in which the investigators found that the acute cardiorespiratory changes following submersion could be divided into three phases (Figure 1). In Stage I, which lasted for an average of 71 seconds, respiration continued while blood pressure and heart rate increased; this was followed by apnea and falling blood pressure (Stage II), which lasted another 60 seconds and then a final phase when there was a precipitated fall in blood pressure to zero (Stage III; average duration 130 seconds). The total time from initial submersion to total cardiac arrest in this study was a mean of 262 seconds. These findings are probably a much closer approximation of what actually happens during human submersion accidents than subsequent studies performed on anesthetized animals, although one would prefer the ethics of the latter. In fact, this data agrees substantially with studies on asphyxia (without drowning) in anesthetized animals, which showed that heart rate and blood pressure increase in the first minute before decreasing, and PaO_2 falls to around 20 mmHg (2.7 kpa) by the time cardiac arrest occurs at around ten minutes (Kristoffersen, Rattenborg, and Holaday, 1967). A more recent study on drowning involving anesthetized dogs showed that following four minutes of submersion all animals were profoundly bradycardic and hypotensive with a PaO_2 of less than 20 mmHg (2.7 kpa) (Conn et al., 1995).

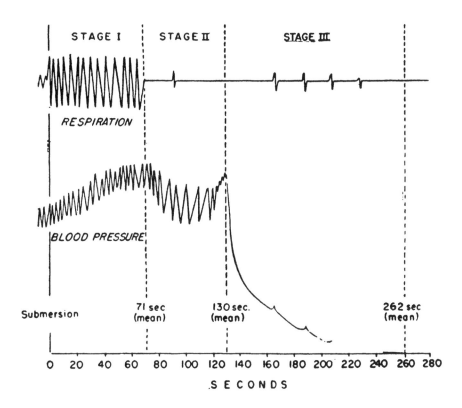

FIGURE 1   Cardiorespiratory changes associated with submersion in experimental animals. (From Fainer, D. C., *J. Applied Physiol.*, 1951. With permission.)

Submersion victims also aspirate water into the lungs. The actual amount, although not precisely known, has been extrapolated from animal experiments and human postmortem studies and used to draw a distinction between "dry" and "wet" drowning. Some authorities suggest that up to 10% of drowning victims do not aspirate water because they develop laryngospasm. This conclusion is based on a study of 91 resuscitated near-drowning human victims reported by Modell (Modell, Graves, and Ketover, 1976), which showed 10% had a PaO_2 of >80 mmHg (10.4 kpa) while breathing 21% oxygen, indicating no significant aspiration, while data from his animal experiments showed that aspiration of as little as 2.2 ml/kg of water results in a fall in PaO_2 to 60 mmHg within three minutes (Modell and Moya, 1966). This belief was reinforced by a postmortem study from the 1930s which found that 10% of drowning victims had no water in their lungs. In actual fact there is no concrete evidence that laryngospasm does occur during submersion while there is good experimental evidence that the breath-hold breaks shortly after submersion (Ramey et al., 1987), and the data shows that unanesthetized animals will continue to breathe while submerged (Fainer et al., 1951).

CENTRAL NERVOUS SYSTEM INJURY

The central nervous system is obviously the most susceptible to damage in any form of hypoxia. In the normal brain the energy substrate required for the preservation of neuronal function is provided by adenosine triphosphate (ATP), the generation of which is fueled by both oxygen and glucose. In the event of either a reduction in supply, as in progressive hypoxia, or complete failure in delivery, as occurs in circulatory arrest, there is a rapid depletion of ATP stores and neuronal damage. Neuronal cells do have a limited ability to maintain ATP levels by anaerobic glycolysis with cerebral blood flow levels as low as 30% of normal (Hossmann, 1983), but below this level there is a rapid accumulation of lactate, which is partly responsible for the development of ischemic cellular edema. The precipitous fall in high energy compound levels causes the breakdown of the cells' ability to maintain the normal gradients between intracellular and extracellular sodium and potassium ions, resulting in a intracellular influx of Na^+ and efflux of K^+. This in turn leads to the cells and mitochondria absorbing water and swelling. There is a well-established window of four–six minutes before irreversible neuronal damage occurs in the presence of complete interruption of oxygen supply to the brain under normothermic conditions (Weinberger, Gibbon, and Gibbon, 1940; Heymans, 1950), although there is preservation of high energy metabolic activity, enzymatic functions and action potentials even after 60 minutes of total anoxia (Hossmann and Kleiheies, 1973). A secondary phase of injury even after the hypoxia is corrected or the circulation restored has been the focus of much research and therapeutic endeavor over the past ten years. It has recently become clear that one of the principal mediators of post-hypoxic/ischemic injury is calcium ion (Ca^{2+}), which is normally required for the preservation of cell membrane integrity. In hypoxic/ischemic injury Ca^{2+} influx has been noted in neuronal (Harris, Symon, and Bronston, 1981) as well as cardiac and smooth muscle cells (Naylor, Poole-Wilson, and Williams, 1979). This sudden influx of Ca^{2+} results in the activation of destructive proteases and phospholipases. Enzymic reactions in turn wreak havoc with intracellular membrane stability and metabolism.

While this chain of events occurs rapidly in the situation of either reduced or absent organ perfusion or hypoxia, the cycle is not interrupted or reversed by simply restoring perfusion. An ongoing period of cell injury that occurs during the re-establishment of circulation, frequently referred to as the "reperfusion injury," is common to all forms of hypoxic/ischemic cellular injury, whether it be neuronal, cardiac, pulmonary, or renal. The key role played by Ca^{2+} in this reperfusion injury, now well established, has led to the considerable recent interest in the potential use of calcium channel blockers in post-hypoxic cerebral injury (White et al., 1983; Deshpande and Wieloch, 1986). Even with restoration of an adequate circulation there will be a prolonged period of cerebral hypoperfusion, despite the fact that the mean systemic pressure perfusing the cerebral circulation has returned to normal. Winegar (Winegar et al., 1983) has shown that cerebral cortical flow approaches zero 90 minutes after reperfusion following a 20-minute cardiac arrest. Furthermore, this state of hypoperfusion is maintained for up to 18 hours after circulatory arrest, while at the same time there was no change in intracranial pressure (ICP). Post-hypoxic cellular injury will also trip the cyclo-oxygenase pathway of the arachidonic acid cascade, producing the vasoactive compounds thromboxane and the leukotrienes (Pichard, 1981). Thromboxane, in particular, is intensely vasoconstrictive. The other major cytotoxic products of ischemic injury are the free oxygen radicals. These are the by-products of high energy metabolism that attack the cell if the normal defense mechanisms, which consist of enzymes and free radical scavengers, fail (McCord, 1985). The role of toxic oxygen radicals in cellular injury has been most clearly defined in the lung in the adult respiratory distress syndrome or acute lung injury, where they have been identified as one of the principal causes of ongoing pulmonary damage (Deneke and Fanburg, 1980; Rinaldo and Rogers, 1982; Davis et al., 1983; Tate and Repine, 1983). This underscores the fact that there is a unifying concept in all forms of hypoxic/ischemic cellular injury. The cycle of events that begins with ATP depletion on through K^+ efflux, cellular edema, reperfusion injury with Ca^{2+} influx through the tripping of the arachidonic acid cascade and the release of toxic oxygen radicals is common to all organs.

The central nervous system injury in near-drowning is analogous to asphyxiation, where the heart continues to circulate blood to the brain that is becoming increasingly desaturated, so there is an ongoing cerebral insult even before the circulation ceases altogether. If the victim is rescued in this period there is a chance that, with effective on-site CPR, effective circulation and oxygen to the brain will be restored. If not, and the period of submersion extends beyond the point of circulatory arrest, the outlook is very much worse, except in the setting of hypothermia. The temperature of the water at the time of the accident has a profound influence on the ability of the brain to withstand hypoxia. It is becoming increasingly clear that near-drownings that occur in icy (<5°C) water conditions have a much more favorable prognosis for cerebral recovery compared to those that occur in warm water pools. There are now many well-documented cases in the medical literature where full neurological recovery has been associated with prolonged submersion times (Kvittengen and Naess, 1963; De Villata et al., 1973; Hunt, 1974; Siebke et al., 1975; Sekar et al., 1980; Young, Zalneraitis, and Dooling, 1980; Montes and Conn, 1980; Bolte et al., 1988; Biggart and Bohn, 1990). In each instance the core temperature shortly after rescue was <30°C; indeed, there seems to be a fairly well-defined cut-off point at around 30°C, above which the prognosis for neurological recovery with prolonged submersion becomes considerably worse. It has been known since Bigelow's experiments in the 1950s that the brain's ability to withstand periods of hypoxia is considerably increased by hypothermia (Bigelow, Lindsay, and Greenwood, 1950). This phenomenon is used to advantage during the repair of complex congenital heart lesions in newborn infants where periods of complete circulatory arrest can be tolerated for up to 60 minutes without neurological sequelae, with brain temperatures as low as 12°C. Although some authorities have suggested that the "diving reflex" is responsible for these remarkable recoveries (Keatinge, 1969; Gooden, 1972), it is far more likely that it is rapid core cooling seen in submersion that is responsible for the preservation of brain function. A series of experiments in anesthetized dogs has shown that temperature drops of up to 6°C occur in one minute following aspiration of icy water compared to only 1°C in dogs who were not allowed to aspirate (Conn et al., 1995). The pulmonary vascular receives the total cardiac output and acts as an extremely efficient heat exchanger in this situation. In this study, respiration continued during submersion, and the serum electrolyte changes confirmed that aspiration had occurred.

IMMERSION AND SUBMERSION HYPOTHERMIA

Many incidents of near-drowning, particularly in high latitudes where water temperatures are cooler, are associated with accidental hypothermia. The degree of hypothermia and the rapidity of onset depend on whether the victim is submerged or merely immersed. Older children or adolescents may be able to maintain flotation until, with the onset of hypothermia, the victim may become increasingly confused, disorientated, stuporous, and finally drown following loss of consciousness. The rapidity of onset of these stages of hypothermia will depend mainly on the water temperature and, to a lesser extent, on factors such as the amount of adipose tissue, type of clothing, and victim's activity while immersed. Even an excellent swimmer cannot expect to survive more than a few minutes in freezing water before severe hypothermia and drowning ensue. At the opposite end of the scale, a skilled swimmer could be expected to survive indefinitely in water temperature above 20°C without developing hypothermia, until drowning following exhaustion (Keatinge, 1969). In high latitudes, sea and lake temperatures seldom rise above 15°C, even in summer months, so hypothermia frequently accompanies near-drowning accidents in this environment.

Profound physiological changes that occur following immersion in cold water (<15°C) have important implications for the individual's ability to survive the incident (Figure 2). Immediately upon immersion there may be a precipitated rise in arterial blood pressure. Goode (Goode, 1976) has recorded a blood pressure of over 200 mmHg in a healthy subject suddenly immersed to the neck in cold water. LeBlanc (LeBlanc, 1976) has shown mean increases of 30–40 mmHg in systolic pressure when either the face or the limbs are immersed in water at 4°C. At the same time, facial immersion causes a reflex bradycardia, the afferent limb of which is the trigeminal nerve and which is independent of baroreceptor function. On the other hand, immersion of a limb into cold water produces a reflex sympathetic discharge, resulting in an increase in heart rate.

The other area where there are major and immediate changes on contact with cold water is the respiratory system. A near instantaneous increase in minute ventilation due to the onset of an involuntary hyperventilation may result in an increase in minute ventilation of up to 90 liters/min in adults for the first few breaths (Cooper, 1976). There is an immediate reduction in $PaCO_2$ and a decrease in cerebral blood flow commensurate with the increase in minute ventilation. The duration of this response varies from individual to individual. Human volunteers may continue to hyperventilate for up to ten minutes in water at 16°C while in other subjects ventilation returns to normal within three minutes in water at 8°C. The magnitude of this respiratory response also depends on the amount of clothing worn by the immersion victim, with gasping and hyperventilation subsiding more quickly when the subject is fully clothed.

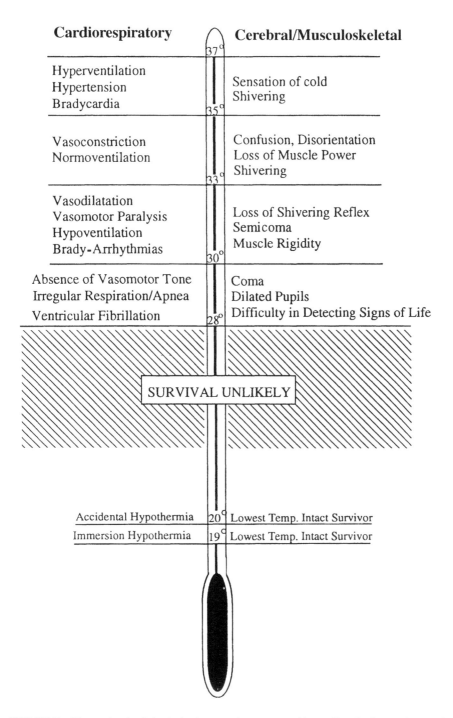

FIGURE 2 The pathophysiological changes that occur with cooling in immersion and accidental hypothermia.

Following the immediate cardiorespiratory responses to immersion in a hypothermic environment, a more gradual adaptation takes place, which depends on the duration of immersion, the water temperature, insulation factors that may decrease heat loss, and, to some extent, the behavior of the immersion victim. As the core temperature decreases to 36–33°C, the body will attempt to defend the victim against further heat loss and restore normothermia by peripheral vasoconstriction, which results in shunting of blood from the periphery to the core. Cardiac output will be maintained, at least initially. At the same time, shivering thermogenesis begins. The involuntary muscle contractions of shivering result in an increase in oxygen consumption and cardiac output. Shivering will be maintained until the core temperature decreases below 33°C, at which time muscle rigidity ensues. Shivering ceases and the decrease in body temperature accelerates. At the same time, the protective peripheral vasoconstrictive reflex wanes with the onset of vasomotor paralysis.

Prolonged immersion in hypothermic conditions inevitably begets vasomotor paralysis, which results in peripheral venous pooling. During immersion, especially if the victim is wearing a flotation device, this venous pooling is counteracted by the effect of the hydrostatic pressure on the dependent parts of the body. In a warm water (25°C) environment, this hydrostatic force may account for up to 35% rise in cardiac output (Arborelius et al., 1972). This observation is more than a physiological curiosity. When the hypothermic immersion victim is removed from the water, the sudden loss of this hydrostatic effect is suddenly released and may result in acute cardiovascular collapse and death. Victims extracted in the vertical position (e.g., helicopter rescue) are particularly susceptible to this phenomenon. This hypothesis for the cause of post-rescue cardiovascular collapse is altogether a more satisfactory explanation than the more time-honored theory of ventricular fibrillation caused by the cold blood returning to the core from the peripheries (Burton and Foholm, 1955) and underlines the dangers of sudden position shifts in hypothermic patients.

At a temperature of around 30°C, complete vasomotor paralysis can be anticipated. Heart rate will decrease with decreasing temperature in the absence of any vigorous activity, such as swimming attempts. As the temperature falls toward 30°C, brady-arrhythmias will develop. The temperature of 28°C is generally accepted as the threshold for the development of ventricular fibrillation in adults, although this has been largely determined from observations made during cardiopulmonary bypass in humans and cannot therefore be applied as precisely to immersion hypothermia. This rule does not necessarily apply to hypothermia in children where a slow sinus rhythm may be preserved at temperatures well below 28°C.

The initial hyperventilation that occurs immediately on immersion in cold water subsides to normoventilation in the core temperature range 33–35°C. Below this temperature it can be anticipated that the victim will hypoventilate. However, at the same time, metabolic rate and hence CO_2 production will diminish (in the absence of physical activity) and therefore $PaCO_2$ may well be normal or even slightly reduced during this phase of cooling. As the temperature falls toward 30°C, respiration becomes irregular and more shallow, with apnea a common feature. Below 30°C spontaneous respiration, if present, may be extremely difficult to detect.

Hypothermia also has important effects on the central nervous system which may result in a delayed drowning. As body temperature decreases below 35°C, the victim becomes increasingly confused and disorientated, which may result in irrational decisions, such as discarding clothing, which further lessen the chances of survival. Below 33°C, a victim becomes semicomatose and can no longer maintain the head clear of the water. A substantial number die from asphyxia and aspiration at this time. At core temperatures of 30°C it may be difficult to distinguish between hypothermia and death as frank coma supervenes. Pupil responses are unreliable, as pupils may become fixed and dilated under severe hypothermic conditions. Below a temperature of 30°C, in an adult, the chances for full recovery with intact cerebral function are poor, although there are reports of full recovery with temperatures as low as 20°C in accidental hypothermia due to exposure (Althaus et al., 1982). The same criteria do not apply to children, however, where full recovery follows submersion, and near-drowning accidents have been reported with temperatures as low as 19°C (Bolte et al., 1988).

The rate of cooling with immersion hypothermia depends on many factors, not the least of which is water temperature. In humans, there is a balance between heat production generated by metabolism and exercise and heat loss to the environment. Normally, when someone is exposed to a thermally hostile environment, behavioral and physiological adaptation occur, which reduce the heat loss, e.g., additional clothing and increased exercise tend to reduce the degree of cooling. Clothing provides insulating properties in accidental hypothermia, as warm air is trapped between layers. Obviously, these same rules do not apply in hypothermic immersion accidents. The victim is frequently inadequately clad in the first place, and even when clothing is worn, its insulating properties are greatly reduced when wet. Despite this, clothing should always be retained following immersion as it has been estimated that the rate of heat loss can be reduced by 50% in such circumstances.

Exercise will also greatly increase heat loss during immersion as it tends to increase blood flow to muscles and thereby accelerate the rate of cooling. During swimming attempts, movements of the arms and legs tend to expose areas of high vascular supply near the skin surface, such as the groins and axillae. The standard teaching is not to try and swim for the shore, unless it is within easy reach, and to minimize the heat loss by adopting the Heat Escape Lessening Position (HELP), a tucked position with the arms by the sides and the legs drawn up (Collis, 1976). In warm water (>20°C) the immersion victim may well be able to maintain normal body temperature with exercise, as the heat production in this instance will balance the heat loss. Keatinge (Keatinge, 1969) has produced survival charts for water at various temperatures, which suggest that in water greater than 20°C the victim's survival is limited only by the capacity to stay afloat, whereas at 10°C the maximum time limit before succumbing to hypothermia and drowning is around three hours (Figure 3).

Finally, the rate of cooling will be profoundly affected by the amount of adipose tissue and the body surface area. The tall, thin person will lose heat much more rapidly than the short, fat individual. The issue of surface area highlights the important differences in cooling between adults and children. The latter, with a large

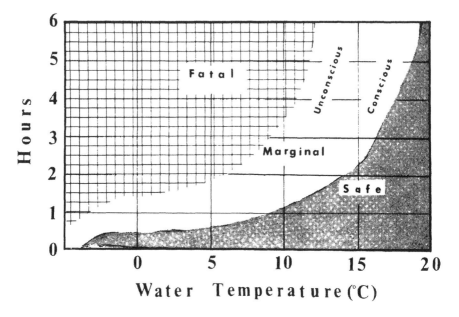

FIGURE 3   Predicted survival times following immersion in water at various temperatures in victims who maintain flotation. (From Keatinge, W., 1969, *Survival in Cold Water*, Blackwell Scientific Publications, Oxford, U.K. With permission.)

surface area to weight ratio, will cool faster. This has important implications in the prognosis for cerebral recovery from hypothermic near-drowning incidents in children, where the rapidity of cooling means that core temperature drops quickly, which undoubtedly confers some degree of cerebral protection during the hypoxia of submersion and helps to explain some of the remarkable recoveries seen after prolonged submersion in children. The core cooling in this situation is so rapid it cannot be accounted for by surface cooling alone, and recent animal studies have shown that the aspiration of cold water (<5°C) sets up a counter-current exchange mechanism within the lungs which accounts for a temperature decrease of up to 6°C within one minute of submersion (Conn et al., 1995) (Figure 4).

RESUSCITATION IN NEAR-DROWNING AND HYPOTHERMIA

Resuscitation at the Scene

Because of the widespread knowledge of techniques of cardiopulmonary resuscitation, most submersion victims arrive at a medical facility having had some sort of resuscitation attempted. The time-honored ABCs (Airway, Breathing, and Circulation) of resuscitation should be applied at the scene. If the victim makes no respiratory effort following clearing of the airway, mouth-to-mouth ventilation should be started immediately. That often results in the resumption of spontaneous respiration, if the immersion period has been of short duration. If no pulses are palpable, chest

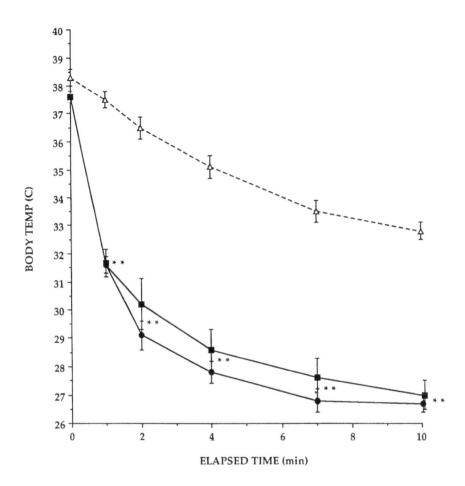

FIGURE 4 Change in core temperature associated with submersion in cold water (5°C). Solid lines represent animals who were anesthetized but not intubated before submersion and aspirated either fresh or salt water. Dashed line represents control animals that were anesthetized, intubated, but not submerged and therefore did not aspirate. (From Conn, A. W. et al., 1995, *Critical Care Medicine*. With permission.)

compressions should be started. If the victim is severely hypothermic, peripheral pulses may be difficult or impossible to detect, but when in doubt, CPR should be started. The reported dangers of causing the hypothermic victim's heart to fibrillate with chest compressions are greatly exaggerated. The victim should be removed as quickly as possible to a hospital, with CPR continued in transit.

If vital signs return with the initial resuscitation maneuvers, the patient should be wrapped in clothing or blankets to minimize further heat loss and be evacuated to a hospital, with care taken to avoid sudden positional changes, which may cause hemodynamic instability in the hypothermic patient.

The most difficult dilemma that faces the on-site rescuer is whether to initiate CPR in the apparently lifeless prolonged submersion victim, especially in the presence of hypothermia. There is no absolute rule in such circumstances but, as a general principle, if the victim has been submerged for less than one hour in hypothermic (icy) conditions, CPR should be started and the decision whether to continue deferred until the patient reaches the hospital. In normothermic near-drowning accidents submersion times of greater than 10 minutes are not associated with normal neurological recovery. Reported submersion times from parents or other witnesses are notoriously unreliable. Quan (Quan and Kinder, 1992) in a series that addressed predictors that could be used to determine survival following aggressive on-site resuscitation following submersion in non-icy water found that there were no neurologically intact survivors in children who had been submerged for more than 10 minutes and who did not have return of a perfusing cardiac rhythm within 25 minutes.

RESUSCITATION IN THE EMERGENCY ROOM

Techniques and duration of resuscitation depend on whether or not the victim is hypothermic and whether or not vital signs are present or absent at the time of arrival. If there is no palpable pulse without chest compression on admission to the emergency room, CPR should be continued according to standard advanced cardiac life support (ACLS) and pediatric advanced cardiac life support (PALS) protocols (*Advanced Paediatric Life Support*, 1993). The importance of administering 100% oxygen to all near-drowning victims, even if they have regained consciousness, cannot be overemphasized. Hasan (Hasan et al., 1971), in a series of 36 near-drowning victims, found that the mean PaO_2 was 55 mmHg, even when breathing supplemental oxygen. Unrecognized and untreated hypoxemia can change a minor hypoxic insult into devastating cerebral damage.

Rectal temperature should be measured with a low-reading rectal thermometer, even if the drowning occurred in warm water. Children, in particular, have the ability to cool rapidly following even a relatively short immersion in non-hypothermic conditions. A brief neurological assessment should be made to evaluate the level of coma, with particular note made of abnormal movements such as decerebrate or decorticate posturing, or seizure activity. Those patients who exhibit these abnormal findings or fail to regain consciousness should be intubated and mildly hyperventilated to a $PaCO_2$ of around 35 mmHg. The other invariable finding in near-drowning is the presence of a metabolic acidosis with a pH of 7.2 or less consistent throughout most published series (Kruss et al., 1979; Modell, Graves, and Kuch, 1980; Frates, 1981; Quan et al., 1990; Biggart and Bohn, 1990). Successful outcomes have been reported with initial pHs of <7.0. Consequently, with the likelihood of acidosis and hypoxemia being present, it is mandatory to obtain arterial blood gases as soon as possible. Empiric treatment of the acidemia with bicarbonate is appropriate if there is a delay in obtaining blood gas analysis. Although there is some current debate about the use of bicarbonate therapy during cardiac arrest in adults, there is no doubt that pediatric patients require relatively large doses for resuscitation (*Advanced Paediatric Life Support*, 1993).

Severe asphyxiation will frequently result in sequestration of large amounts of fluid from the intravascular space, the so-called "leaky capillary syndrome." Replacement of these third space losses frequently necessitate that large amounts of colloid be given in the initial resuscitation period in order to obtain an adequate systemic and cerebral perfusion pressure. Failure to respond to intravascular replacement (20mls/kg) of colloid should be an indication to start inotropes.

Acidemia will tend to antagonize the effect of catecholamine drugs, as will hypothermia, although a recent study has shown that dopamine will increase cardiac output even under hypothermic conditions (Nicodemus, Chancy, and Herold, 1981). Even with the best of resuscitation it is unlikely that sinus rhythm and cardiac output can be restored in the patient with a fibrillating heart and a core temperature of <30°C; hence, a rewarming protocol should be commenced in hypothermic patients. The choice of rewarming technique depends on the degree of hypothermia and, to some extent, whether or not circulation is intact.

REWARMING TECHNIQUES

The modes of rewarming can be divided into those that use the body's own endogenous heat production and those that require the application of external or internal heat sources to raise body temperature. Whether rewarming is rapid or slow is also considered.

Passive rewarming results from the prevention of excessive heat loss. The patient is placed in an ambient temperature of 21–23°C and covered with warm blankets. The technique relies on the patient's ability to raise body temperature by endogenous heat production while at the same time minimizing further heat losses to the environment. The respiratory tract evaporative losses can be minimized by breathing warmed humidified oxygen (40–45°C) and intravenous fluid infusions are warmed by passage through a heating coil. For passive rewarming to be effective it is essential that the shivering mechanism be preserved. Below 30°C shivering is suppressed and little benefit is gained by slow passive rewarming at these temperatures. The temperature increase using this technique is about 1°C/hr (Edsall, 1980).

Active rewarming relies on heat transfer from an exogenous heat source to the patient through the skin or via the core. In the former this may take the form of external surface rewarming by a heated water mattress or a radiant heat source. This technique is useful in mild hypothermia (32–35°C), but care must be exercised with the use of all topical heating as thermal injury to the skin is a real possibility. Meticulous attention to maintaining an adequate circulating volume and oxygenation are crucial during rewarming, since the onset of vasodilation is accompanied by major fluid shifts which may lead to cardiovascular collapse and death.

Active core rewarming is the most rapid and efficient of all rewarming techniques as heat is delivered in close proximity to the central circulation. Methods of active core rewarming include: (a) airway rewarming; (b) warmed intravenous fluids; (c) peritoneal dialysis with warmed dialysate fluid; (d) gastric lavage; (e) colonic lavage; (f) bladder irrigation; (g) mediastinal and pleural lavage; and (h) partial cardiopulmonary bypass. The most accessible and least invasive of all forms of active core rewarming is through heating the inspired gas delivered by an endotracheal tube. Increasing the temperature of the inspired gas to 40–45°C with high relative humidity is an efficient method of increasing temperature. By exposing the extensive capillary network of the pulmonary vascular bed to humidified heated gases, this technique reduces the net heat loss from the respiratory tract to zero. Humidification of the respiratory tract will also have beneficial effects on micociliary transport. If a heated water bath humidifier is unavailable a condenser humidifier (Swedish nose) or a Waters canister will provide heating of inspired gases in the intubated patient. The condenser humidifier is simply a gauze screen which allows expired water vapor to condense. The moisture then evaporates and warms the inspired gases. The efficiency of this device for the conservation of temperature and the reduction of respiratory tract heat loss has been demonstrated in the operating room environment (Steward, 1976). A Waters canister that was formerly used for CO_2 absorption of exhaled gases during anesthesia is also useful for airway rewarming. The CO_2–soda lime reaction produces heat which then raises the temperature of the inspired gases. While neither device is as efficient in the hypothermic patient as heated water bath humidifiers, both are readily portable and ideal for resuscitation in the field or use during patient transport. Lloyd (Lloyd, 1973) has described a portable version of the Waters canister complete with mask and breathing circuit for use in the field. In unintubated, spontaneously breathing patients raising the temperature of the oxygen delivered by mask will also have a beneficial effect on core temperature, although it will be less efficient compared to that delivered by an endotracheal tube.

There are several reports in the literature of central core rewarming by the irrigation of body cavities and the gastrointestinal tract (Linton and Ledingham, 1966; Coughlin, 1973; Johnson, 1977; Soung et al., 1977; Ledingham and Mone, 1978; Reuler and Parker, 1978; Jessen and Hagelsten, 1978; Ledingham and Mone, 1980; Miller, Danzl, and Thomas, 1980; Ledingham et al., 1980; Mahajan, Myers, and Baldini, 1981; Schissler, Parker, and Scott, 1981). Rewarming the peritoneum and abdominal organs with rapid exchanges of warmed peritoneal dialysis fluid has proven successful in resuscitating severely hypothermic victims. The technique is to use isotonic dialysate with 1.5% dextrose warmed to 45–50°C with exchanges every 40 minutes (Johnson, 1977). Temperature rises of up to 2°C/hr have been reported using this approach. Careful monitoring of serum potassium and blood sugar is necessary, as hyperglycemia and hypokalemia may occur with rapid fluid exchanges.

Heat also may be transferred to the body by intragastric or intracolonic infusions of warm fluid which will indirectly transfer heat to the core. There are several reports of the use of intragastric lavage techniques in the literature, commonly combined with peritoneal dialysis (Reuler and Parker, 1978; Miller et al., 1980). Ledingham (Ledingham et al., 1980) has recently described a modified Senstaken tube with a continuous flushing system for lavage of the esophagus and stomach. Colonic rewarming is technically more difficult as the proper positioning of the tube is uncertain, and there is always the possibility of damage to the colonic mucosa. Direct warming of the heart and mediastinum through a thoracotomy has been described (Coughlin, 1973; Althaus et al., 1982). A less invasive but equally effective method is direct blood rewarming using partial cardiopulmonary bypass and a heat exchanger. There are several case reports of the successful use of this technique in severe nonimmersion hypothermic accidents associated with cardiac arrest (Towne et al., 1972; Truscott, Firor, and Clein, 1973; Wickstrom et al., 1976; Althaus et al., 1982). Partial bypass is typically established from femoral or iliac veins to femoral artery. Wickstrom (Wickstrom et al., 1976) has described three patients with ventricular fibrillation and temperatures <25°C who were rewarmed to normal temperatures in less than one hour, two of whom survived without sequelae. Althaus (Althaus et al., 1982) described a truly remarkable series of successful resuscitations using partial bypass in three adult avalanche victims. All had core temperatures of <25°C and were in ventricular fibrillation, yet survived intact, although one had been buried for five hours.

There is little doubt that partial cardiopulmonary bypass is the "Rolls Royce" of rewarming techniques and is the most rapid and effective method of rewarming the arrested patient. The technique is invasive, requires heparinization, and can be done only in large centers where the equipment and personnel are available. Although there have been some remarkable recoveries using this technique in severe accidental hypothermia, the outcome is less likely to be successful in submersion hypothermia because of the timing of cerebral hypoxia in relation to cooling. The two situations are not comparable as the "dry" hypothermia victim cools gradually before the hypoxic insult, while the cerebral insult is instantaneous and frequently devastating in near-drowning. Having said that, Bolte (Bolte et al., 1988) has reported full neurological recovery where extracorporeal rewarming was used in the resuscitation of a two-and-a-half-year-old child who was submerged for 66 minutes in freezing water and had a core temperature of 19°C at the time of rescue. Letsou reportedly (Letsou et al., 1992) had two children submerged for more than 30 minutes with temperatures of less than 25°C and good neurological recovery.

CHOICE OF REWARMING TECHNIQUES

Despite an improvement in diagnosis and treatment of hypothermia in the past decade there is still debate in the medical literature whether rewarming should be by the slow passive technique or by the rapid active technique. Proponents of the slow passive technique advocate its use as it causes the least hemodynamic disturbance and fluid shifts. They cite an increased incidence of "afterdrop" and cardiac arrhythmias during rapid active rewarming (Emslie-Smith, 1958; Eruehan, 1960; Duguid, Simpson, and Stowers, 1961; Savard et al., 1985). Most of the negative experiences with rapid active rewarming were in the late 1950s and early 1960s when resuscitation as we know it was in the earlier phases of development and little was understood about fluid shifts associated with hypothermia. Most deaths that occurred could be more properly ascribed to the unmasking of hypovolemia and hypoxemia during rewarming.

There has been a more critical look recently at the theory of "afterdrop" causing further core cooling and cardiac standstill during rewarming. The theory is based on the suggestion that the periphery dilates during rewarming and there is a return of cold blood to the core that causes further central cooling and cardiac rhythm disturbance. However, Savard (Savard et al., 1985) has shown that the "afterdrop" in core temperature precedes peripheral dilation in human volunteers exposed to

HYPOTHERMIA 33–36°C

- Warm IV fluids
- Warm blankets
- Heated water mattress
- Heated, humidified oxygen

HYPOTHERMIA <33°C

INTACT CIRCULATION   NO CIRCULATION

- Warm IV fluids   - CPR
- Heated humidified gases by ETT   - Warm IV fluids
- Peritoneal lavage   - Heated humidified gases by ETT
- Gastric/rectal lavage   - Peritoneal lavage
                                       - Gastric/rectal lavage
                                       - Extracorporeal rewarming

FIGURE 5   Rewarming protocol for immersion or accidental hypothermia. The approach depends on the degree of hypothermia and the presence or absence of circulation.

hypothermia and, furthermore, at the time of maximal peripheral dilation, core temperature has already started to rise. There seems little reason, therefore, to advocate the use of slow passive rewarming for anything but mildly hypothermic patients. There is now a considerable body of evidence, albeit often anecdotal, to support the use of rapid active rewarming in serious hypothermic injury, and several large series attest to the successful use of the technique where heartbeat and cardiac output are maintained (O'Keefe, 1977; Ledingham and Mone, 1978; Miller et al., 1980; Edsall, 1980). In the situation where there is no spontaneous circulation, body temperature *must* be increased by active core rewarming. The current recommendations are that passive external rewarming be used in mild hypothermia (32–35°C), rapid active rewarming at temperatures below this, and rapid internal core rewarming in every instance in which there is no circulation (*Advanced Paediatric Life Support*, 1993). The current recommendations for rewarming are summarized in Figure 5.

DURATION OF RESUSCITATION

Perhaps the most difficult decision facing the physician in the emergency department is how long resuscitation efforts should be continued in the presence of no cardiac output, especially when hypothermia is present. The recent publicity given to some remarkable recoveries in children who have survived intact following prolonged hypothermic immersion accidents has led to some very protracted resuscitation efforts lasting several hours. The problem is compounded by the fact that there is some difficulty in distinguishing between death and hypothermia at <30°C. Therefore, CPR and rewarming are continued until either a temperature of >33°C is established, at which stage resuscitation is abandoned if there is no cardiac output, or until a sinus rhythm is restored.

TABLE 1
Intact Neurological Survival Associated with Prolonged Submersion

Reference	Temp °C	Age (Years)	Submersion time (min)	Duration of CPR
Siebke (1975)	24	5	40	1.75 hrs
Kvittengen (1963)	24	5	22	2.5 hrs
Hunt (1974)	27	5	30	2. hrs
Young (1974)	27	7	15	2.5 hrs
De Villata (1973)	28	16	—	1 hr
Sekar (1980)	29	23	25	45 min
Bolte (1988)	19	2.5	66	2 hrs

Unfortunately, there is no easy answer to this dilemma. A review of the literature reveals that the longest period of submersion associated with intact survival is now 66 minutes (Bolte et al., 1988) and that this was associated with a core temperature of 19°C in a child (Table 1). There is, then, a rational basis for pursuing aggressive resuscitation in children following a hypothermic submersion of 60 minutes duration in very cold water, as there have been successful outcomes following hypothermic arrests with periods of CPR greater than two hours. However, one should bear in mind that these are isolated case reports and only the dramatic recoveries, rather than the heroic failures, are published. We hold the view that failure to increase core temperature after 60 minutes of appropriate rewarming and resuscitation techniques probably truly indicates death.

In contrast, the prognosis for intact survival in pediatric victims of warm water drowning who present to the emergency room with absent vital signs is worse than hypothermic submersion. The outcome is probably as bad as from any other form of hypoxic cardiac arrest since victims uniformly remain dead or survive with devastating neurological damage (Nichter and Everett, 1989; Biggart and Bohn, 1990). The decision on the duration of CPR should be made in light of the knowledge that although it may be possible with aggressive resuscitation to restore a sinus rhythm, the outcome is likely to be a severely brain-damaged patient. The results of prolonged resuscitation in this group of patients would not justify continuing with CPR for more than 20 minutes.

IN-HOSPITAL TREATMENT OF NEAR-DROWNING

As a rule all patients who have suffered a submersion accident, even if relatively trivial, should be admitted to hospital for a minimum of 24 hours of observation. At the end of this period, those patients who have had a relatively brief submersion and who are neurologically normal with no respiratory symptoms may be discharged. The treatment of more severe near-drowning accidents is based on the severity of the cerebral hypoxic insult and the degree of pulmonary damage. A neurological assessment based on the level of consciousness should be made following resuscitation.

Those patients with posturing movements, seizures, or persistent coma should be admitted to ICU and electively ventilated mechanically for at least 24 hours, as these abnormalities indicate a significant hypoxic insult. Any patient who regains consciousness following resuscitation but who has signs of pulmonary edema with a significant degree of ARDS (tachypnea, cyanosis, grunting, etc.) should be admitted to ICU for 24 hours of ventilation. Those with lesser degrees of pulmonary involvement (mild ARDS) may require only diuresis and monitoring of blood gases, not ventilation.

NEAR-DROWNING TREATMENT PROTOCOL

The current treatment protocol for near-drowning victims who have restoration of cardiac output is based on the attempt to decrease secondary cerebral injury factors and the treatment of pulmonary complications, which can aggravate cerebral injury and lead to death from hypoxemia.

TREATMENT OF CEREBRAL INJURY

The treatment of the hypoxic cerebral insult in near-drowning consists of avoiding factors that will increase cerebral edema in the already injured brain. These factors include overhydration seizures, hyperthermia, hypercarbia, and hypoxia. Consequently, those patients who remain comatose after resuscitation from near-drowning are treated with the following protocol:

1. **Hyperventilation** to a $PaCO_2$ of 35 mmHg: where the patient exhibits abnormal posturing movements, muscle relaxants should be used to abate presumed rises in ICP.
2. **The maintenance of oxygenation:** a PaO_2 of >90 mmHg with PEEP >5 cm H_2O if the FiO_2 requirement is above 0.5.
3. **The maintenance of cerebral perfusion pressure:** a mean systemic pressure (MAP) >50 mmHg is necessary to provide an adequate cerebral perfusion pressure. In the event that MAP remains <50 mmHg, dopamine 5–20 µg/kg/min should be started.
4. **Free water restriction** to 30% normal maintenance fluid for the first 24 hours with addition diuretics added to treat pulmonary edema or to avoid a positive fluid balance.
5. **The treatment of seizure activity** with phenobarbitone 5–10 mg/kg/day up to a dose of 20 mg/kg/day if seizures are intractable.
6. **Temperature control:** strict attention to the avoidance of a rise in temperature in the first 24–48 hours (above 37°C) is vital. The tendency is for the temperature to rise above normal after CNS injury. Increases in temperature above 37°C will aggravate cerebral injury and should be treated with paralysis and surface cooling. Experimental evidence also indicates that a mild (35°C) degree of hypothermia may help to protect against secondary injury in this situation.

This regimen should be maintained for 24 hours, at the end of which a repeat neurological assessment should be made with specific note taken of the depth of coma and the presence of abnormal movements. Those patients who show an improvement in neurological findings should be weaned from the respirator over a 24–48 hour period depending on the degree of cerebral insult and the extent of pulmonary involvement. Those patients who remain persistently comatose, especially with flaccidity or abnormal posturing movements, should have an electroencephalogram (EEG) and evoked potentials to establish baseline cerebral activity. If the EEG is done sooner, i.e., immediately after resuscitation, the result may be misleading as cerebral activity is frequently very depressed following prolonged hypoxia, especially when associated with hypothermia. In the event the patient remains persistently comatose, treatment should be continued for a further 24 hours and the assessment repeated before a decision is made to discontinue aggressive support. Somatosensory-evoked potentials and brainstem auditory-evoked responses provide useful information on neurological outcome with bilaterally absent SEPs indicating persistent vegetative survival (Goodwin, Friedman, and Bellefleur, 1991; Fisher, Peterson, and Hicks, 1992).

TREATMENT OF PULMONARY COMPLICATIONS

Immersion accidents are frequently accompanied by the development of ARDS triggered by the aspiration of water into the lungs. This may vary in degree from relatively trivial involvement with minimal respiratory symptoms such as a slight increase in respiratory rate and a slightly increased alveolar to arterial oxygen difference (A-aDO$_2$) to florid pulmonary edema with profound hypoxemia and opacification of the lungs on X-ray. Fortunately, most minor immersion incidents fall into the former category and are the pathological equivalent of the beginning of the exudative phase of early ARDS. Good response to diuretics and fluid restriction is expected. At the other end of the severity scale, the degree of acute lung injury may require positive pressure ventilation with high peak airway pressures and high levels of PEEP (up to 20 cm H$_2$O). This is the pathological equivalent of a florid exudative phase of ARDS, which may eventually evolve into the proliferative phase with damage to epithelial cells, dense hyaline membrane formation, the invasion of fibroblasts, and the development of pulmonary fibrosis (Glauser and Smith, 1975). Death may result from progressive hypoxemia. Although pulmonary aspiration is the trigger for the development of ARDS, hypoxic damage to multiple organs and sepsis may contribute significantly to the ongoing acute lung injury. It is now well established that oxygen therapy plays a major role in the development of ARDS through the generation of toxic oxygen radicals (Frank, 1985). Therefore, the same principles of treatment apply to the treatment of pulmonary involvement in neardrowning as in any other form of ARDS, namely to attempt to maintain an arterial saturation of >90% (PaO$_2$ >60 mmHg) with an FiO$_2$ <0.5 using the lowest peak inspiratory pressure possible.

The major underlying mechanical change in ARDS is a decrease in lung compliance and functional residual capacity (FRC). This "stiffening" of the lung caused by filling of the interstitial space with a protein-rich exudative fluid can be reversed by the application of PEEP, which will result in the re-recruitment of lost lung volume and a rise in FRC. With respect to PEEP, the objective is to apply sufficient PEEP to increase the PaO_2 to reduce the FiO_2 less than 0.5 and simultaneously avoid hemodynamic compromise (so called "best PEEP") (Suter and Fairley, 1975). Septic complications should be identified and vigorously treated as septicemia, a common problem in near-drowning that will maintain the cycle of lung injury. More recently, the successful use of ECMO for the treatment of ARDS secondary to near-drowning has been reported (O'Rourke et al., 1993), although this addresses only the issue of the reversal of the pulmonary, not the cerebral injury. The majority of those patients with severe hypoxemia who cannot be managed with conventional ventilation also have irreversible cerebral injury (Bohn et al., 1986).

INFECTIOUS COMPLICATIONS OF NEAR-DROWNING

There is a high incidence of septic complications following severe near-drowning accidents that may manifest as either a pneumonitis or septicemia. Bacterial invasion may come from a variety of sources. In the first instance, the victim may inhale a significant quantity of water that may be contaminated by a variety of usually nonpathogenic organisms. There also may be severe ischemic damage to the gut mucosa resulting in bloody diarrhea, following severe asphyxia in near-drowning. Loss of integrity of the GI tract may result in bacterial invasion and septicemia. Recent conclusive evidence shows hypothermia itself may result in diminished immunity to bacterial invasion in the hypoxic host. Bohn et al. (Bohn et al., 1986) have found a high incidence of life-threatening septicemia in hypothermic near-drowning victims associated with marked reductions in the number of circulating polymorphonuclear leukocytes (PMNs); indeed, septicemia combined with hypoxia was the most frequent cause of death in this series, although all patients who died had severe cerebral hypoxia. In a series of animal experiments, the same group showed that under hypothermic conditions (30°C) there is a reduction not only in the number of circulating PMNs, but also in production and release by the bone marrow (Biggart et al., 1983; Biggart et al., 1984). Near-drowning victims, especially those who are hypothermic, are thus greatly at risk for developing septic complications from external invading organisms, nosocomial infections, and auto infection from their normally nonpathogenic bacteria. Oakes (Oakes et al., 1982) has reported a 40% incidence of positive sputum cultures in 40 near-drowning victims despite the use of prophylactic antibiotics. Our policy has not been routine use of antibiotic prophylaxis, but rather identification of septic events by daily cultures of sputum, urine, and blood and subsequent treatment with the appropriate antibiotic.

OUTCOME

With improved on-site resuscitation and advances in intensive care management, there has been an increase in the number of near-drowning victims who survive both with and without neurological sequelae. There are only three possible outcomes from drowning: death, survival with severe neurological damage, and intact survival. Very few, if any, children seem to survive with mild neurological deficits except in hypothermic submersion accidents (Bell, Ellenberg, and McComb, 1985); however, reliable statistics on outcome following submersion accidents are difficult to interpret. Published figures for bad outcome (death or severe neurological damage) vary from 6% to 100% (Hasan et al., 1971; Hunter and Whitehouse, 1974; Peterson, 1977; Conn et al., 1978; Kruss et al., 1979; Pearn, Bart, and Yamaoka, 1979; Kruss et al., 1979; Modell et al., 1980; Montes and Conn, 1980; Frates, 1981; Dean and McComb, 1981; Dean and Kaufman, 1981; Pfenninger and Sutter, 1982; Oakes et al., 1982; Jacobsen et al., 1983; Frewin et al., 1985; Bell et al., 1985; Nichter and Everett, 1989; Quan et al., 1990; Biggart and Bohn, 1990; Quan and Kinder, 1992). Because the incidence of devastating neurological deficit, especially in children, tends to be very high, it is important that prognostic factors be used to identify poor quality survivors as early as possible after resuscitation so that aggressive support may be discontinued.

The principal prognostic factor affecting outcome prior to resuscitation in the drowning victim without vital signs is the water temperature. There is no doubt that the victim of a hypothermic immersion (water temperature <5°C), especially a child, has a greater chance of surviving intact than the near-drowning victim from the warm water backyard pool. The medical literature contains reports of prolonged submersion times of up to 40 minutes associated with intact survival. For this reason alone it is worthwhile pursuing a course of aggressive resuscitation in hypothermic near-drowning. The details of successful resuscitations of hypothermic (<30°C core temperature) near-drownings with intact survival are given in Table 1.

The other variable that may influence outcome in the prehospital period is the adequacy of on-site resuscitation. Many victims who are rescued following brief submersion (less than five minutes) will be cyanotic and apneic but with a preserved spontaneous heart beat that may be difficult to palpate because of profound bradycardia. Efficient CPR will frequently result in the return of a palpable pulse and spontaneous respiration, which will make all the difference to the outcome. The series published by Quan have shown that in non-icy water drownings where advanced life support resuscitation is rapidly available on site, good outcomes can be achieved in children without vital signs if the duration of submersion is less than ten minutes (Quan et al., 1990; Quan and Kinder, 1992). Nussbaum (Nussbaum, 1985) in a series of warm-water drownings found that estimated submersion times of less than nine minutes were associated with a higher incidence of good outcomes. Although the duration of submersion is obviously important in determining outcome, observer estimates of the time elapsed tend to be rather inaccurate. Frates (Frates, 1981) reviewed pre-hospital prognostic factors and correlated these with outcome using multivariant analysis. The "best" correlation with poor outcome was fixed dilated pupils on admission, followed by persistent coma and the absence of vital signs on admission. In warm-water drownings Frates was unable to show any statistical significance between duration of submersion and survival.

When attempting to judge the prognosis following resuscitation one should attempt to separate neurological and non-neurological assessment of prognostic indicators, although these overlap to some extent. The non-neurological assessment

TABLE 2
Coincident Diseases and Precipitating
Causes for Near-Drowning Accidents

Head Injuries
Air Embolism
Cervical Spine Injuries
Cardiovascular Disease
Seizure Disorders
Drug and Alcohol Abuse
Hypoglycemia
Child Abuse

should include complications such as the severity of the lung injury and hypoxemia which in the worst cases may result in the death of a neurologically intact survivor. One should also be alert to the fact that a considerable number of near-drowning victims have co-incident diseases or trauma that may have been the underlying cause for the submersion accident. A published series of near-drowning accidents in adults has shown that 50% have a significant medical history that may have contributed to the accident (Hunter and Whitehouse, 1974). Principal among these are seizure disorders, cervical spine injuries from diving into shallow water, and drug and alcohol abuse (Table 2).

The assessment of prognosis for neurological outcome after resuscitation has proved more difficult. Some accurate method of assessing cerebral damage in these patients after the restoration of cardiac output is important not only to determine subsequent treatment but also to evaluate the efficacy of cerebral protection protocols. Factors that would indicate a poor prognosis are the absence of spontaneous respiration, except in the presence of hypothermia. Jacobsen (Jacobsen et al., 1983) has reported a 100% mortality in children where spontaneous respiration has not returned following resuscitation. Lavelle (Lavelle and Shaw, 1993) found that unreactive pupils in the emergency room and a GCS of 5 or less on arrival in ICU indicated a poor prognosis. Both Modell (Modell et al., 1980) and Conn (Conn and Barker, 1984) have devised a scoring system based on whether the patients are awake (A), have a blunted sensorium (B), or are comatose (C) following resuscitation. In Modell's series those patients in group A have 100% survival, while mortality increases to 10% in group B and 34% in group C. Orlowski (Orlowski, 1979) has devised a scoring system for pediatric near-drowning victims using patient age, initial pH, submersion time, pupillary response, and the effectiveness of resuscitation. Although these scoring systems may be a helpful guide in determining prognosis in the immediate post-resuscitation period, we feel that a more definitive estimate can be made after a period of 12–24 hours has elapsed, when the continuation of a comatose state indicates a poor prognosis.

The near-drowning victim who remains in a coma without spontaneous limb movements and who exhibits abnormal brain stem function 24 hours after the accident will have a poor neurological outcome (Bratton, Jardin, and Morray, 1994).

A modification of the Glasgow coma score has become a widely accepted criteria for evaluating neurological injury (Dean and Kaufman, 1981; Jacobsen et al., 1983), with a GCS of 5 or less associated with a greater than 80% mortality in Dean's series (Dean and Kaufman, 1981). Abnormal posturing or seizure activity in the immediate post-resuscitation period, however, do not necessarily indicate a poor prognosis. In a review of 49 near-drowning incidents in children Bell (Bell et al., 1985) found that the presence of any motor activity was associated with a significantly greater incidence of intact survival. However, if posturing movements persist or recur after the first 12–24 hours, there is a high probability of severe brain damage. Similarly, flaccidity and fixed dilated pupils are associated with a high mortality. In Bell's series reactive pupils at the time of admission discriminated between fatalities and intact survivors but could not distinguish intact and vegetative survivors (Bell et al., 1985). Caution should be exercised in interpreting pupillary responses in the immediate post-resuscitation period as large amounts of adrenaline (epinephrine) or hypothermia may cause dilation of the pupils.

There is general agreement that the absence of a heartbeat on admission to a hospital is a universally poor prognostic sign. The finding of asystole in the emergency room is invariably associated with death or PVS (Nichter and Everett, 1989; Biggart and Bohn, 1990; Lavelle and Shaw, 1993), the exception being when the victim is hypothermic ($<33°C$) following submersion in icy ($<5°C$) water. Nichter (Nichter and Everett, 1989) has shown a universally bad outcome in near-drowning victims who present without a perfusing cardiac rhythm in the emergency room. Biggart's series of 27 victims presenting to the emergency room without spontaneous circulation contained only three intact survivors (Biggart and Bohn, 1990). All three were hypothermic ($<33°C$). An important distinction must be drawn between those victims who are hypothermic because of prolonged submersion and cardiac arrest in warm water, and who have a bad prognosis, and those victims who are hypothermic because of submersion in cold water, and who have the possibility of a good recovery.

REFERENCES

Althaus, U., Aeberhard, P., Schupbach, P., Nachbur, B. H., and Mishlemann, W., 1982, "Management of profound accidental hypothermia with cardiorespiratory arrest," *Annals of Surgery*, 195, 492.

The American Academy of Pediatrics and The American College of Emergency Physicians, 1993, *Advanced Paediatric Life Support*, 2nd edition.

Arborelius, M., Balldin, U. I., Lilja, B., and Lundgren, C. E., 1972, "Haemodynamic changes in men during immersion in head above water," *Aerospace Medicine*, 43, 592.

Bell, T. S., Ellenberg, L., and McComb, J. G., 1985, "Neuropsychological outcome after pediatric near drowning," *Neurosurgery*, 17, 604.

Bigelow, W. G., Lindsay W. K., Greenwood, W.F., 1950, "Hypothermia: Its possible role in cardiac surgery. Investigation of factors governing survival in dogs at low temperatures," *Annals of Surgery*, 132, 849.

Biggart, W. D., Bohn, D. J., Kent, G., Barker, C., and Hamilton, C., 1983, "Neutrophil circulation and release from bone marrow during hypothermia," *Infection & Immunology*, 40, 708.

Biggart, W. D., Bohn, D. J., Kent, G., Barker, C., and Hamilton, C., 1984, "Neutrophil migration *in vitro* and *in vivo* during hypothermia," *Infection & Immunology*, 46, 857.

Biggart, W. D. and Bohn, D. J., 1990, "The influence of hypothermia on outcome following near-drowning accidents in children," *Journal of Pediatrics*, 117, 179.

Bohn, D. J., Biggar, W. D., Smith, C. R., Conn, A. W., and Barker, G. A., 1986, "Influence of hypothermia, barbiturate therapy, and intracranial pressure monitoring on morbidity and mortality after near drowning," *Critical Care Medicine*, 14, 529.

Bolte, R. G., Black, P. G., Bowers, R. S., Thorne, J.K., and Corneli, H. M., 1988, "The use of extracorporeal rewarming in a child submerged for 66 minutes," *JAMA*, 260, 377–379.

Bratton, S. L., Jardin, D. S., and Morray, J. P., 1994, "Serial neurological examinations after near drowning and outcome," *Journal of Pediatric Adolescent Medicine*, 148, 167–170.

Burton, A. C. and Foholm, O. G., 1955, *Man in a Cold Environment*, Edward Arnold, London.

Collis, M. L., 1976, "Survival behaviour in cold water immersion," in *Proceedings of the Cold Water Symposium*, The Royal Life Saving Society of Canada, Toronto, ON.

Conn, A. W. and Barker, G. A., 1984, "Fresh water drowning and near-drowning — an update," *Canadian Anaesthetists Society Journal*, 31, S38.

Conn, A. W., Edmonds, J. F., and Barker, G. A., 1978, "Near drowning in cold fresh water: Current treatment regimen," *Canadian Anaesthetists Society Journal*, 25, 259.

Conn, A. W., Miyasaka, K., Katayama, M., Fujita, M., Orima, H., Barker, G. A., and Bohn, D. J., 1995, "A canine study of cold water drowning in fresh vs. salt water," *Critical Care Medicine*.

Cooper, K. E., 1976, "Respiratory and thermal responses to cold water immersion, in *Proceedings of the Cold Water Symposium*, The Royal Life Saving Society of Canada, Toronto, ON.

Coughlin, F., 1973, "Heart warming procedure," *New England Journal of Medicine*, 288, 326.

Davis, W. B., Rennard, S. I., Bitterman, P. B., and Crystal, R. G., 1983, "Pulmonary oxygen toxicity: Early reversible changes in human alveolar structures induced by hyperoxia," *New England Journal of Medicine*, 309, 878.

De Villata, D., Barat, G., Peral, P., et al., 1973, "Recovery from profound hyothermia with cardiac arrest after immersion," *British Medical Journal*, 2, 394.

Dean, J. M. and Kaufman, N. D., 1981, "Prognostic indicators in paediatric near drowning: The Glasgow coma scale," *Critical Care Medicine*, 9, 536.

Dean, J. M. and McComb, J. G., 1981, "Intracranial pressure monitoring in severe paediatric near drowning," *Neurosurgery*, 6, 627.

Deneke, S. M. and Fanburg, B. L., 1980, "Normobaric oxygen toxicity of the lung," *New England Journal of Medicine*, 303, 76.

Deshpande, J. K. and Wieloch, T., 1986, "Flunarizine, a calcium entry blocker, ameliorates ischemic brain damage in the rat," *Anesthesiology*, 64, 215.

Duguid, H., Simpson, R. G., and Stowers, J. M., 1961, "Accidental hypothermia," *Lancet*, 2, 1213.

Edsall, D. W., 1980, "Treatment of hypothermia," *JAMA*, 244, 1902.

Elsner, R., Franklin, D. L., Van Citters, R. L., and Kenney, D. W., 1966, "Cardiovascular defence against asphyxia," *Science*, 153, 941–947.

Emslie-Smith, D., 1958, "Accidental hypothermia. A common condition with a pathognomic electrocardiography," *Lancet*, 2, 492.

Eruehan, A. E., 1960, "Accidental hypothermia," *Archives of Internal Medicine*, 106, 218.

Fainer, D. C., Martin, C. G., and Ivy, A. C., 1951, "Resuscitation of dogs from fresh water drowning," *Journal of Applied Physiology*, 3, 417–426.

Fisher, B., Peterson, B., and Hicks, G., 1992, "Use of brainstem auditory-evoked response testing to assess neurologic outcome following near drowning in children," *Critical Care Medicine*, 20, 578.

Frank, L., 1985, "Oxidant injury to the pulmonary endothelium," in *The Pulmonary Circulation and Acute Lung Injury*, Said, S. A., Ed., pp. 283–305, Futura Publishing, New York.

Frates, R. C., 1981, "Analysis of predictive factors in the assessment of warm-water near drowning in children," *American Journal of Diseases of Childhood*, 135, 1006.

Frewin, T. C., Sumabat, W. O., Han, V. K., Amacher, A. L., Del Maestro, R. F., and Sibbald, W. J., 1985, "Cerebral resuscitation therapy in paediatric near drowning," *Journal of Pediatrics*, 106, 615.

Glauser, F. L. and Smith, W. R., 1975, "Pulmonary interstitial fibrosis following near drowning and exposure to short term high oxygen concentrations," *Chest*, 68, 373–375.

Goode, R. C., 1976, "Acute responses to cold water," in *Proceedings of the Cold Water Symposium*, The Royal Life Saving Society of Canada, Toronto, ON.

Gooden, B. A., 1972, "Drowning and the diving reflex in man," *Medical Journal of Australia*, 2, 583.

Goodwin, S. R., Friedman, W. A., and Bellefleur, M., 1991, "Is it time to use evoked potentials to predict outcome in comatose children and adults?" *Critical Care Medicine*, 19, 518.

Harris, R. J., Symon, L., Bronston, N. M., et al., 1981, "Changes in extracellular calcium activity in cerebral ischaemia," *Journal of Cerebral Blood Flow & Metabolism*, 1, 203.

Hasan, S., Avery, W. G., Fabian, C., and Sackner, M. A., 1971, "Near-drowning in humans: A report of 36 patients," *Chest*, 59, 191.

Hayward, J. S., Hay, C., Matthews, B. R., Overweel, C. H., and Radford, D. D., 1984, "Temperature effect on the human dive response in relation to cold water near-drowning," *Journal of Applied Physiology*, 56, 202–206.

Heymans, C., 1950, "Survival and revival of nervous tissue after arrest of the circulation," *Physiology Review*, 30, 375.

Hossmann, K. A., 1983, "Neuronal survival and revival during and after cerebral ischaemia," *American Journal of Emergency Medicine*, 1, 191.

Hossmann, K. A. and Kleiheies, P., 1973, "Reversibility of ischemic brain damage," *Archives of Neurology*, 20, 375.

Hunt, P. K., 1974, "Effect and treatment of the 'diving reflex,'" *Canadian Medical Association Journal*, 111, 1330.

Hunter, T. B. and Whitehouse, W. M., 1974, "Fresh water drowning: Radiological aspects," *Radiology*, 112, 51.

Jacobsen, W. K., Mason, L. J., Briggs, B. A., Schneider, S., and Thompson, P. C., 1983, "Correlation of spontaneous respiration and neurological damage in near drowning," *Critical Care Medicine*, 11, 487.

Jessen, K. and Hagelsten, J. O., 1978, "Peritoneal dialysis in the treatment of profound accidental hypothermia." *Aviation Space Environmental Medicine*, 49, 426.

Johnson, L. A., 1977, "Accidental hypothermia: peritoneal dialysis," *Journal of the American College of Emergency Physicians*, 6, 556.

Keatinge, W., 1969, *Survival in Cold Water*, Blackwell Scientific Publications, Oxford, U.K.

Kristoffersen, M. B., Rattenborg, C. C., and Holaday, D. A., 1967, "Asphyxial death: The roles of acute anoxia, hypercarbia and acidosis," *Anesthesiology*, 28, 488–497.

Kruss, S., Bergstrom, L., Suntarinen, T., and Hyvonen, R., 1979, "The prognosis of near-drowned children," *Acta Pediatric Scandinavia*, 68, 315.

Kvittengen, T. D. and Naess, A., 1963, "Recovery from drowning in fresh water," *British Medical Journal*, 1, 1315.

Lavelle, J. M. and Shaw, K. N., 1993, "Near drowning: Is emergency department cardiopulmonary resuscitation or intensive care unit cerebral resuscitation indicated?" *Critical Care Medicine*, 21, 368.

LeBlanc, J., 1976, "Physiological changes in prolonged cold stress," in *Proceedings of the Cold Water Symposium*, The Royal Life Saving Society of Canada, Toronto, ON.

Ledingham, I. McA. and Mone, J. G., 1978, "Accidental hypothermia," *Lancet*, 1, 391.

Ledingham, I. McA. and Mone, J. G., 1980, "Treatment of accidental hypothermia: A prospective clinical study," *British Medical Journal*, 280, 1102.

Ledingham, I. McA., Routh, G. S., Douglas, I. H. S., and MacDonald, A. M., 1980, "Central rewarming system for the treatment of hypothermia," *Lancet*, 1, 1168.

Letsou, G. V., Kopf, G. S., Elefteriades, J. A., Carter, J. E., Baldwin, J. C., and Hammond, G. L., 1992, "Is cardiopulmonary bypass effective for treatment of hypothermic arrest due to drowning or exposure?" *Archives of Surgery*, 127, 525–528.

Linton, A. L. and Ledingham, I. McA., 1966, "Severe hypothermia with barbiturate intoxication," *Lancet*, I, 24.

Lloyd, E. L., 1973, "Accidental hypothermia treated by central rewarming through the airway," *British Journal of Anaesthesia*, 45, 41.

Mahajan, S. L., Myers, T. J., and Baldini, M. G., 1981, "Disseminated intravascular coagulation during rewarming following hypothermia," *Journal of the American Medical Association*, 245, 2517.

McCord, J. M., 1985, "Oxygen derived free radicals in postischemic tissue injury," *New England Journal of Medicine*, 312, 159.

Miller, J. W., Danzl, D. F., and Thomas, D. M., 1980, "Urban accidental hypothermia: 135 cases," *Annals of Emergency Medicine*, 9, 456.

Modell, J. H., Graves, S. A., and Ketover, A., 1976, "Clinical course of 91 consecutive near-drowning victims," *Chest*, 70, 231.

Modell, J. H., Graves, S. A., and Kuch, E. J., 1980, "Near drowning: correlation of level of consciousness and survival," *Canadian Anaesthetists Society Journal*, 27, 211.

Modell, J. H. and Moya, F., 1966, "Effects of volume of aspirated fluid during chlorinated fresh water drowning," *Anesthesiology*, 27, 662.

Montes, H. E. and Conn, A. W., 1980, "Near-drowning: An unusual case," *Canadian Anaesthetists Society Journal*, 27, 172.

Naylor, W. G., Poole-Wilson, P. A., and Williams, A., 1979, "Hypoxia and calcium," *Journal of Molecular Cellular Cardiology*, 11, 683.

Nichter, M. and Everett, P. B., 1989, "Childhood near-drowning: Is cardiopulmonary resuscitation always indicated?" *Critical Care Medicine*, 17, 993.

Nicodemus, H. F., Chancy, R. D., and Herold, R., 1981, "Hemodynamic effects of inotropes during hypothermia and rapid rewarming," *Critical Care Medicine*, 9, 325.

Nussbaum, E., 1985, "Prognostic variables in nearly drowned, comatose children," *American Journal of Disease in Childhood*, 139, 1058–1059.

Oakes, D. D., Sherek, J. P., Maloney, J. R., and Charters, A. C., 1982, "Prognosis and management of victims of near-drowning," *Journal of Trauma*, 22, 544.

O'Keefe, K. M., 1977, "Accidental hypothermia: A review of 62 cases," *Journal of the American College of Emergency Physicians*, 6, 491.

Orlowski, J. P., 1979, "Prognostic factors in paediatric cases of drowning and near drowning," *Journal of the American College of Emergency Physicians*, 8, 176.

O'Rourke, P. P., Stolar, C. J. H., Zwischenberger, J. B., Snedecor, S. M., and Bartlett, R. M., 1993, "Extracorporeal membrane oxygenation: Support for overwhelming pulmonary failure in the pediatric population. Collective experience from the Extracorporeal Life Support Organization," *Journal of Pediatric Surgery*, 28, 523.

Paulev, E.-P., et al., 1990, "Facial cold receptors and the survival reflex diving bradycardia in man," *Japanese Journal of Physiology*, 40, 701–712.

Pearn, J. H., Bart, R. D., and Yamaoka, R., 1979, "Neurological sequelae after childhood near drowning: A total population study from Hawaii," *Pediatrics*, 64, 187.

Peterson, B., 1977, "Morbidity of childhood near-drowning," *Pediatrics*, 59, 364.

Pfenninger, J. and Sutter, M., 1982, "Intensive care after fresh water immersion in children," *Anesthesia*, 37, 1157.

Pichard, J. D., 1981, "Role of prostaglandins and arachadonic acid derivatives in the coupling of cerebral blood flow to metabolism," *Journal of Cerebral Blood Flow & Metabolism*, 1, 361.

Quan, L. and Kinder, D., 1992, "Pediatric submersions: prehospital predictors of outcome," *Pediatrics*, 90, 989.

Quan, L., Wentz, K. R., Gore, E. J., and Copass, M. K., 1990, "Outcome predictors in pediatric submersion victims receiving prehospital care in King County, Washington," *Pediatrics*, 86, 586.

Ramey, C. A., Hayward, D. N., and Hayward, J. S., 1987, "Dive response of children in relation to cold water drowning," *Journal of Applied Physiology*, 63, 665–668.

Reuler, J. B. and Parker, R. A., 1978, "Peritoneal dialysis in the management of hypothermia," *JAMA*, 240, 2289.

Rinaldo, J. E. and Rogers, R. M., 1982, "Adult respiratory distress syndrome: Changing concepts of lung injury and repair," *New England Journal of Medicine*, 306, 200.

Savard, G. K., Cooper, K. E., Veale, W. L., and Malkinson, T. J., 1985, "Peripheral blood flow during rewarming from mild hypothermia in humans," *Journal of Applied Physiology*, 58, 4.

Schissler, P., Parker, M. A., and Scott, S. J., 1981, "Profound hypothermia: Value of prolonged cardiopulmonary resuscitation," *South Medical Journal*, 74, 474.

Sekar, T. S., MacDonnell, K. F., Namsirikul, P., and Herman, R. S., 1980, "Survival after prolonged submersion in cold water without neurological sequelae; report of two cases," *Archives of Internal Medicine*, 140, 775.

Siebke, H., Rod, T., Breivik, H., and Lind, B., 1975, "Survival after 40 mins. submersion without sequelae," *Lancet*, 1, 1275.

Soung, L. S., Swank, L., Ing, T. S., Said, R. A., Goldman, J. W., Perez, J., and Geiss, W. P., 1977, "The treatment of accidental hypothermia with peritoneal dialysis," *Canadian Medical Association Journal*, 117, 1415.

Steward, D. J., 1976, "A disposable condenser humidifier for use during anaesthesia," *Canadian Medical Association Journal*, 23, 191.

Suter, P. M. and Fairley, H. B., 1975, "Optimum end-expiratory airway pressure in patients with acute pulmonary failure," *New England Journal of Medicine*, 292, 284.

Tate, R. M. and Repine, J. E., 1983, "Neutrophils and the adult respiratory distress syndrome," *American Review of Respiratory Disease*, 128, 552.

Towne, W. D., Geiss, W. P., Yanes, H. O., and Rahimtoola, S. H., 1972, "Intractable ventricular fibrillation associated with profound accidental hypothermia: successful treatment with partial cardiopulmonary bypass," *New England Journal of Medicine*, 287, 1135.

Truscott, D. G., Firor, W. B., and Clein, L. J., 1973, "Accidental profound hypothermia. Successful resuscitation by core rewarming and assisted circulation," *Archives of Surgery*, 106, 216.

Weinberger, L. M., Gibbon, M. H., and Gibbon, J. H., 1940, "Temporary arrest of the circulation to the central nervous system; I Physiological effects," *Archives of Neurological Psychology*, 43, 615.

White, B. C., Winnegar, C. D., Wilson, R. F., and Krause, G. S., 1983, "Calcium blockers in cerebral resuscitation," *Journal of Trauma*, 23, 788.

Wickstrom, P., Ruiz, E., Lilja, G. P., Hinterkopf, J. P., and Haglin, J. J., 1976, "Accidental hypothermia. Core rewarming with partial bypass." *American Journal of Surgery*, 131, 622.

Winegar, C. D., Henderson, O., White, B. C., et al., 1983, "Prolonged hypoperfusion in the cerebral cortex following cardiac arrest and resuscitation in dogs," *Annals of Emergency Medicine*, 12, 471.

Young, R. S. K., Zalneraitis, E. L., and Dooling, E. C., 1980, "Neurological outcome in cold water drowning," *JAMA*, 244, 1233.

6 Water Rescue Methods for Emergency Service Providers

John R. Fletemeyer

This chapter has two objectives: (1) to provide emergency service providers (including police and fire and EMS personnel) with information about the etiology of drowning and victim identification techniques and (2) to provide guidelines for effective water rescue intervention methods that do not require a high level of swimming proficiency or formal lifeguard training.

Considering that the professional and technical requirements of job performance within the emergency provider industry have increased significantly over the years, it is understandable that more and more training time is needed to master these requirements. Just ask any training officer, and he or she will testify that training time is always at a premium. Because water rescue training has traditionally assumed a low priority, it is not surprising that very little (if any) training is devoted to this subject. Consequently, most emergency service providers are ill-equipped to handle most water-related emergencies. This is true even in areas with large water bodies and a history of aquatic-related mishaps involving human life.

The general lack of water rescue training within the industry puts a victim at an increased risk regarding his or her chances for survival and places the provider at a disadvantage as well. All too often during a highly emotionally charged aquatic accident, an emergency provider arriving at the scene will disregard his or her personal safety and try to effect a rescue, even without the benefit of any water rescue training. Such a scenario often invites tragedy: the loss of life of both the victim and rescuer. There are numerous accounts of a firefighter or policeman diving headfirst into a lake or river to save a victim, only to drown.

Records maintained by the Policeman's Memorial Foundation in Washington, DC testify to the seriousness of this problem. This organization reports that 121 officers have drowned during active duty, most after making a heroic yet fatal attempt to dive in after a drowning victim. Based on over 15 years of training police officers and firemen, this author is convinced that many people would be alive today if only they had been able to call upon some basic water rescue training received in the course of their department's training program.

This belief provides the focus for this chapter. To reiterate, it is crucial that every policeman, firefighter, and paramedic receive some basic water rescue training. As first responders, sooner or later, they probably will be confronted with an aquatic emergency of some kind. Any department failing to provide this training must be considered negligent.

DROWNING: AN OVERVIEW

In Chapter 3 of this book, Dr. Christine Branche notes that 5,000–6,000 people drown in the United States each year. As Dr. Samuel Freas noted in Chapter 1, since many drownings are labeled otherwise, e.g., a boat-related drowning is a boating fatality and not a drowning, it is likely that the number of drownings is much greater than statistics reveal. Regardless of whether we consider the statistics accurate, drowning is still one of the leading causes of accidental death. Among individuals between the ages of 5–44, drowning is the second leading cause of accidental death. In states such as water-bound California, Florida, and Hawaii, drowning is the leading cause of accidental death in those aged 5–44.

The significance of drowning takes on even greater importance when we consider the statistics for near-drowning. It has been estimated that for every person who dies by drowning, 14 others are treated in emergency rooms and countless more receive emergency medical treatment at the accident scene from emergency service providers and lifeguards. These numbers translate into millions of dollars in emergency care treatment and hospital care, and into a problem that no first responder agency can ignore.

It should be pointed out that a drowning can occur almost anywhere: from a backyard pool, river, lake, or quarry, to a seemingly benign water source such as a bathtub, toilet, or bucket of water. Consequently, it is nonsense for an agency to believe that it does not need to provide water safety training for its personnel because it does not have a major body of water within its jurisdiction.

Other statistics about drowning reveal that about four times more men than women drown. Blacks are twice as likely to drown than whites, and alcohol is implicated in at least 50% of all drownings.

Surprisingly, most drownings occur within 10 ft of safety and within 50 ft of shore. This suggests that most water rescues can be performed without having to enter the water, either by reaching a victim with an extension object such as a pole or by throwing a buoyant object capable of supporting a victim above the surface. Only in rare cases, when a victim has been submerged or is suffering from a serious injury, is it necessary for a rescuer to enter the water. Later in this chapter, I will provide information recommending actively entering the water only after other methods have failed.

Contrary to popular belief, and as Dr. Jerome Modell notes in Chapter 2, drowning is not an instantaneous event. Most drownings do not result in a period of uncontrollable panic causing the victim to end up in a floating, face-down position in the water. Instead, most drownings involve a relatively lengthy and progressive process consisting of a number of medically defined, relatively easily recognizable stages.

By learning these stages and their behavioral and physiological correlation, an emergency responder is more likely to make the right decision and thus be less likely to become a needless drowning statistic.

THE PHYSIOLOGY OF DROWNING

Drowning reduced to its simplest definition is death by suffocation when submerged in the water. Unfortunately, many medical professionals have expanded this definition to include any death occurring in the water. This more generic definition confuses drowning with other forms of death occurring in aquatic environments, such as physical trauma, drug overdose, and disease. Adding to the confusion are deaths resulting from secondary complications that are sometimes wrongly labeled as drownings by some medical professionals. These secondary complications usually involve infection or occult damage to the respiratory or cardiovascular systems. Examples of this are adult respiratory distress syndrome (ARDS) and pulmonary edema. Infection results from the victim ingesting water that carries a viral form of bacteria into the lungs.

To understand the mechanics and physiology of drowning, we must first regard drowning as an evolving process usually associated with four stages: (1) **initial apnea**; (2) **dyspnea**; (3) **terminal apnea**; and (4) **cardiac arrest**. Although these stages can be defined by a number of characteristics, they are not always mutually exclusive (Table 1). For example, Stage 3, terminal apnea, and Stage 4, cardiac arrest, can occur either independently or together. Contrary to popular belief, most drownings do not occur at a rapid rate, progressing from a state of controllable panic to a state of unconsciousness — the point when a victim slips below the surface. Since most drownings occur over a relatively long period, many lifesaving textbooks often refer to a two-minute window of opportunity, which represents the time a rescuer has to recover a victim who is not breathing and begin resuscitation. As we will see later, and as Dr. Desmond Bohn elaborates on in Chapter 5, this time period can be significantly extended if the drowning occurs in cold water.

While most drownings progress through the stages summarized in Table 1, some do not. Those that do not usually are associated with some form of severe trauma that renders the victim unconscious, such as drug overdose, seizure, electrocution, or heart attack. In such cases, the two-minute window of opportunity obviously ceases to apply to the rescue intervention scenario, and the rescuer must initiate a response as quickly as possible.

TYPES OF DROWNING

Developing an understanding of drowning is further complicated by the fact that there are different types of drowning, based on the victim's physiological responses to being submerged. Every emergency responder should have an understanding of these types, so that a victim can be provided with the most appropriate first aid and medical care.

TABLE 1
Stages of Drowning and Their Physiological Characteristics

Stage/Title	General Description	Physiological Characteristics
I. Initial Apnea	A reflex reaction causes the victim's glottis to close. Breathing stops.	• Blood pressure rises; adrenaline flow increases if the victim panics. • Victim swallows water resulting in less buoyancy and a diminished capacity to breathe. • As victim becomes less buoyant, the head can no longer be held above the water. • The brain begins to experience degeneration because of lack of oxygen. • Acidosis begins due to the buildup of excess waste chemicals in the blood.
II. Dyspnea	The victim is usually in a semiconscious state, but begins to swallow more water. In most cases water enters the lungs, causing a deterioration of the alveoli and damage to the surfactant. This condition increases the ability for the lungs to exchange oxygen and carbon dioxide.	• Aspiration of water into the lungs usually due to failure of the swallow reflex. • Vomiting occurs. • Frothing at the mouth occurs due to the mixture of surfactant and water in the lungs. • Brain hypoxia continues to evolve; acidosis continues to cause a severe imbalance in the victim's blood chemistry.
III. Terminal Apnea	As soon as the victim becomes unconscious and stops breathing the victim is considered to have entered this stage.	• Brain hypoxia and acidosis continue. • In some cases tonic convulsions may occur, in which the victim's entire body becomes rigid, causing involuntary jerking. • The victim's sphincter muscles may relax, resulting in uncontrolled urination and/or defecation in some cases.
IV. Cardiac Arrest	The victim's heart ceases to pump blood to the brain and other vital organs. Depending on the circumstances, the third and fourth stages may begin simultaneously, meaning that the heart and lungs stop at approximately the same time. However, quite often the heart will continue to beat for some time after breathing stops.	• Heart stops beating, resulting in the loss of circulation. • Brain and other vital organs are no longer supplied with blood. • Brain damage occurs along with other significant and usually irreversible cellular damage unless CPR is begun soon after.

WET DROWNING

The vast majority of drownings are wet drownings (Kringsholm, 1991). In a wet drowning, water enters the victim's lungs upon relaxation of the initial laryngeal spasm. If the drowning occurs in salt water, the victim's blood plasma diffuses through the membranes of the alveoli because the salt (sodium) content of the water is higher than that of the water in the blood. Because sodium attracts water, the water plasma is drawn out of the blood and into the lungs. In extreme cases, the victim's blood volume can drop almost 40%, resulting in a thickening of the blood and a shrinkage of the red blood cells. Consequently, the red blood cells lose their capacity to deliver oxygen to the tissues. Although oxygen therapy should always be considered, it is especially crucial to provide it to a victim who has aspirated salt water.

In a freshwater drowning, the opposite occurs. Water enters the victim's lungs and is then drawn through the membranes of the alveoli into the blood. This occurs because the sodium content of the blood is higher than that of fresh water. In extreme cases, the victim's blood volume has been known to double, which may cause a condition called hemolysis. Hemolysis results when the red blood cells rupture as a result of their water volume from fresh water. Another problem associated with freshwater drownings is an imbalance in the victim's blood chemistry. An imbalance of electrolytes, for example, results in ventricular fibrillation in an estimated 80% of freshwater drownings (YMCA, 1988).

DRY DROWNING

A dry drowning occurs when the victim fails to aspirate, so water is not aspirated into the lungs. This occurs when the victim undergoes laryngospasm while submerged and cardiac arrest ensues without the victim taking an intervening breath. In his discussion of dry drowning episodes in Chapter 2, Dr. Jerome Modell notes that approximately 10% of drowned victims are thought to have drowned without aspiration; however, he also notes that the actual incidence of drowning without aspiration may be lower since such a diagnosis can be confused with cases of victims of foul play who enter the water.

VICTIM IDENTIFICATION

Victim identification is the first step to a successful rescue. In Chapter 16, Dr. Tom Griffiths and associates discuss some of the visual scanning methods lifeguards should use when trying to identify a drowning subject. These methods can be learned by any emergency responder in a relatively short time and should be incorporated into an agency's training program (Figure 1a).

For scanning to be effective, it is important that the first responder become familiar with some of the behaviors that a victim in the active stages of drowning commonly exhibits. Having observed more than 500 near-drowning events over the past 20 years and having conducted a survey involving 284 near-drownings that occurred on South Florida beaches between 1988 and 1995, I am impressed by the fact that most behavior associated with drowning is usually subtle and inconspicuous in nature, especially to a nonprofessional not versed in victim detection. It is indeed ironic that some of these signs are so subtle that even the victim is not aware that he or she is drowning. This is perhaps why many victims pulled in by lifeguards on surf beaches sometimes remark, "Why did you rescue me? I was OK!"

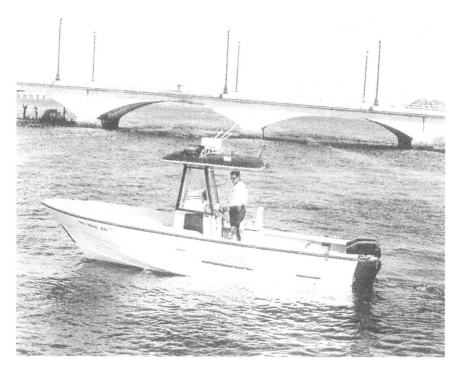

FIGURE 1a   Every emergency first responder should have some basic water rescue training. Here a marine unit trained in water rescue responds to a boating accident.

Contrary to popular belief, most victims do not yell or wave for help, and most do not experience a period of intense thrashing and controllable panic before disappearing below the surface. Among a sample of 248 near-drownings used in a drowning behavior study conducted by Fletemeyer (1966), approximately one third (31%) of the victims remained passive, providing the lifeguard with little or no indication that they were in trouble. Most of the near-drowning victims were facing toward the shore, and most were attempting (usually unsuccessfully) to swim to shallow water or to a point of safety.

Other behaviors the near-drowning victims commonly displayed in the study included hyperventilating or gasping for air, the head maintained low in the water, and the head bobbing up and down (Figure 1b). It should be noted that other investigators have identified behaviors other than those just mentioned. Table 2 represents a relatively complete inventory of the behaviors most commonly associated with drowning. Every emergency provider should become familiar enough with these behaviors so that he or she can identify them when they occur.

EMERGENCY INTERVENTION

Emergency intervention involving a water rescue requires considerable skill, knowledge, good judgment, and usually a high level of swimming ability. Unless an

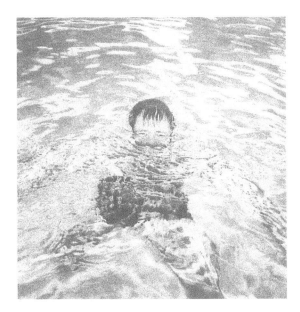

FIGURE 1b   Typical drowning posture.

TABLE 2
List of Behaviors Commonly Associated with a Drowning or Near-Drowning

- Head low in the water, mouth at water level.
- Head tilted back with mouth open.
- Eyes glassy and empty, unable to focus.
- Eyes closed.
- Hair over forehead and in the eyes.
- Hyperventilating, gasping for air, irregular breathing.
- Shouting for help.
- Waving hands.
- Trying to swim to a particular direction (usually to shore) but not making any headway.
- Trying to cling to any supporting object such as a buoy, piling, rope, or even another bather.
- Trying to roll over on the back to float.
- Uncontrollable movement of arms and legs, sometimes called "thrashing" or "panic."

---

emergency first responder has had a background in swimming and has received certification in a lifeguard training course, going into the water after a victim is not recommended.

The fact that most near-drownings occur within 10 ft of safety and within 50 ft of shore makes it possible to perform other types of land-based water rescue intervention methods that do not require the need for any active water rescue and that do not normally compromise the safety of the first responder effecting the rescue.

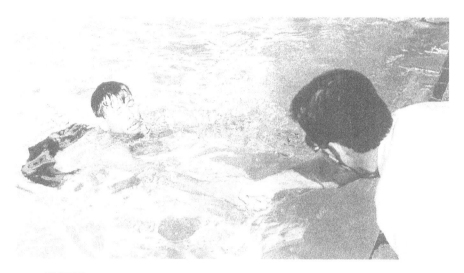

FIGURE 2a   A version of the reach rescue using the arm to reach the victim.

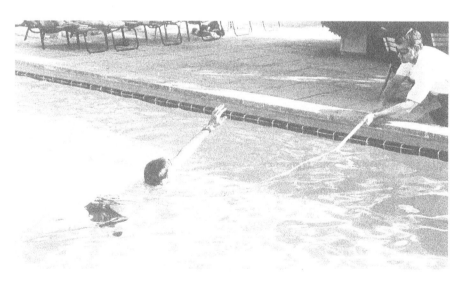

FIGURE 2b   A version of the reach rescue using an extension object, such as a pole, to reach the victim.

Performing a land-based rescue is relatively simple, provided there is careful planning and certain precautions are taken. The simplest and perhaps most effective land-based rescue is the **Reach Rescue** (Figures 2a–c). This rescue involves reaching out to the victim with either a hand or an extension object while remaining on land. One particularly excellent extension object is a "shepherd's hook," which can be found in the immediate vicinity of most swimming pools.

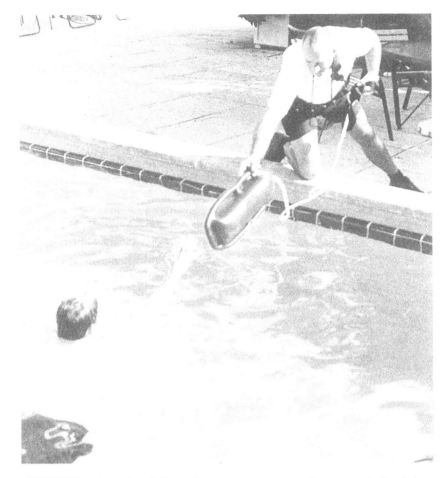

FIGURE 2c   A version of the reach rescue using a rescue buoy to reach the victim.

When performing a land-based rescue, the rescuer must exercise care to avoid either slipping into the water or being accidentally pulled in by the victim. Considering this danger, it is recommended that the rescuer lie in a prone position when reaching or lock hands with a second rescuer.

When performing the reach rescue, these recommendations should be followed:

- Talk to the victim and urge the victim to remain calm. Do not do or say anything that encourages panic.
- If the victim cannot be reached by extending a hand, locate a suitable extension object such as a rake handle, a two-by-four, or a sturdy tree branch.
- Extend your arm or the extension object to the victim's hand and instruct the victim to firmly take hold.
- Slowly draw the victim back to shore, being careful not to jerk the object from the victim's grip.

- When performing this rescue, always stay away from the water's edge to avoid being pulled into the water.
- Sometimes it may be possible to wade into shallow water to further extend your reach; however, always enter the water cautiously to avoid being caught in a current or stepping off into a sudden drop-off or deep water.
- If possible, have a spotter nearby ready to assist in the event of an unanticipated problem.

A second land-based rescue method is the **Throw Rescue** (Figure 3). This rescue is useful when a victim cannot be readily reached with a hand or an extension object. It involves throwing a floating object that is capable of supporting the victim's body weight. Objects that can be used in this capacity include an empty water jug, a beach ball, a personal flotation device (life preserver), and an inner tube.

Even better to use is a throw ring or bag attached to a long line, usually 75–100 ft in length. Recently a throwing disk was introduced with the potential of being thrown over even greater distances than the conventional bag or buoy, but some practice is needed before it can be used effectively. Figure 4 shows some of the throwing rescue devices available to emergency responders.

When using a throw bag, disk, or buoy, the following recommendations should be heeded:

- Hold the device with the throwing hand.
- Hold the end of the line with the non-throwing hand.
- Position yourself at the water's edge, away from any object that might present an obstacle to your throwing motion.
- Make two or three trial throws without actually throwing the device. Try to account for factors that might affect the accuracy of your throw, such as wind direction and velocity, current direction, and wave action.
- Throw the device past the victim's head and shoulder and then slowly draw the device back to the victim while instructing the victim to grasp the bag, buoy, or rope.
- Once the victim has taken hold, slowly begin to reel the victim back to shore.

While this rescue equipment works well in the majority of cases, at least two factors limit its use. The first is cold water. In some cases when the victim is suffering from severe hypothermia, he or she may lack the neuromuscular coordination needed to grab a buoy or bag tossed to him. In still other cases, the victim may be panicking and therefore unable to understand the need to grab a buoy or throw bag.

The final rescue method is the **Active In-Water Rescue.** As stated earlier, many first responders may not have the swimming ability and rescue skills needed to make an active in-water rescue. Ultimately this determination must be made by each individual, hopefully prior to being forced into a rescue situation when rational judgment may not prevail.

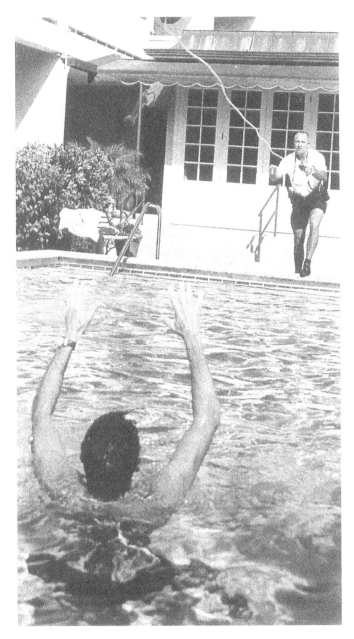

FIGURE 3 A demonstration of the throw rescue.

When conducting an active in-water rescue, a lifesaving can or buoy should always be used (Figure 5). These rescue aids have two functions; they can effectively be used to secure the victim, and they can be used as a flotation aid in the event the rescuer becomes fatigued and needs to rest. When conducting an in-water rescue, the following recommendations should be considered:

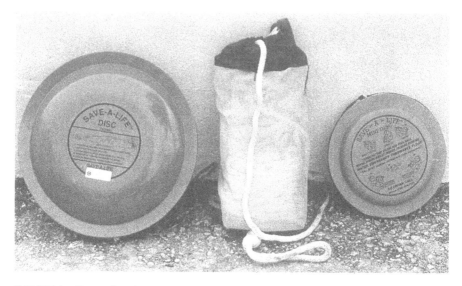

FIGURE 4 Types of equipment commonly used in the throw rescue — aerial disk (left and right) and throw buoy (center).

- Remove all loose clothing and shoes.
- A police officer who responds should lock his or her gun in the trunk of the car or give it to a responsible adult. Only as a last resort should a gun be left on the ground.
- Designate a spotter if additional help is immediately available.
- Enter the water carefully with the lifesaving buoy harness properly secured across the chest and shoulder. Never dive headfirst into the water because this could cause serious head or neck injury.
- Approach the victim with the buoy between you and the rescuer.
- Place the buoy against the victim's cheek and instruct the victim to grab the buoy. Never establish direct physical contact with the victim unless the victim is unconscious.
- Once the victim has the buoy, begin returning to shore while offering the victim verbal reassurance that he or she will be OK.
- If the victim is alert and not injured, instruct the victim to assist the rescue effort by kicking.

A variation of this method involves the use of two rescuers — one remains on land and feeds out line, and the other swims out a line and a buoy to the victim. Usually this variation requires the use of at least 300 ft of 3/8-in diameter, polypropylene line.

When a long landline is use, the land-based rescuer feeds out the line as the water rescuer swims to the victim. Once the water rescuer reaches the victim and secures the buoy around the victim, he gives a signal to the land-based rescuer. At this time the land-based rescuer slowly begins to pull in both the rescuer and the victim.

In some cases, two or three line pullers can be used, especially if a current makes the pulling difficult.

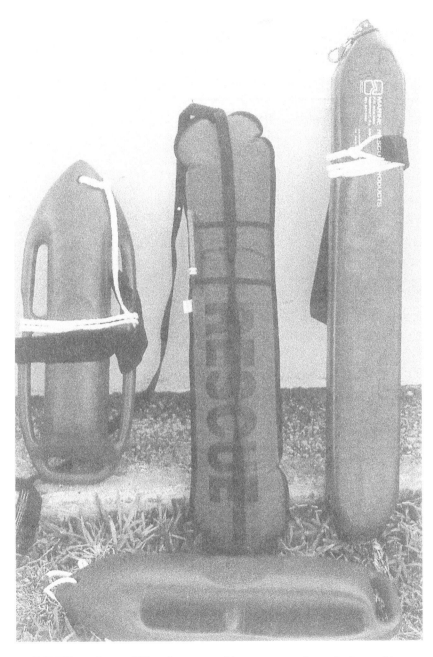

FIGURE 5   Types of lifesaving cans and buoys commonly used when making an in-water rescue.

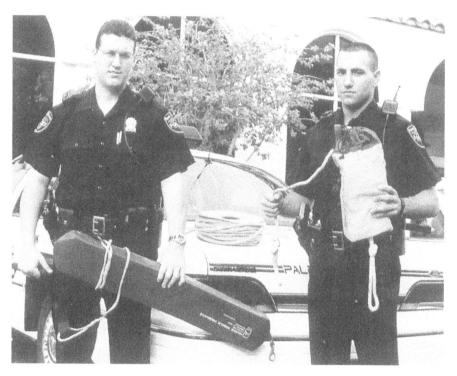

FIGURE 6 Two patrol officers with recommended standard rescue equipment, including a buoy, 300 ft of 3/8-in polypropylene line, a throw bag, and a spring-loaded pin punch (shown in Figure 7).

EQUIPMENT RECOMMENDATIONS

Some basic equipment is necessary to perform the three rescues just described. This equipment is relatively inexpensive and easily transportable and should be made available to each and every emergency responder (Figure 6). The equipment inventory should include:

- A throw bag, buoy, or disk attached to at least 100 ft of polypropylene line.
- A lifesaving can or buoy.
- A spool of at least 300 ft of 3/8-in yellow polypropylene line.
- A spring-loaded pin punch
- Mask, fins, and snorkel (optional but recommended)
- A neoprene wet suit (optional but recommended in areas with cold water)

Before issuing this equipment, each agency should establish guidelines regarding its care, maintenance, and use. This equipment should be incorporated into the training program recommended in this chapter.

ADDITIONAL CONSIDERATIONS

The rescue methods described thus far will likely be useful in the vast majority of rescue situations encountered by an emergency first responder. There are, however, a few rescue scenarios that may require some special considerations.

In a rescue involving a submerged car, it is recommended that the rescuer not enter the vehicle to extricate a victim or victims. Instead, a victim should be removed from the outside by reaching in. In cases when the windows are closed and the glass is not broken from the impact of the crash, a spring-loaded pin punch can be used effectively to break a window in a matter of seconds (Figure 7). To obtain practice using a spring-loaded pin punch, it is recommended that a training session be conducted at a local wreck yard.

When confronted with a submerged vehicle, extreme caution must always be taken, because a car under water can represent a death trap. As a car sinks, it can easily turn upside down because of the buoyancy factor caused by the tires and gas tank. When this happens, the rescuer can easily be pinned beneath the car.

Once a car settles to the bottom, time is critical. Even if an air pocket is created, it will quickly be lost due to the water pressure and the air attempting to escape. The rescue should begin by identifying certain landmarks that will help determine the exact location of the car before it sank. In some cases, if time and conditions permit, a line with a float can be attached to the car bumper. As one can imagine, trying to fix the location of a submerged car becomes exceedingly more complicated if the accident occurs at night or if water conditions are extremely murky.

Another factor exacerbating a submerged vehicle rescue is current. If a vehicle has plunged into a river or swift-moving stream, the rescuer must exercise extreme caution when trying to extricate the occupants. Although it may be easier to break a window or open a car door on the downstream side of the vehicle, this practice is dangerous because the current may shift the car, causing it to pin the rescuer to the bottom, a boulder, or a submerged tree.

Cars that fall through the ice require other measures, including rescuer use of thermal protective wear, safety ropes and lines, and, in some cases, heavy-duty lifting equipment such as cranes, tractors, or semi-towing trucks.

Other situations that require special action involve aquatic accidents associated with fuel spills. Such accidents represent a special concern when aviation fuel — a very volatile and high caustic agent — is involved. When spills occur, the rescuer should not enter the water without protective gear. Scuba-diving equipment, including a protective dry suit, is essential. Because the availability of this equipment is unlikely in most emergencies requiring an immediate response, this type rescue should not be considered as a course of action. A rescue operation becomes a search-and-rescue operation when local dive teams mobilize and bring their specialized equipment to the accident scene.

It is not possible in the limited scope of this chapter to provide any additional information on underwater rescues. Such information generally is provided in advanced certification courses taught by many of the national scuba organizations

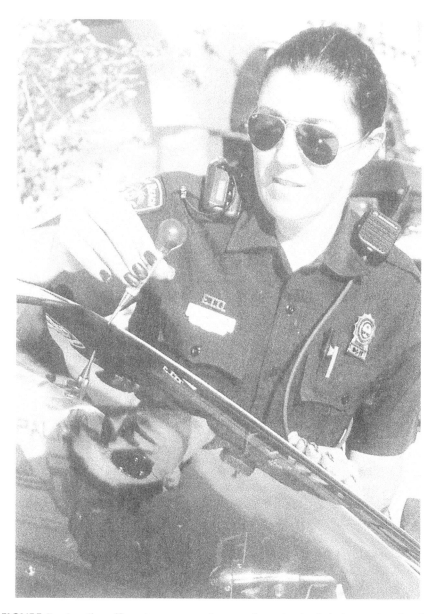

FIGURE 7   A police officer demonstrates the use of a spring-loaded pin punch to break a car window.

such as the National Association of Underwater Instructors, the Professional Association of Diving Instructors, and the YMCA. Any area with a history of vehicle accidents involving water should establish an underwater dive team trained to respond to some of the types of underwater emergencies mentioned previously.

SPINAL INJURY MANAGEMENT

In responding to any aquatic emergency, a spinal injury always must be suspected. This is especially true if any of the following circumstances occur:

- The emergency occurs in shallow water.
- The victim dove headfirst into the water.
- The emergency occurs where there are bottom conditions.
- The emergency occurs in an area where there is structure that might be responsible for the injury, such as pile, groin, pier, etc.
- The emergency is related to some activity that might lead to a spinal or head injury, such as surfing, water skiing, jet skiing, etc.

While the above might lead one to suspect a head or neck injury, the victim's condition will ultimately determine whether he or she has sustained such an injury. All emergency first responders should become familiar with the following signs and symptoms:

- Complaints by the victim of severe pain or pressure in the head, neck, and/or back area.
- Tingling or loss of sensation in the hands, fingers, feet, and/or toes.
- Unusual bumps or depressions on the head or in the spinal area.
- Blood or other fluids in the ears and nose.
- Heavy external bleeding of the head, neck, or back.
- Evidence of seizures.
- Nausea, vomiting, headache, and/or loss of balance.
- Bruising of the head, especially around the eyes and behind the ears.

Providing first aid to a victim suffering from a head or spinal injury in the water requires special training and is beyond the scope of this chapter. The American Red Cross (1993: 88) recommends the following:

- Minimize movement of the head and spine.
- Maintain an open airway.
- Check for consciousness and breathing.
- Control any external bleeding.
- Keep the victim from becoming chilled or overheated.

The need to minimize the movement of the head and spine, is exceedingly difficult to accomplish in the water because of waves and currents. Perhaps the most effective way of accomplishing this procedure is by using a cervical collar and a spine board (Figure 8). Cervical collars come in different sizes and must be fitted

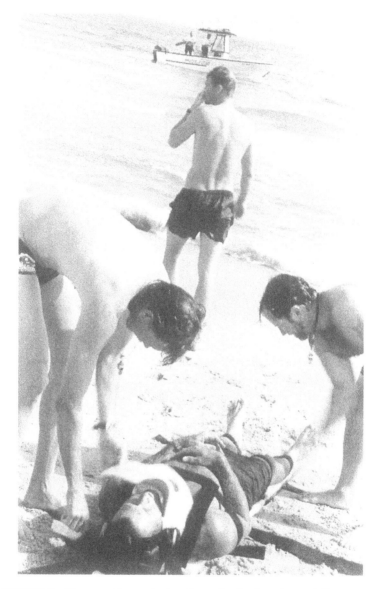

FIGURE 8   The use of a cervical collar and spine board to stabilize a water accident victim.

to the victim according to his or her weight and height. A collar that is too small may cause additional physical trauma to the victim. Any emergency responder who uses collars should be given appropriate training.

Spine boards, commonly used in conjunction with cervical collars, stabilize the victim's head, neck, and spine and prevent movement and additional injury during transport. In water emergencies, spine boards that are designed to float are generally easier to use than models that are negatively buoyant. Spine boards fitted with Velcro

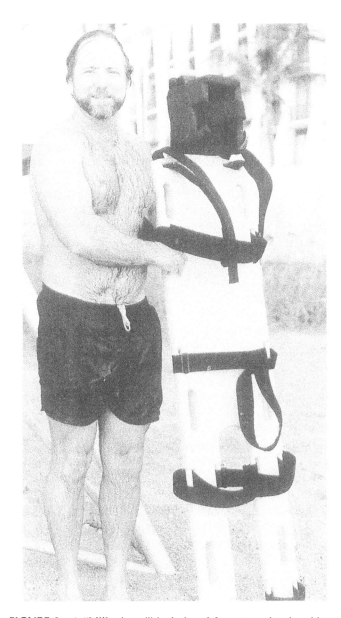

FIGURE 9 A "Miller board" is designed for water-related accidents.

straps are more efficient to use than those with buckles or some other type of securing mechanisms (Figure 9).

In certain water emergencies, it may not be possible to use a spine board; a spine board may not be readily available or the emergency is so life threatening that there is no time to apply a cervical collar and to secure a victim on a spine board. Examples of emergencies when the use of a spine board might not be practical include:

- The victim has a lacerated artery and requires immediate transport to shore to control bleeding.
- The victim is not breathing and does not have a pulse.
- The victim is trapped in a submerged vehicle and requires immediate extrication.

In examples such as these when the victim must be taken to shore immediately, steps should nevertheless be taken to secure the head and neck. One method of accomplishing this is to use the hands and forearms to form a splint that supports the head and neck. The rescuer carefully approaches the victim from the rear and carefully slides hands and forearms under the victim's arms alongside the neck and toward the ears and mandible (Figure 10). Care must be taken by the rescuer to keep the forearms straight to serve as a splint and not to twist the head and neck in any way when swimming or wading back to shore. This technical procedure requires training and some hands-on practice.

COLD WATER RESCUE

Dr. Desmond Bohn notes in Chapter 5 that the effects of cold on the human body significantly increase the chances of survival — especially among children — even after a prolonged submersion in cold water.

It is important to dispel the widespread belief that cold water rescues and associated longer survival times occur only in northern areas. Since the typical body temperature of an individual is approximately 98.6°F and water, even in the tropics, often falls below this temperature, cold water can be encountered almost anywhere. The increased survival time frequently cited during northern winters can occur almost anywhere.

Cold water rescues require special considerations and precautions. Even a conscious victim may be unable to respond to a reach or throw rescue because he or she lacks the neuromuscular coordination required to reach for a pole or hang onto a buoy or line.

Similarly, a first responder attempting an in-water rescue might be completely disabled upon entering frigid water. If a cold water rescue is attempted, it is critical for the rescuer to take certain measures to prevent the loss of body heat. This can be accomplished in a number of different ways: wearing a neoprene wet suit, a dry suit, or wool clothing. Warm clothing, however, can easily become water logged and negatively buoyant in a very short time, making swimming impossible, so clothing might not be considered as an option.

Perhaps the easiest and most effective way to retain body heat is to keep the head and neck above the water. These two areas of the body are usually the first to dissipate heat when immersed in cold water.

If the rescuer begins to suffer from hypothermia, he or she should get out of the water immediately. If this is not possible, body heat may be conserved by assuming the Heat Escape Lessening Position (HELP). This position is maintained by floating

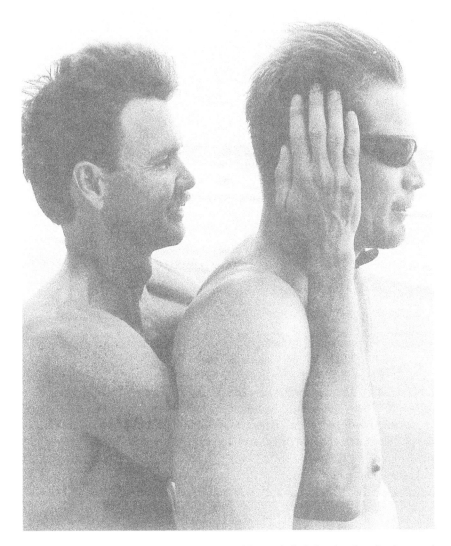

FIGURE 10   Demonstration of a method to stabilize a victim's head and neck when a spine board and cervical collar are not available or practical to use.

with the head out of the water and the body in a fetal tuck position (Figure 11). All emergency first responders should learn how to perform this maneuver by practicing it in a pool.

CURRENTS, WAVES, AND TIDES

With the exception of a swimming pool, most bodies of water will be affected by waves, currents, or tides, or a combination thereof. Ocean beaches, for example, sometimes have dangerous rip currents responsible for more deaths than the

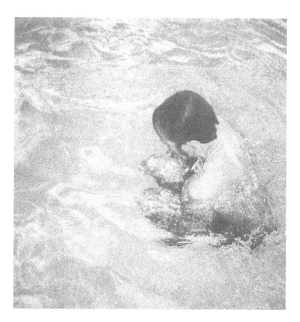

FIGURE 11.   Assuming the "HELP" position.

combination of hurricanes, tornadoes, and floods, while some fast-moving rivers have potentially lethal currents called strainers and hydraulics.

Space does not permit discussion of these conditions, but suffice it to say that every emergency first responder should conduct a survey of his or her area to identify potentially dangerous conditions such as those just mentioned. In some cases, it might be prudent to contact a professional to conduct a survey since many water hazards may not be readily apparent to a novice unfamiliar with the area.

SUMMARY

This chapter provides an overview of drowning, emphasizing that it is a process with a number of characteristic stages rather than a spontaneous event without rhyme or reason. It also presents information about water rescue methods that can be used by most emergency first responders, even those who lack background in lifeguard training or high levels of swimming proficiency. These methods require training. Because emergency first responders — whether they represent the police, fire, or EMS — will likely be among the first to arrive on the scene of a drowning event, these agencies must provide water rescue training to their staffs. Failure to do so not only puts a victim at an increased risk of serious injury, even death, but endangers the rescuer as well.

REFERENCES

American Red Cross, 1993, *American Red Cross Standard First Aid*, Mosby Lifeline Publishers, St. Louis, MO.

Fletemeyer, J., 1995, *Florida Beach Patrol Chiefs Association Water Rescue Survey Study*, 1–8.

Forsten, D. and Murphy, M., 1986, *On Guard: The YMCA Lifesaving Manual*, Human Kinetics Publishers, Champaign, IL.

Kringsholm, B., 1991, "Autopsied Causes of Drowning in Denmark, 1987–1988," *Forensic Science International* 52: 85–95.

DISCLAIMER

The author has made every attempt to provide accurate and reliable information about drowning and water rescue intervention methods. The author and related parties disclaim responsibility for any adverse effects resulting from the recommendations stated in this chapter. Because of the uncertainties surrounding water rescues, the author strongly recommends that each individual employed as an emergency first responder receive training in this area from qualified professionals with lifeguarding and lifesaving backgrounds.

7 The YMCA Perspective on Drowning Prevention

Laura Slane

THE IMPORTANCE OF AQUATIC SAFETY

The interest in aquatic activities has exploded over the past few decades. Greater access to swimming facilities and water parks makes it easier to include aquatic activities in recreation and fitness routines. Enthusiasts are found on the water, rafting, canoeing, sailing, and boating; in the water, in recreational and competitive swimming, synchronized swimming, and water polo; under the water, skin and scuba diving; and even above the water, parasailing. The popularity of aquatic activities has generated a new awareness of the need for aquatic education and safety for all age groups.

For those without awareness and proper training, the aquatic environment can be as dangerous as it is fun. Even those who do not participate in water sports need water safety knowledge. Drowning is the fourth-leading cause of death in the United States, claiming about 4,000 lives each year. In addition to those who die by drowning, untold numbers are injured in accidents in open-water areas and at public, private, and residential pools. Carelessness, rough play, and unsafe headfirst entries can lead to injury on pool decks, near starting blocks, and on or around diving boards.

YMCAs have been involved in drowning prevention for well over 100 years. Through swimming classes, lifeguard training programs, and camps that offer water-front and boating activities, YMCAs promote water safety.

This chapter explores the reasons for the YMCA's involvement in aquatic safety, the history of that involvement, and the different methods the YMCA uses today to teach people to be safer in and around water environments.

THE YMCA

As in any organization, each segment, division, or program must reflect and support the basic purpose of the organization. The YMCA aquatic program philosophy must be in keeping with the overall purpose of the YMCA.

The YMCA mission is to put Christian principles into practice through programs that build healthy spirit, mind, and body for all.

YMCAs offer programs based on seven objectives: grow personally, clarify values, improve personal and family relationships, appreciate diversity, become better leaders and supporters, develop specific skills, and have fun. Although learning

111

a skill may be the central and visible activity, the real focus of YMCA programs is on promoting participants' growth and development and building the values of caring, honesty, respect, and responsibility.

This overall philosophy is the basis for how YMCA programs are developed. Programs are the tools Y staff and volunteers use to accomplish the Y mission. In aquatics, by teaching swimming and water safety, the Y helps people live safer, healthier, and more fulfilling lives.

Another unique dimension of the YMCA is that it is an association of people working together for the common good. People may initially make contact with the Y to participate in one program or activity, but, as they participate, they and their families are drawn into other YMCA experiences. Relationships develop among members, staff, and volunteers. People are offered opportunities to serve others through volunteer leadership roles.

YMCAs are community based. Their work is carried out under the direction of policy-making volunteers who serve as members of boards and committees. Programs are run by paid and volunteer leaders and staff.

YMCAs are at work in more than 130 countries worldwide. The Ys are as different as the communities they serve, but they are bound together in common purpose and mutual support.

U.S. YMCAs serve more than 14 million people each year at over 2,000 locations in 49 states. YMCAs are for people of all ages, incomes, abilities, races, and religions. Half of the YMCA's constituents are under 18, and half are female.

WATER SAFETY AND THE YMCA

YMCAs are in a unique position to address water safety: They own and manage about 2,100 pools across the country, not including those that are rented and/or leased and those YMCA sites on waterfronts, lakes, and oceanfronts. About 77% percent of YMCAs offer aquatic programs at their facilities, resident camps with waterfronts and pools, backyard pools, colleges, and community and city pools.

The YMCA has a comprehensive approach to water safety, including:

- awareness and education of program participants
- community awareness and education
- staff and volunteer training

Professional development of staff, risk management, and aquatic facility assets are all reasons for the YMCA's concern about the need to be continually involved in aquatic safety. The YMCA of the USA develops guidelines and takes positions on issues relating to water safety and aquatic program operation as part of its comprehensive approach to water safety.

The role of the YMCA of the USA is to help local YMCAs deliver the mission. The staff at the YMCA of the USA addresses program development needs by assessing information from local YMCAs, and societal, educational, and industrial trends. The YMCA of the USA researches and evaluates good local programs and then encourages the replication of those programs at other YMCAs.

YMCAs integrate other components into their aquatic programs, such as environmental issues, character development, safety, health, wellness, and nutrition. Environmental components might focus on learning about the areas in which people enjoy the water, being safe, and protecting the environment. Character development is about demonstrating positive values and making decisions based on the values of caring, honesty, respect, and responsibility. Programs include discussions and activities on leading a healthy life. These program components enhance participants' learning and development.

Collaboration — both internal and external — is used to reach out and expand the YMCA aquatic programs and to spread the YMCA's message on aquatic safety. Externally, YMCAs expand their work by collaborating with other community organizations and offering programs outside their buildings. YMCAs collaborate with schools, parks and recreation departments, cities, colleges, hospitals, and many other community-based organizations to offer programs that meet community needs.

YMCAs work to support and strengthen families of all shapes and sizes. They offer a wide range of aquatics programs for families and educate both parents and children on water safety.

The YMCA of the USA program training and certification system offers almost 200 training courses for staff and program volunteers in different program disciplines and leadership development areas. Program areas include active older adults, aquatics, camping, community development, childcare, family, health and fitness, international, sports, and teen leadership. Leadership courses relate to management and professional development. Our largest certification area is aquatics, with more than 30 national aquatic certification courses plus a variety of scuba courses. A quality control system maintains consistency and quality of the courses and includes a sanction process that verifies that all instructors and trainers are certified to teach. National trainers are required to submit training records to the YMCA of the USA for processing, and in return they receive verifications of those they have certified.

Participants receive certification cards and can obtain transcripts. YMCA of the USA training courses are tools used to assist local Ys in delivering consistent, high-quality programs.

Training courses are offered at local Ys through coordination of training among a group of Ys in a regional area and at national training events. This way, training is close to home, convenient, and affordable. Most training is led by Y staff members who volunteer to educate others in their fields of expertise.

YMCA programs are updated on a regular basis. Through research and communication with instructors, trainers, and YMCA staff, information is collected and reviewed prior to aquatic program revisions. In addition, by communicating with other aquatic professionals and keeping in touch with industry trends, the YMCA stays abreast of new and innovative methods.

Quality is a primary concern, and policy-making volunteers are involved in ensuring that quality. Aquatic and/or program committees meet regularly and are involved in evaluating and monitoring the quality of Y programs. If program quality is high, then YMCAs will also have good risk management procedures in place. Local YMCAs look to the YMCA of the USA aquatic guidelines to evaluate aquatic programs.

Another tool at the YMCA's disposal is peer review. The Ys invite assessment teams of staff from other Ys to evaluate their programs based on the YMCA of the USA aquatic guidelines and local policies.

HISTORICAL INVOLVEMENT IN AQUATIC SAFETY

The YMCA has been teaching people to swim for more than 100 years. YMCAs entered the field of lifesaving between 1885 and 1890. The first indoor YMCA swimming pool was built in 1885 in Brooklyn. By 1909, there were 293 YMCA pools.

In 1906, William Ball of the Detroit YMCA invited George Corsan of Toronto to come to Detroit and provide swim instruction for one week. Corsan's methods included the teaching of crawl stroke to beginners, the use of "water wings," and mass teaching procedures. In subsequent years, Corsan visited other YMCAs, with similar results. These were the first successful YMCA learn-to-swim campaigns for drowning prevention.

In 1909, Dr. George J. Fischer conceived the idea of a national swimming effort. Soon thereafter, the YMCA was the first organization to employ national representatives to carry out a national education program for water safety and lifesaving, which helped broaden the scope of YMCA aquatics. By 1917, YMCA leaders had taught 376,000 people to swim and dive. From 1909–1963, more than 17 million people learned to swim and more than 1.5 million were certified in lifesaving at the YMCA. In 1909, the American Red Cross and the YMCA also entered into an agreement to promote first aid on a national basis and to grant joint certificates for standardized first aid courses. In 1910, William Ball and the Red Cross' Major Lynch discussed Red Cross instruction in swimming and particularly in lifesaving.

By 1911, lifesaving work was established at the YMCA College in Springfield, Massachusetts. The YMCA lifesaving program was created by William Ball, Dr. James McCurdy, George Affleck, and Dr. George J. Fischer. The first American book on lifesaving was written by George Goss as a thesis, *Aquatic First Aid,* at Springfield College, and a few years later the manual was published. In 1912, a National YMCA lifesaving service was organized. In 1916, the first aquatic school to train leaders in swimming was established at the Boston YMCA. Dr. Peter Karpovich, Thomas Cureton, Donald Stone, and Charles Silvia continued to research swimming and lifesaving methods and techniques until a new program was developed. Cureton and Silvia developed a program that included the physiology of drowning, comparison of resuscitation techniques, methods of respiration, hygienic effects of water on individuals, and a wide assortment of practical methods.

From 1930–1936, Cureton developed a program for teaching swimming to children. Dr. John Brown invited Cureton to conduct a study in making the program adaptable to the YMCA. By 1932, the YMCA reported more than a million swimmers a year in YMCAs.

The first national YMCA aquatic conference in 1937 led to the first progressive program, including a complete reorganization of the instructional materials, scientific testing to determine progress, appropriate recognitions of achievement for both sexes and all ages, and specific standards for volunteer and professional leadership. In 1938, the new YMCA aquatic literature was released. It was the first progressive program of graded aquatic tests, charts, and worksheets based on extensive research and the use of scientific measuring techniques. Levels in the YMCA Progressive Swimming program — Minnows (beginners), Fish (intermediate), and Sharks (advanced) — were born. The first national plan for certifying aquatic directors and instructors on a professional basis was begun.

From 1939–1945, the aquatics emphasis centered on aquatic survival techniques and warfare aquatics. During the war period, scuba diving made significant advances. In 1943, Cureton published *Warfare Aquatics* which was used in YMCA Institutes during this period.

In 1949, Silvia's text, *Manual of Lifesaving and Water Safety Instruction*, was published, citing supporting research for the methods used. This was first lifesaving and water safety text to advocate the use of mouth-to-mouth resuscitation. Silvia coined the term "lifesaving through watermanship" to impress upon the teacher and student the importance of basing lifesaving training on the principles of watermanship. Thorough understanding of these principles resulted in the development of techniques to eliminate waste motion and to improve mobility.

During the 1950s, the YMCA aquatic program was broadened to include boating, water ballet, water polo, skin and scuba diving, and programs for the disabled. In 1956, the YMCA introduced national Learn to Swim Month. In 1958, Harold Friermood published the *New YMCA Aquatic Workbook*, which described the complete YMCA aquatic program. In 1959, the YMCA was the first organization to test and certify instructors in skin and scuba diving based on the recent issue of *The New Science of Skin and Scuba Diving* by the Council for National Cooperation in Aquatics.

The prime objective of the YMCA aquatic program was *Teach America to Swim* and to encourage every swimmer to be a lifesaver.

In 1960, Dr. Richard Pohndorf completed his book, *Camp Waterfront Programs and Management*, an expansion of his 1946 work, which dealt with important aspects of water safety. The book was published for the YMCA for its work in camping programs across the country.

In 1969, 20 study groups were organized and charged with the research, development, and formation of new aquatic programs, as well as recommendations for changes in existing programs. Their work was validated through field testing in local Ys. In 1970, the study groups presented their findings at the National YMCA Aquatic Conference in Fort Lauderdale, Florida. This was followed by the implementation of the programs in 1972. The new YMCA aquatic program had a new philosophical orientation for progressive swim instruction; a training, certification, and recognition program for aquatic leadership; the Tadpole preschool swimming program; a swimming program for the handicapped; and a synchronized swimming program. The testing of skills in the progressive program was streamlined by combining skills and by removing some of the emphasis on testing. The new program expanded objectives from just swimming skills to include endurance, personal safety, and lifesaving. The YMCA Aquatic Safety and Lifesaving program was launched — the first lifesaving program that divided lifesaving into three levels: aquatic safety, advanced aquatic safety, and lifesaving. The YMCA was the first organization to develop a lifeguard training and certification program, released in 1974 with different certifications for pool, lake and river, and surf lifeguards.

In 1986, Aquatic Facility Manager and Aquatic Instructor Trainer certifications was released at the National YMCA Centennial Aquatic Conference in New Orleans. The Aquatic Facility Manager course was designed for staff members who manage aquatic programs and require training in how to teach swimming, supervision and training of swimming instructors and lifeguards, budgeting, communications, problem solving, and program development. The new Aquatic Instructor Trainer certification replaced the Aquatic Director certification designed for trainers for instructors in the YMCA programs. *On the Guard — The YMCA Lifeguard Manual* was released as the new lifeguard program.

In 1987, *Y SKIPPERS — An Aquatic Program for Children Five and Under* and *Parent's Guide to Y SKIPPERS* were published, the basis for a boating safety and aquatic safety education program for parents and their young children. In 1989, the *Teaching Boating Safety* manual was released. Both the manual and program were funded through grants from the United States Coast Guard. The manual was designed to aid instructors in presenting safe boating principles to first-time or casual boaters, as part of the effort to meet the need for increased boater education.

In 1994, Trainer level certifications for each specialist instructor course replaced the Aquatic Instructor Trainer certification. The Principles of YMCA Aquatic Leadership course replaced the Basic Aquatic Leadership course. The Pool Operator on Location course was also updated. New programs and instructor training were developed or released including YMCA On the Guard II, YMCA Water Polo/Wetball, YMCA Synchronized Swimming, YMCA Prenatal Exercise (Land and Water), YMCA Healthy Back (Land and Water), and YMCA Active Older Adults Land/Water Exercise. In 1996, the new YMCA Splash PROGRAM was released, the updated "Learn to Swim" program. "Fun, Function, and Safety: Improving and Expanding Your YMCA Aquatic Center" will soon be available to YMCAs. This paper addresses planning and improving your aquatic center, safety considerations for today's pool equipment, and renovating and building new aquatic facilities.

The YMCA has been a leader in water safety and aquatic education for over 100 years and is committed to continuing this role, well into the future.

YMCA AQUATICS TODAY

Swim instructional programs are a cornerstone of YMCA programming. Five of the ten most popular programs in YMCAs are aquatics. YMCA instructional swim programs are a primary focus of pools. The Y offers a variety of programs for all ages that stress water safety, including lifeguarding, youth and adult instructional swim classes, parent/child and preschool classes, and the community-based learn-to-swim campaign, which are components of other YMCA programs, such as camping, childcare, and family programs. Learning to swim and basic water safety are important life skills that everyone should know and continue to be priorities for YMCAs. These programs, available to the thousands of communities where Ys are located, demonstrate the YMCA's annual impact on millions in the areas of water safety and drowning prevention. The programs described in the next section show how the YMCA makes a significant contribution to water safety in America.

In 1992, after a comprehensive review of the YMCA aquatic program with trainers, YMCA aquatic directors, and external consultants it was decided to add or expand the following features in the revision of *On the Guard*:

- detailed training program for lifeguard instructors and trainers
- comprehensive program to provide lifeguards with the basic training needed for any water environment
- provide new lifeguards with enough information to ask the right questions to find the right job
- help young people build job skills
- prevention as a priority, not just reaction
- equipment-based training
- training to help lifeguards make good decisions on and off duty
- training to help lifeguards deal with members and participants in a friendly and professional manner

Experts in the field were enlisted to assist the YMCA with the development. Through the use of current research and technical experts, the group evaluated the information based on what local YMCAs and their communities needed.

The new YMCA lifeguarding and aquatic safety program includes three programs: On the Guard II, the YMCA Lifeguard program; Aquatic Safety; and Aquatic Personal Safety and Survival — a broad-based approach to educating a variety of age groups on how to be safe in and around aquatic environments.

A four–six hour introductory course on water safety that requires no previous training or swimming ability is designed to be adapted to the needs of individuals in different aquatic settings, from corporate fitness to a backyard family pool. Course topics include history and philosophy of YMCA aquatic safety and lifeguarding training, personal aquatic safety, accident prevention principles, basic first aid and rescue breathing, and nonswimming rescues.

An eight-hour course that trains participants in personal safety and survival skills in and around aquatic environments includes the same information as the Aquatic Safety course, plus general aquatic information and basic survival skills. This course requires the ability to swim 300 yards. Many participants are junior high and high school students who want to prepare to be lifeguards and learn more about water safety.

On the Guard II, the YMCA's lifeguard training manual, presents a comprehensive education centered on preventing accidents. It focuses on the practical aspects of what lifeguards need to know to prevent accidents and to react to emergency situations in water environments, such as swimming pools, lakes, rivers, and oceans. This training program helps participants learn and apply safety principles in their own lives, develop leadership skills, maintain a healthy lifestyle, and improve their decision-making skills. The goal of the YMCA lifeguard program is to develop lifeguards who not only know a lot, but who also care a lot, about lifeguarding and about those they are trained to serve.

Based on sound decision making, proper use of rescue equipment, knowledge of water safety, and proficiency in rescue skills, this course builds the knowledge and skills needed to perform the lifeguard duties. This 28-hour course is a prerequisite to all other aquatic specialist instructor courses and includes classroom and pool sessions. Prior to starting the course, class participants must have CPR (adult, youth, and infant) and first-aid certification and pass a swim test.

Besides being advanced-level swimmers, YMCA lifeguard candidates should be caring, strong, quick to respond, confident, fit, and intelligent, with good interpersonal skills. The YMCA welcomes and involves everyone in their programs, but the hazardous duty of a lifeguard may disqualify some candidates with certain physical or mental conditions from being certified. Those who do not qualify may participate in the program, but certification is not available. To qualify for certification, an individual must be able to:

- remain alert, with no lapses in consciousness
- sit for extended periods, including in an elevated chair
- move to various locations, including in and around an elevated chair
- communicate verbally, including projecting the voice across distances
- hear noises and distress signals
- observe all areas of the water area
- perform all needed rescues and survival skills
- think in the abstract, solve problems, make decisions, instruct, evaluate, supervise, and remember

After the completion of the training, lifeguards need facility-specific training and orientation. The equipment-based lifeguard training program stipulates that each lifeguard have a rescue tube/buoy when on duty.

Trainees are educated on the safety and survival skills every swimmer must know. They learn how to guard, pool dangers, and suggested rules to protect the swimmers' safety, followed by information on dealing with emergencies, including rescue skills, emergency systems, first aid in aquatic environments, and spinal injury management. The program covers what lifeguards need to know for outdoor lifeguarding through discussions of weather, open-water dangers, and the precautions to take against them. The course also includes specialized knowledge required for basic open-water lifeguarding. The training program reviews some of the job responsibilities of lifeguards, beginning with basic legal terms and proceedings that might be relevant if they become involved in lawsuits against an aquatic facility. Basic pool management concerns, such as pool chemistry, filtration, and safety inspections are covered. The program also includes guidance on how to seek and obtain a lifeguarding position and ideas for further training.

The program strives to give lifeguard candidates enough knowledge to ask the "right" questions of potential employers and to evaluate potential hazardous situations. The Y training not only teaches lifeguards how to serve and protect those they are responsible for but also helps them to grow and develop.

Every classroom session includes an opportunity to discuss the material in the manual and apply it to lifeguarding situations. Through group work based-training and experiential learning activities, participants review the material. To increase retention levels, participants have five interactions with the material. They read the manual, answer the review questions, apply and learn the material in class, address the issues in the water, and are tested on the material. The course addresses the "why" not just the "how." In addition, throughout the course, there are value discussions that relate to how lifeguards react in difficult situations; for instance, do they follow the same rules as they enforce when on duty? Is helping others still their job when they are not on duty? The pool sessions allow time for training and conditioning to increase speed and endurance, especially development of leg strength. Once the rescue skills have been learned in the water, they are applied in situations that arise on the job. Lifeguard candidates complete a two-hour practical session with experienced lifeguards prior to certification.

To be certified, participants must pass 80% of each section of the written test, plus perform all skills in the practical skills test. Certification may also include the instructor's subjective judgment on the candidate's maturity, attitude, and classroom participation demonstrated throughout the course. YMCA certification is valid for two years with the requirement that CPR and First Aid must be kept current to maintain a current certification. The YMCA lifeguard certification has long been accepted by states and many organizations.

Comprehensive lifeguard instructor and lifeguard trainer courses have been developed to complement the basic program. The lifeguard instructor course is an 18-hour program to train candidates to teach the YMCA lifeguard and aquatic safety programs. An instructor manual and video are used to provide consistency in courses throughout the country. Lifeguard instructor certification is valid for three years. YMCA Lifeguard, CPR, and first aid must be kept current to maintain certifications. The lifeguard trainer program is 23 hours and allows participants to train and certify lifeguard instructors and lifeguards.

YMCA SPLASH is the new community-based learn to swim program, which was released in March 1996. The primary purpose of this program is to help people of all ages, especially children and families, learn how to be safer around water. It is designed to meet community needs and to fit into YMCA's program scheduling.

YMCA SPLASH includes a core five-day pool or classroom program, plus specialty courses on boating safety, beach safety, and backyard pool safety. The core program is a daily adventure combining a water environment, swimming skills, and character development. Detailed lesson plans have been developed for the 30–45 minute classes. Class adaptations are included for preschoolers, adults, and teens.

The program includes basic swimming skills, tips on beach safety, pool safety, boating safety, backyard pool safety, water park safety, beach safety, character development activities, and environmental awareness, family activities, and parent education. For Ys it offers an opportunity to meet needs of families, collaborate internally and externally, expand work in underserved communities, involve volunteers, and meet a pressing community need.

The YMCA of the USA has designated May as YMCA SPLASH Month. The Ys offer special programs at this time, but the program can also be offered at any other time throughout the year. YMCAs offer it in the classroom at many of the after-school care program sites, and work with schools, apartment complexes, youth groups, and other community organizations to offer the program either in the pool or a classroom.

The YMCA Progressive Swimming program is a seven-level program designed for children and adults. Each level builds on the preceding one.

The instructors are crucial to the success of the program and are taught a basic understanding and respect for the uniqueness of each student. Student-centered teaching methods are used. They are designed to build on each participant's potential, encourage safety awareness, and develop skills.

In the YMCA Progressive Swimming program health and physical fitness is a springboard for building self-confidence, self-esteem, and values like respect and caring. As swimmers learn to take care of themselves in the water, they also learn to help others, work together, and strive to be the best they can be.

Physical, mental, and spiritual growth are stressed at each level. Physical development is introduced through the teaching of aquatic sport skills, including competitive swimming, diving, and synchronized swimming, and each class session includes time for sustained swimming. Teaching styles challenge and develop the student's cognitive abilities. The program provides the tools and information students need to solve problems and helps them find their own solutions. They learn to think beyond rote memorization and response. The positive, personal growth that occurs from this may be understood through "I can, I am, I will" philosophy: I can accomplish these things and achieve; I am a worthy person because I have achieved success and I am liked by my instructor; and I will be able to solve future problems, perhaps not immediately, but eventually. Spiritual development is achieved in the program in a number of ways. The choices people make about their own behavior and the way they perceive others is a reflection of their values. Instructors facilitate discussions about positive values and making good choices within each session. Classes explore good ways to handle situations, to work together, and to help others.

At each level of the program, participants are involved in activities related to five components: personal safety, stroke development, water sports and games, personal development, and rescue.

The YMCA's goal is for every student participating in the progressive swimming program to become safety conscious around water. The information learned in these classes form the basis for accident prevention. Role-playing is one method used to demonstrate personal safety, and it helps the student understand the importance of what is being taught. Safety and survival skills students learn include floating, treading, swimming, and relaxation techniques necessary for supporting themselves.

When students are building endurance and working on perfecting their strokes, encouragement and goal setting are important. An important part of learning strokes is understanding how and why they work. Instructors explain why a principle of physics applies to the stroke, or why a certain concept of exercise physiology works the way it does.

To give students a well-rounded aquatic background, they are provided with opportunities to participate in recreational and competitive aquatic activities to help them develop a lifelong interest in aquatic sports and activities.

Water games are included at all levels; these games develop confidence, stamina, skills, and a cooperative attitude. Aquatic sports skills for synchronized swimming, competitive swimming, and diving are also introduced. Underwater swimming adds an element of excitement and exploration. The proper and safe use of a mask and fins helps the students discover the underwater environment. An introduction to small craft and boating opens new possibilities for recreational activities.

The program gives people the sense of accomplishment that strengthens self-esteem. They learn about values and think about consequences of choices in order to close the gap between stated values and actual behavior. They interact with others so their values are tested.

With proper training, even young children can perform basic, nonswimming rescues and provide simple, aquatic emergency care. At each level, participants are introduced to skills that prepare them to respond to emergencies.

YMCA SKIPPERS program includes two programs: Infant Water Enrichment, a water adjustment class for children six months through 3 years of age, and the Revised Tadpole program, water adjustment and beginning swimming skills for children 3–5 years of age. The objectives of these programs are fun, exercise, parent education, water adjustment, boating safety, use of personal flotation devices (PFD), and safety education.

Aquatic safety is not limited to the time spent in the class; as a result of the program, aquatic safety becomes a way of life for everyone involved. Safety begins with knowledge and is taught by example and encouraged by a well-established routine. Away from the Y, parents are encouraged to know the location of water (lakes or pools) near their homes or even in their homes. They learn that they should always accompany their child, or the child should not have access to water area. The keys to safety are planning ahead by establishing a routine, similar to the one used at the Y which helps to diminish the probability of a child's entering the water without adult supervision.

The under-3 program follows the infant aquatic guidelines that are recommended by the American Academy of Pediatrics for those who choose to participate in these programs. It is a water orientation class directed to the parents, who can then help their children learn to swim when they are ready. Safety is best taught by example and parents and children who are exposed to a caring environment where safety is practiced are likely to continue these practices in other environments. The water activities, which focus on water adjustment, may include blowing bubbles, kicking, and jumping. Activities are fun, encourage laughter, and demonstrate trust and caring between parent and child. Parents learn about accident prevention, basic rescue techniques, boating safety principles, and how to respond in an emergency. Home activities are encouraged by the instructor, and families practice the games, songs, and activities done in class. Educational handouts are distributed on a variety of topics such as health, family enrichment, boating, and swimming pool safety. Classes are appropriate for children's developmental stages.

The program for children 3–5 years of age is designed to teach children the fundamentals of swimming and water and boating safety. The skills they learn become a foundation for a later lifelong involvement in swimming to promote good health.

An important aspect of the program is teaching boating and water safety. Children learn to respect the water and to exercise caution when in or near it. They develop an awareness of their own bodies, acquire a feeling of independence, gain a sense of success, and increase their self-esteem. They also learn how to perform elementary nonswimming rescue skills. These skills can help them to save their own or someone else's life. Parents and caregivers are reminded not harbor a false sense of security because children will continue to need constant supervision in or near water.

Most classes are held without parents in the water, although some Ys run this program with parents in the water. Parents are involved through parent education sessions that teach aquatic safety skills, offer information on child development and parenting, and discuss how to help children practice the skills they learn in class.

The classes are divided by ability into four skill levels. Children learn beginning skills such as water adjustment, blowing bubbles, kicking, and floating. They also learn advanced skills, such as swimming lengths of crawl stroke with rotary breathing, elementary backstroke, back crawl stroke, and diving. They learn how to use PFDs, get in and out of a boat, perform surface dives, tread water, and learn synchronized swimming skills. Skills are taught through games, songs, and adventures.

In their swimming classes, lifeguard training programs, and day and resident camps, the Ys have long been concerned about boating safety. The YMCA Boating Safety program was developed to meet the need for more boating education. It is designed for YMCAs to use as a separate course or as part of other programs, including camping and family programs. It provides an orientation or a review of safe boating principles to first-time or casual boaters and includes information on safety basics and boating basics.

The YMCA is committed to continue its work in water safety and drowning prevention. Through consistent education of people of all ages in all communities, YMCAs will continue to help prevent tragic accidents and drownings and to help people lead safe and healthier lives.

SUMMARY

The YMCA is one of the country's largest advocates for water safety and drowning prevention. With over 100 years of experience in teaching people swimming, boating safety, and lifeguarding, and supporting and strengthening families through a variety of programs, YMCAs have the ability to reach people of all ages, incomes, backgrounds, and abilities with their water safety messages.

The YMCA of the USA offers more than 200 training courses for staff and program volunteers in different program disciplines and leadership development; a number of these courses are in aquatics. The national program training and certification systems monitors the consistency and quality of these courses nationwide.

Four YMCA programs have a particularly strong impact in teaching people how to be safe in and around water: YMCA Lifeguard, YMCA community learn to swim program, YMCA Progressive Swimming program, and the YMCA SKIPPERS program. On the Guard II, the YMCA Lifeguard program, teaches the knowledge and skills needed to perform the duties of a lifeguard. Through sound decision making, proper use of rescue equipment, knowledge of water safety, and proficiency in rescue skills, lifeguard candidates will not only know a lot but also care a lot about lifeguarding and those they are trained to serve.

YMCA community learn to swim program goal is to teach people of all ages, especially children and families, how to have fun and be safe in and around water. The program includes basic swimming skills; information and safety tips for pools, boating, beaches, backyard pools, and water parks; character development activities; environmental awareness; family activities; and parent education.

YMCA Progressive Swimming is a seven-level swim instruction program for children and adults. Each level builds on the skills learn in the preceding one, and addresses five components through skills and activities: personal safety, stroke development, water sports and games, personal development, and rescue.

YMCA SKIPPERS is a water orientation and instructional swim program for children under the age of 5. The objectives are fun, exercise, parent education, water adjustment, boating safety, use of personal flotation devices, and safety education. For parents of children under 3 years, a water orientation class is offered that teaches parents how to help their children adjust to the water environment. The parents learn about accident prevention, basic rescue techniques, boating safety principles, and how to respond in an emergency, plus water games, songs, and activities that help children feel comfortable in the water. The program for children 3–5 years is designed to teach children the fundamentals of swimming and water and boating safety. The children learn to respect the water and exercise caution when in or near it. They develop an increased awareness of their own bodies, acquire a feeling of independence, plus learn swimming skills and basic rescue techniques. Parents are involved through parent education sessions that teach aquatic safety, offer information on child development and parenting, and discuss how to help children practice the skills they learn in class.

The YMCA is committed to continued work in water safety and drowning prevention. Through consistent education of people of all ages in all communities, YMCAs will continue to help prevent tragic accidents and help people lead safer, healthier lives.

REFERENCES

Schultz, Paul, December 1970, *History and Philosophy of YMCA Aquatics: A Brief Summary Background.*

Silvia, Charles E., 1965, *Lifesaving and Water Safety Today,* National Board of Young Men's Christian Association, Association Press, New York.

YMCA of the USA, 1994, *On the Guard II, the YMCA Lifeguarding Manual,* Human Kinetics Publishers, Inc., Champaign, IL.

YMCA of the USA, 1994, *On the Guard II, the YMCA Lifeguard Instructor Manual,* Human Kinetics Publishers, Inc., Champaign, IL.

YMCA of the USA, 1989, *Teaching Boating Safety,* Human Kinetics Publishers, Inc., Champaign, IL.

YMCA of the USA, 1984, *Y Basics: Yesterday, Today and Tomorrow,* Human Kinetics Publishers, Inc., Champaign, IL.

YMCA of the USA, 1987, *Y SKIPPERS, An Aquatic Program for Children Five and Under,* Human Kinetics Publishers, Inc., Champaign, IL.

YMCA of the USA, 1992, *YMCA Progressive Swimming,* Human Kinetics Publishers, Inc., Champaign, IL.

8 Drownings on the Beaches of Brazil

David Szpilman

INTRODUCTION

Brazil, with a continental extension of 8,511,996.3 sq km, occupies the largest part of South America. The country is divided into one federal district and 26 states, 10 of which have ocean access. This vast beach area of 7,408 km has tropic, subtropic, and temperate climates and an average water temperature of 20°C (Figure 1).

This coastal region has various beautiful landscapes with beaches of world-renowned beauty (Figure 2). More than 90% of these beaches show levels of bacterial contamination below 10 CFU/ml (units of formed colonies per ml^3), which indicates excellent conditions for the leisure beach visitor.

These inviting elements are major reasons why Brazilians are so inclined to water sports and why tourists decide to stay in Brazil permanently. It is also the reason why Brazil's beaches are famous vacation and relaxation spots.

Sports such as surfing, wind surfing, jet skiing, scuba diving, swimming, racing, soccer, and volleyball are avidly pursued (Figure 3). The sandy beaches are also perfect natural settings for aquatic sport competitions and for cultural events such as concerts and dances.

Although Brazil is a country experiencing widespread problems due to socio-economic differences and the diversity of ethnic groups, the beach still represents a unifying force and functions as an important vehicle for socialization and community.

As Brazil's social and economic conditions gradually improve, aquatic activities play a greater role in social progression. The number of pools used for relaxation and athletic training purposes in clubs, condominiums, and homes has increased, as has the number of teams in official aquatic competitions.

The most popular water sports in Brazil, in descending order, are: swimming, fishing, surfing, scuba diving, rowing, canoeing, water skiing, water biking, jet skiing, water polo, synchronized swimming, diving, and others. An estimated 5–10 million people practice some form of water sport either for fun or for a serious workout. A total of 100,000 athletes belong to aquatic organizations and compete at various levels nationwide.

A recent study of 100 swimmers on the beaches of Rio de Janeiro produced the statistics shown in Figures 4 and 5. Another study done in January 1996 by the Marketing and Communication Institute (MCI) for the Ministry of Sports shows:

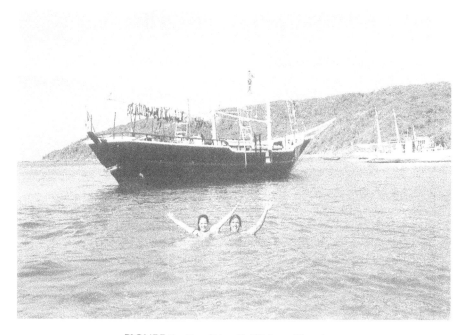

FIGURE 1   Brazil has 7,408 km of beaches.

1. Swimming is the number one preferred sport, with walking second.
2. Soccer rates as the most popular sport among men.
3. Three out of ten Brazilians consider themselves regularly active athletes or at least practice some sport three times per week.
4. Youth 16–24 years of age like swimming the best, with 21% in favor of the sport. Soccer was second with 18%, and volleyball was third with 14%.
5. In the age group 25–39, 19% shows a connection with swimming and soccer.
6. Men prefer swimming, 18%; walking, 10%; other sports, 39%.
7. Women prefer swimming, 23%; walking, volleyball, and gymnastics, 18%; aerobics, 11%; other sports, 27%.

THE HISTORY OF LIFESAVING IN BRAZIL

Brazil's history of aquatic lifesaving started in Rio de Janeiro (Figure 6). Rio is a modern city with incomparable natural beauty surrounding its beaches. Climate and tropical splendor entice thousands of tourists as well as natives to come and enjoy the ocean year round, but the clear blue water and sandy beaches are blinders for possible dangers to the unsuspecting bather. Strong currents have the potential to turn into treacherous situations and even cause death, making Rio de Janeiro one of the leading regions of Brazil for water rescues (Figure 7).

Learning of these conditions, Commodore Wilbert E. Longfellow came to Rio de Janeiro (then the capital of Brazil) in 1914 and began the Service of Lifesaving

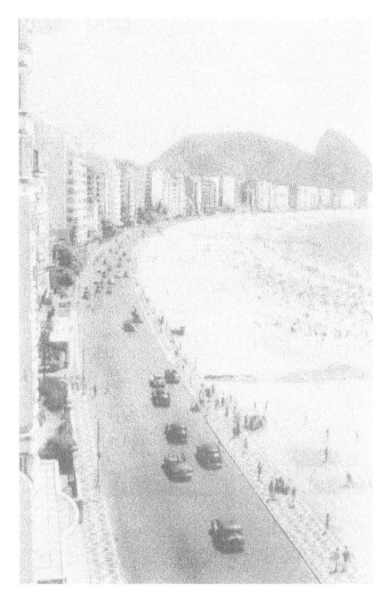

FIGURE 2   The beach at Rio de Janeiro in an earlier era.

of the American Red Cross. The goal was to organize and train lifeguard volunteers to stand guard on all the beaches of Brazil. Recognizing the inefficiency of this strategy, a national campaign was implemented to attempt to educate and alert everyone about the potential dangers on all Brazilian beaches. The slogan was: "Each person should know how to swim and each swimmer should know how to save lives."

On May 10, 1917, Prefeito Amaro Cavalcante decreed that Corpo Maritimo de Salvamento (CMS) (maritime rescue) would function under the rescue services of

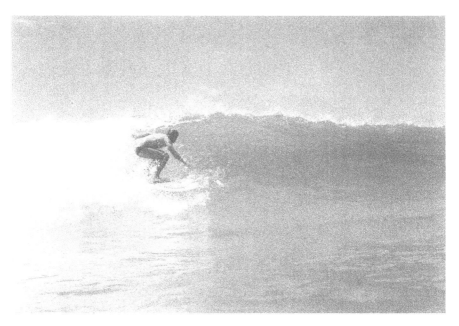

FIGURE 3   Surfing is a popular sport in Brazil.

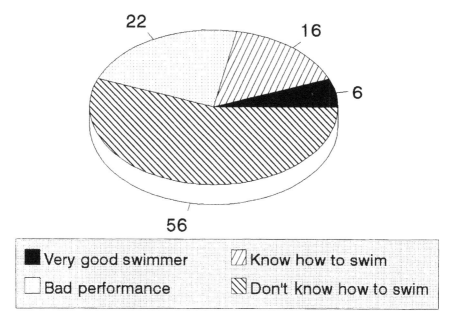

FIGURE 4   Results of a 1993 survey of 100 bathers on Rio de Janeiro beaches about swimming knowledge.

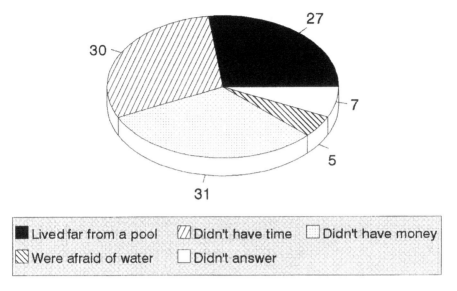

FIGURE 5   Results of a 1993 survey of 100 bathers on Rio de Janeiro beaches about why they are poor swimmers or do not know how to swim; 86% indicated they wanted to learn.

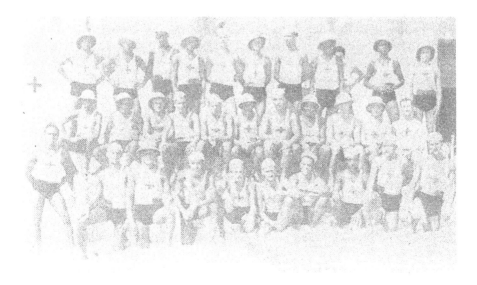

FIGURE 6   Brazil's history of lifesaving started in Rio de Janeiro.

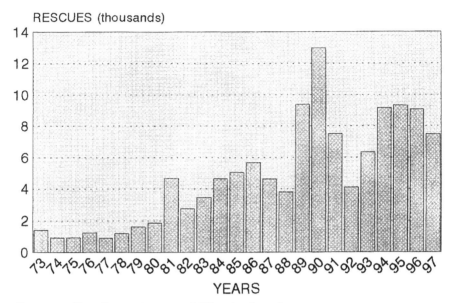

RESCUES (thousands)

YEARS

Source: Fire Department of Rio de Janeiro

FIGURE 7 Grupamento Martimo (GMAR) in Rio de Janeiro made 120,070 beach rescues between 1973 and 1977.

the Red Cross on Copacabana Beach. In 1939 this post was transformed into the Ismael Gusmao Rescue Station in honor of its founder (Figure 8).

Explosive demographic growth, intense immigration to Rio, and an improved standard of living in the 1950s increased contact between people and the sea, alerting the authorities to the need to create a system of lifesaving specializing in aquatic accidents. In 1963, the Corpo Maritimo de Salvamento (Salvamar) under the Secretary of Public Safety was initiated. A small group of people with either an affinity for or experience with beach rescue was recruited and, by 1967, the Training Center for Rescue and Lifeguards was approved and created by the Secretary of Public Safety (Figures 9 and 10).

To respond to the need for the quickest and most efficient medical attention, in 1968 the first Centers for Recuperation of Drownings (CRA) were inaugurated. The first three, on the beaches of Ramos, Copacabana, and Barra da Tijuca — on the shores of Rio — were all equipped to provide emergency medical assistance in drowning cases. Today, these CRAs are equipped with all necessary emergency medical equipment and staffed with doctors and nurses who have available ambulances and boats to access the scene of an accident (Figure 11). Modern equipment and the latest rescue techniques facilitate rapid response to water accident scenes and treatment of victims.

In 1975 the Secretary of Public Safety mandated that Salvamar become a part of the Department of Civil Defense.

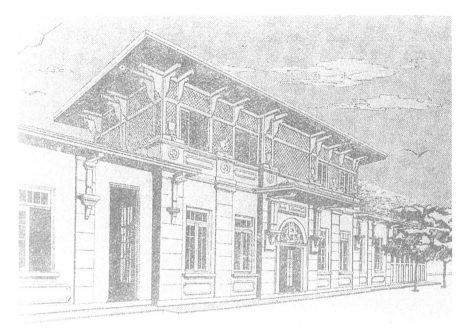

FIGURE 8   The Ismael Gusmao Rescue Station.

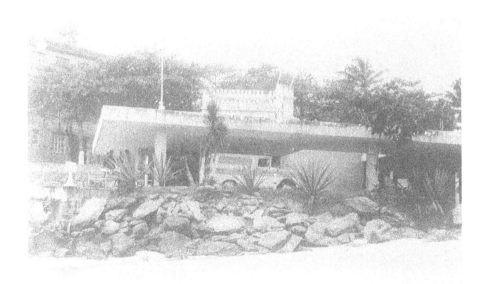

FIGURE 9   The Training Center for Rescue and Lifeguards.

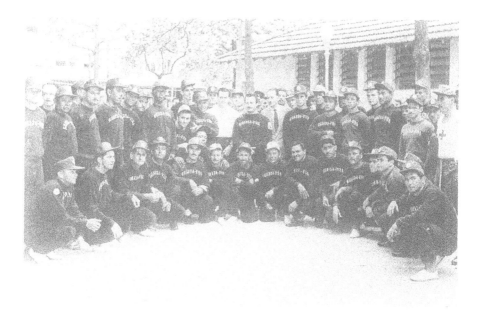

FIGURE 10   Trainees at the Training Center for Rescue and Lifeguards.

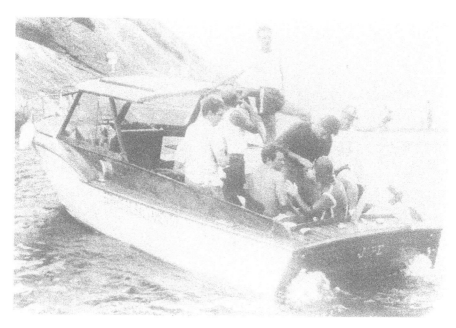

FIGURE 11   Doctors and nurses have rescue boats available.

In 1984 Salvamar passed the fire department's requirements and on October 16, 1984, Grupamento Martimo (GMAR) was activated, with headquarters in Botafogo. Three other satellite stations followed the same guidelines as the principal CRA to establish and stabilize the link between first responders and doctors.

This managerial transition of rescue service was an arduous task because of the need to train all the specialized military personnel as well as transfer the now extinct Salvamar to its new department. After training the military personnel for their new function, some elements remained permanent protocol for GMAR.

The early years were characterized by great sacrifice on the part of instructors and some lifeguards. As the years passed, rescues increased and deaths decreased on the beaches of Rio, confirming that the decision to form a highly professional water rescue system was a wise choice.

With the enormous Brazilian coast spanning 7,408 km, it was natural that a phenomenon in Rio would eventually spread to other areas as well. As the former capital, Rio remains the economic, political, and cultural center of the country, as well as the pioneer in the water rescue movement. As the years passed, the heightened level of expertise transformed this city into the nucleus for all forms of water rescue training. Lifeguards, instructors, doctors, and specialized paramedics were among those personnel trained to better serve the public.

SOBRASA

The Brazilian Water Rescue Society (SOBRASA) (Figure 12) is a nonprofit, civil entity founded in March 1995 by a group of professionals with a common objective and organizational philosophy: to achieve high standards of water safety and rescue. This is the only organization in Brazil not affiliated with the military that dedicates efforts to water rescue. Its principal function is unification of all Brazilian rescue services.

DROWNING STATISTICS

Drowning rates are high in Brazilian waters. Some factors that contribute to the large number of drownings are:

Brazil's geographic location and its tropical climate
Narrow temperature range throughout the four seasons
Large territorial extension — 8,511,996.3 sq km
Atlantic coastal extension — 7,408 km
Average water temperature — 20°C
Densely populated coastal regions
Constant influx of tourists
Brazilians' strong attraction to the ocean and ocean activities
Increase in oceanic industries

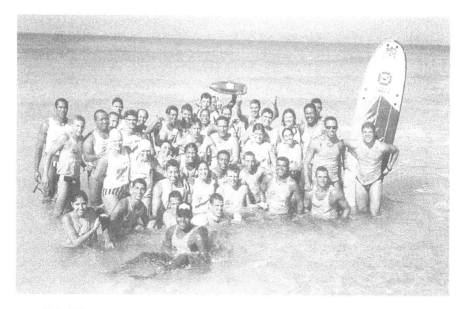

FIGURE 12   Members of the Brazilian Water Rescue Society (SOBRASA).

Constant increase in nautical and aquatic oriented sports
Large nonswimming proportion of the population
Large number of currents

The incidences of death by drowning between 1981 and 1991 were few, but the Brazilian population has suffered an annual 2% increase in drownings. Comparing the number of deaths per 100,000 inhabitants, we observe an increase between 1981 and 1983, but also a gradual decline until 1988, while maintaining the same course with small variations until 1991. In 1995, out of 150 million inhabitants, there were 6,727 deaths, an average of 4.5 per 100,000 (Figure 13).

The country of Brazil has one federal district and 26 states, 10 of which have coastal areas and long rainy seasons. Figure 14 shows the number of deaths in each state in 1988 and 1995. The number of deaths per 100,000 people varies greatly from state to state. The three states with the greatest number of drowning deaths in 1995 have no coastline. The state of Acre had the highest incidence, 19.93 deaths per 100,000 people. In contrast, Fernando de Noronha had no drownings, and Goias had only 1.2 per 100,000. Sao Paulo had the most people and the highest total number of drownings for both years analyzed, 5.2 and 5.0 per 100,000, ranking it eleventh in deaths per 100,000. The total number of cases was 1,659.

Of the drownings in Brazil, 83.5% are males with an average age of 16. There are important variations in the sexes and ages of the victims. The average age of those who drown in the ocean is 22 years, and 74.2% of these victims are males. Freshwater drownings, predominately in private pools, claim the lives of both sexes under 5 years of age.

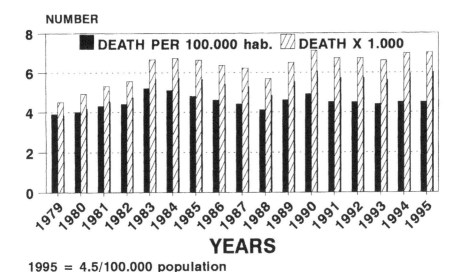

FIGURE 13   A comparison of drownings, 1979–1995.

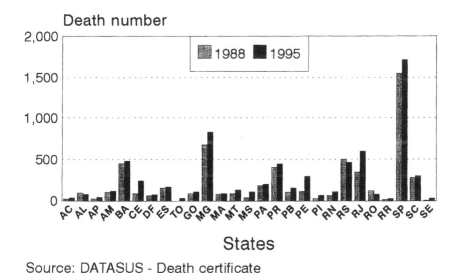

FIGURE 14   A comparison of drownings by state, 1988 and 1995.

These statistics, collected for research by the Ministry of Health, include drownings of victims at their residences. Some drownings may have occurred at locations outside of the victims' states of residence.

SPECIAL HAZARDS

Upon entering the water, a human being's natural defense mechanism can be both a safety valve and a serious danger. Marine life such as sharks and jellyfish often touch off a state of panic and loss of control that causes a victim to drown.

SHARKS

Brazil has close to 70 species of shark, which may range from 2–18 m in length. Only 12 of those species are dangerous and may attack bathers, fishermen, and divers. Hammerheads and tintureiras, the most common attackers, are known to be aggressive hunters that usually bite whatever appears in front of them.

Until a few years ago, shark attacks were uncommon. Occasionally, these animals stray from their habitat in search of prey and find themselves closer than usual to the shoreline. Between 1955 and 1992, 51 attacks were reported, 10 of which were fatal. During that time, the frequency of attacks on bathers increased.

In Sao Marcos Bay in Maranhao, during Summer 1992, there were three attacks in three months. During that same period, on Boa Viagem Beach, Pernambuco, another attack occurred. All of the victims were surfers who lost feet, legs, and arms. Surfers dangle these body parts over the side of their boards into the water, presenting to a passing shark a sight that looks like a tasty marine mammal.

What is the reason for this sudden increase in shark attacks? The sharks have always been there, but in recent years, more people go to the beach and surf on coastal areas that were not previously popular. Since surfing became popular, 50 attacks have been reported on the Pernambuco Coast, 7 attacks in 1995 alone.

JELLYFISH

The jellyfish is a timid creature that floats on the surface of the warm waters of the Brazilian coast, usually appearing during the fall and winter months. The aurelia family is very common to the Brazilian coast. Its tentacles can reach up to one meter in length and may inflict serious lesions that cause intense irritation, pain, and dermatitis. The lack of awareness of the risk involved with this animal can result in death. Cause of death may be difficult to detect.

Fortunately, the species of the cianea and chironex families, considered to be the most deadly jellyfish in the world, are not found on the Brazilian coast.

OTHER DANGEROUS MARINE LIFE

Other types of fish known to take a bite out of a fisherman's hand include barracuda, moray eel, blowfish, bicuda, bicudinha, enchova, swordfish, and vermelho-dentao.

AQUATIC RESCUE SERVICES

GRUPAMENTO MARITIMO DO RIO DE JANEIRO (GMAR–CBMER)

In 1984, the Rio de Janeiro firefighters, as GMAR, assumed the responsibility of managing and executing all rescue activities on state beaches. GMAR had an operational base in the Rio suburb of Botafogo, with three subgroups (SGMAR) in Copacabana, Barra da Tijuca, and Sepetiba, serving the entire shoreline of the state, approximately 90 km.

This preventative work, security, and rescue, are practiced daily, year-round, from 7 A.M. to 7 P.M. during peak hours of beach usage, when the majority of rescues occur (Figure 15). After hours, GMAR remains on call.

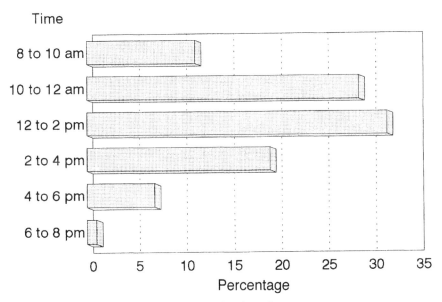

Source: Fire Department of Rio de Janeiro

FIGURE 15   A comparison of water rescues by time period.

GMAR is made up of 900 lifeguards, professional military personnel, and first responders, a sufficient number to cover an extension of beaches that spans 90 km. One or more guards are distributed every 500 m in rescue towers to observe patrons and prevent accidents. During peak beach season, signs are posted warning patrons about the dangers of the area and where drownings are most prevalent. Each lifeguard is equipped with a portable radio to remain in contact with headquarters and other towers, in the event the guard must leave the tower to attempt a rescue or when backup is required. Depending on the severity of the rescue and the distance to the closest operational base, an ambulance or a helicopter responds to the lifeguard's call.

Each subgroup has CRA and medical equipment, radio, two ambulances, two jet skis, one ultra light, and access to boats and two helicopters that serve the first responder and transport the attending doctor.

When weather conditions are most hazardous, a helicopter is provided to assist the rescue personnel. This helicopter serves all the municipal beaches of Rio. It is equipped with a large basket to safely carry a victim to the shore or to the nearest medical station. Another helicopter with medical supplies is on standby, if needed.

A lifeguard attends to the drowning victim, and, if medical attention is necessary, the victim is transported to the nearest station.

DROWNING RECUPERATION CENTER (CRA)

The primary function of the CRA is to provide medical attention to the victim during the early stage of rescue until the victim can be stabilized and sent to the hospital. CRA personnel are trained in advanced life support and work as a team to provide specialized emergency medical attention. A doctor and two nurses are on duty daily from 7 A.M. to 7 P.M. This team is present at beach rescues and is responsible for all reports registered at the CRA.

It is the lifeguard's responsibility to make the principal evaluation of the patient's vital signs and type of drowning and also provide basic life support until the medical team reaches the scene. This evaluation is very important and aids in the efficacy of care given in transport to the CRA.

A detailed report is written, beginning with the environmental conditions when the drowning occurred and actions taken by the lifeguard and the medical team. The relationship between lifeguard and the CRA medical team is extremely important because it ensures that high quality care is given consistently at each step of the process.

ATTRIBUTES OF GMAR

Attributes of GMAR include:

- Continual prevention and safety measures in all bodies of water for the sake of preserving human lives.
- Approval and enforcement of safety measures during all types of beach events.

- Promoting proper and safe ways to enjoy water sports or leisure bathing.
- Executing protection services.
- Establishing a safety system for public pools.
- Planning and executing guidelines for drowning prevention, rescue, and first response to drowning victims.
- Planning and execution of rescue guidelines.
- Training of ocean and pool guards.
- Teaching basic life support to the community.
- Looking for and being responsible for lost children. Each day an increasingly large number of children misplace their spots on the beach with their parents. Since the beginning of this institution, every lost child has been reunited with his/her parents.
- Working in conjunction with all governmental facets that deal with search and recovery, exercises pertaining to parachuting, underwater activities enveloping ships, and safety of planes during maritime exercises.
- Responsibility for rescue of populated islands during flooding.
- Acting as an integral part of the safety plan for nuclear cities like Angra dos Reis.
- Responsibility for the transportation of accident victims or corpses from local islands.

GMAR is highly respected and recognized as a fundamental part of the community throughout Brazil. Training, technical efficiency, and the professionalism of its members are just a few of the reasons for its popularity. A 1994 study of the citizens of Rio showed that 95% agreed that lifeguards are accepted as highly credible professionals.

RESCUE SERVICES IN OTHER STATES IN BRAZIL

The more advanced states like Sao Paulo, Santa Catarina, Parana, and Rio Grande do Sul have rescue services similar to GMAR. Rio remains the center for aquatic rescue and the model for form and efficiency for the entire country. Rescue personnel from all over Brazil frequently come to GMAR for diverse technical training.

Sao Paulo's rescue service, based in Santos, is recognized as the most advanced. The other states in the east, northeast, north, and the midwest are in a phase of rapid construction of these types of services.

THE BRAZILIAN WATER RESCUE SOCIETY (SOBRASA)

SOBRASA is a nonprofit, civil entity that acts as a national coordinator of all civil institutions and the military that participate in rescue services; organizes aquatic sports, private business, syndicates, and the general public; and organizes research, studies, and projects that promote aquatic awareness, safety, and prevention.

SOBRASA is funded by a group of professionals with water rescue backgrounds who are concerned about the number of drownings and deaths resulting from aquatic accidents. One director and 18 members who represent diverse entities involved in different water rescue activities collaborate to guide the society.

ACTIVITIES OF SOBRASA

The following is a list of SOBRASA activities.

- First responder classes (six levels)
- Water rescue classes (three levels)
- Summer camps and recreational activities
- Professional rescue team training
- Water rescue competitions
- Junior lifeguard training
- Volunteer lifeguard training
- Prevention and safety education
- Support for scientific and athletic projects
- Bulletins on the Internet
- Unification of all rescue services offered in Brazil
- Lectures and symposiums about prevention and safety

LIFEGUARDS

There are two types of professional, full-time lifeguards:

THE OCEAN GUARD

Ocean guards are professional military lifeguards whose job is prevention, rescue, and initial treatment of victims. Because of the intense demands of the job, they receive specialized training, and they are in higher demand. There are about 2,800 active guards on the coast, rivers, lakes, etc.

The lifeguards are members of the low to lower middle classes who enlist in the firefighter branch of the military. They are then selected to receive the eight-month general firefighter training specializing in aquatic prevention and rescue, called the ocean rescue course. The course is also taken by military personnel from other states.

THE POOL GUARD

Pool guards generally are not from the military and are autonomously employed. Their work is basically drowning prevention and pool security. Their training is less extensive than that of ocean guards — a 45-day course given by GMAR.

There are about 5,300 pool guards. Official rescue organizations like GMAR are the only legal entities that train these professionals. Six courses are given each year, producing 100–200 guards.

In recent years there has been a rise in the number of pools constructed in condominiums, clubs, aquatic parks, schools, etc. This has been followed, unfortunately, by a significant rise in fatal accidents. This prompted a vigilant application of legislation resulting in strict rules, which has made the pool guard into an integral part of the maintenance and safety of pools.

For a country with continental dimensions, vast coastal regions, and a large population, Brazil still has an insufficient number of guards. The majority of guards work on their days off.

WATER SAFETY RESEARCH

The following statistics relate to the number of drownings in 1991:

- There were 6,727 deaths in 150,000,000 habitants.
- There were 4.5 deaths per 100,000 habitants.
- The state of Acre ranked highest, with 19.9 deaths per 100,000 inhabitants.
- There were no drownings in the state of Fernando de Noronha.
- 83.5% of drowning victims were men.
- The average drowning victim was 16 years of age.

DEFINITIONS OF RESCUE AND DROWNING

Rescue — A victim is rescued from the water and presents ability to breathe on his/her own. These cases do not need medical attention. The cases where there is no physical contact between victim and guard are usually not recorded as rescues.

Drowning — The guard finds the victim with breathing difficulties and/or coughing. These cases receive medical treatment.

CHARACTERISTICS OF RESCUES

The following is noted about the 41,279 rescue cases between 1972 and 1991:

- An average of 5.5% (2,304 cases) needed medical attention upon arrival at a CRA.
- There were 286 deaths (7%).
- 92.6% were ocean and pool rescues made by the guards, and 7.4% were rescues by bathers who happened to be near the victims.
- 90% of the time the drownings were transported to the CRA by the medical team. The remaining 10% were transported by private cars, helicopters, and boats, when the situation was close to a CRA.
- The victims of freshwater accidents were transported to the CRA by friends or relatives.
- In all cases, the lifeguard administered basic life support except in freshwater drownings.

- 60% of rescues occurred between 10 A.M. and 2 P.M.
- 67% of rescues occurred in the summer months.
- When the person was rescued in his or her own residential locale, 10% were in coastal regions, 79.3% were in areas other than coastal areas, 7.9% were in other cities, and 2.8% were in other neighborhoods.

Classifications of Drownings

For the last 23 years rescue teams and medical services from the CRA have classified four levels of drownings. A study of statistics from 2,304 drowning cases made it possible to construct these levels (Szpilman 1994). A new six-level classification was developed from the evaluation of the chemical sign verified right after the accident while still at the scene which determines the treatment and prognosis at each level.

Measures of Prevention

In the last 20 years the mortality rate on the beaches of Rio has declined 0.7%, proving that the intervention of lifeguards has been successful and that prevention efforts are producing results.

Analyzed Factors of First Responder and Mortality

To establish a prognosis of drownings, diverse factors were evaluated pertaining to the location of the accident and the cause of death. This facilitates the best understanding of the level of seriousness of drowning.

Factors that demonstrate $P<0.05$:

- Cardiac respiratory arrest — 93%
- Respiratory arrest — 44%
- Pulmonary edema with hypotension or shock — 19.4%
- Lucid, confused, or dizzy state — 5%
- State of coma — 73%
- Sexes: Male — 14.9%; Female — 3%
- Abdominal distention: Visible — 54.3%; Nonvisible — 1.7%
- Response of pupils: Normal — 0.7%; Abnormal — 85.7%
- Motor skills response: Normal — 0.3%; Abnormal — 81.6%
- Age: 11–30 years — 6.6%; 31–50 years — 10.4%; over 50 years — 17.2%
- Marital status: Single — 6.2%; Others — 12.5%
- Incidences of shock: 85.4%

Factors that demonstrate P>0.05 (insignificant):

- Where the drowning occurred
- The victim's swimming ability
- Alcohol consumption
- What the victim ate three hours prior to the accident
- Whether the victim was vomiting
- Hypothermia
- Hypotension and blocked arteries

SECONDARY DROWNINGS

A total of 13% of all drownings are classified as secondary drownings where the victim actually suffers the effects of drowning after being rescued from the primary incident. The mortality rate of secondary drowning is 13.4%.

FRESHWATER AND SALT-WATER DROWNINGS

Of all drownings, 16.7% occur in fresh water and 12.3% in salt water, which shows there is little significant variation between the two.

POST-RESCUE FOLLOW-UP

The following post-rescue follow-up data has been compiled.

- 94.5% of rescues are released at the scene of the accident.
- 5.5% are transported to a CRA.
- 78.2% are released and sent home.
- 10.7% die at the CRA.
- 11.1% must be transported to the hospital.
- 10.2% die in the hospital.
- 89.8% are released and able to go home.
- Mortality of total rescues is 0.7%.

OTHER POINTS OF INTEREST

Of the victims rescued, 100% who required medical attention showed signs of hypothermia (body temperature <35°C or <95°F).

When is it necessary to provide CPR? CPR is administered in every case in which the exact time of the accident is unknown or the time of the accident is under one hour, except if the body is rigid and decomposing. In Summer 1994, there were four patients who had been underwater for more than ten minutes in a water temperature of more than 15°C. Two died in six hours and two survived. One of the survivors suffered severe neurological deficiencies.

THE PREVENTION OF DROWNINGS

Prevention is the most efficient measure a rescue service can take. In Brazil several forms of aquatic prevention are used.

ON THE BEACH

Lifeguards — The presence of the lifeguard is a fundamental factor in prevention. The lifeguard observes water conditions, the quality of the water, and the motion of the water. The lifeguard makes the public aware of potential danger, posts signs that describe water conditions, foresees possible danger, and prevents people from putting their lives and the lives of others at risk.

Signs — Posted to identify signs of dangers and to warn bathers.

Flags — Used to indicate general ocean conditions on a daily basis.

A red flag means swimming is prohibited.

A white flag means conditions are good for swimming.

Buoys — Used to mark off limitations in a given area for ships, planes, jet skis, boats, etc. These protect the physical well-being of swimmers. These buoys generally are placed 200 m away from the area of focus.

Support for ships, helicopters, and jet skis — These units are activated when ocean conditions are dangerous and unfavorable for the public to frequent the beach.

Beach supervision — The beach is supervised on a daily basis to identify areas most likely to be conducive to drownings.

THE POOLS

The pool guard — The presence of the pool guard is of great importance to pool patrons. They verify water conditions, check emergency equipment, remain attentive to all activities in and around the pool area, pay special attention to children, and are alert to potentially dangerous situations before they occur.

Observation — The guards are stationed at poolside stands to ensure a panoramic view of the area of responsibility.

Inflatable buoys — Used by small children who are not able to swim.

Levels of protection — Mandatory laws govern the safe practices of all pools.

Nets — At night, nets are set in place to provide protection.

GENERAL INFORMATION

Newspaper, television, and radio advertisements frequently alert the public to the danger of drowning and how to prevent it.

Activities to bolster beach awareness are offered constantly.

COMMUNITY EDUCATION — PREVENTION

Diverse programs are offered to the community, with the goal of reducing accidents on our shores.

BASIC LIFE SUPPORT CLASSES (BLS)

Since 1968, the high rate of aquatic accidents in Brazil has worried all those participating in the rescue services. The pioneer of these services, Corpo Maritimo de Salvamento do Rio de Janeiro, offers BLS classes in Rio. Other organizations give similar classes throughout the country to prepare members of the community to provide first responder services at accident scenes, to help prevent unnecessary death and drowning, and to provide adequate care.

SOBRASA offers courses that train the instructor to teach the various levels to the public regardless of background knowledge, economic status, and profession. These measures all help to reduce the number of aquatic-related deaths.

First responder courses offered by SOBRASA are:

Non-Professional

Courses offered to the non-professional include First Aid, open to all ages; CPR, one- and two-person CPR open to all ages; and First Responder, which teaches technical use of emergency equipment.

Professional

First Aid Instructor, First Responder Instructor, and Course Instructor Trainer courses are offered to professionals.

WATER RESCUE COURSES FOR CHILDREN

A course created in 1964 by Corpo Maritimo de Salvamento has been augmented by GMAR for the benefit of children. A summer camp on the beaches of Rio allows 1,500 children to learn through planned activities, games, and actual situations where drowning is possible. They learn prevention and how to defend themselves in emergency situations.

SOBRASA is considered an important educational and social organization with goals of dispersing knowledge, awareness, and prevention of drowning throughout the country.

WATER RESCUE CLASSES

The objective of these courses is to provide the lay person with basic knowledge so that in the event of a drowning the simplest means of rescue, such as throwing a flotation device and towing the victim to safety, can be effectively used. These courses also introduce students to the ocean and pools and makes them aware of potentially dangerous situations that may occur. Courses taught include self rescue, second- and third-party rescue, and professional rescue.

BLS AND WATER RESCUE VIDEOS

SOBRASA makes videos about BLS and water rescue available to schools, condominiums, clubs, gyms, and businesses during times of instruction.

WATER RESCUE COMPETITIONS

Water rescue competitions are held to increase public interest in aquatic activities.

SEMINARS ON THE PREVENTION OF AQUATIC ACCIDENTS

All entities involved with aquatic activities meet to discuss the best means of rescue techniques, prevention, and medical treatment.

SUPPORT FOR SCIENTIFIC AND SPORT PROJECTS

Brazil supports the interchange of data between science and sports relating to rescue and any other information that benefits the cause in and outside the country.

MEDICAL AND WATER RESCUE MANUALS

A medical manual and other water rescue manuals were updated and given to all associated with the subject of water rescue.

9 Contemporary Ocean Safety and Lifeguard Rescue Service on Oahu, Hawaii

Ralph S. Goto

> *The battle is not to the strong alone;*
> *it is to the vigilant, the active, the brave.*
>
> — *Patrick Henry*

> *Mai huli o'e I kokua o ke kai!*
> *Never turn your back to the sea!*
>
> — *Hawaiian Proverb*

TOURISM, THE MILITARY INDUSTRIAL COMPLEX, AND THE BEACHBOY

Contemporary lifeguarding in Hawaii is rooted in island cultural history, economy, and lifestyle.

The first inhabitants of Hawaii made great use of the surrounding ocean. It was a source of survival, providing food for daily sustenance. It was a source of recreation and health, a place of gods and legend.

The first inhabitants of Hawaii were great water persons from the *Kahviki Ula* (Tahiti and the Polynesias) and later the Marquesas. Arriving about 500 A.D., they found the Hawaiian Archipelago, a beautiful chain of 150 volcanic islands arising from the middle of the Pacific Ocean.

It was, however, the in-migration of tourists and the military — persons unfamiliar with oceans — that further shaped and refined ocean safety services. The influence of the tourism industry is considered by many to be the driving force that shaped the advancement and development of organized ocean-safety services. The roots of Hawaii's lifeguard system can be traced to the beachboy system that existed from the early days of the tourism industry on Oahu.

Hawaiian beachboys were renowned for their ocean recreation prowess and aquatic abilities. They served as major-domos of the beaches, who provided instructional and safety services. After World War II, a formal, municipal lifeguard service was established on Oahu in 1946 to ensure that organized safety services would remain available to the growing tourism industry. These services are currently offered by the Water Safety Division of the City and County of Honolulu's Department of Recreation.

Tens of millions of dollars are spent annually to lure tourists to Oahu from mainland America, Canada, Europe, and the Far East, particularly Japan.

This pitch for tourism has even made its way to cyberspace. The Hawaii Visitors' Bureau described Oahu as follows (from the following Internet URL: <http://www.visit.hawaii.org/islands/oahu/island.html>):

> You could search the whole world over and never find another island like Oahu. It's an island of magnificent panoramas, ringed with white sand beaches, capped by towering volcanic peaks, and in between the mountains and the ocean lies the playground of the Pacific ...
>
> Oahu is "the gathering place." It has more hotels, more restaurants, and more major attractions than all of the other islands put together. Our major city, Honolulu, is here. So is the "world's best beach" at Waikiki.
>
> Honolulu is sophisticated, lively, and as breathtaking as the Banzai Pipeline. It has more in the way of arts, culture, and entertainment. It has an abundance of galleries, nightclubs, and museums, a major zoo, aquarium, Iolani Palace (the only royal palace on U.S. soil), Pearl Harbor, the Arizona Memorial ... the list goes on and on.
>
> But the best of Oahu is its natural setting. No matter where you turn, there's a new vista waiting to be discovered. Miles of beaches. Dramatic peaks. Palm trees swaying in the gentle trade winds.
>
> No other American city could offer you the opportunity to surf the world's biggest waves, snorkel a lagoon, hike into a dormant volcano, golf at a dozen championship courses, and catch the sunset from a five-star restaurant. All within an hours drive of your hotel room.
>
> The key to enjoying Oahu, as with most of the islands, is mobility. The bus circles the island for only a dollar. Or rent a car and get out to see the "real" Hawaii ... the gentle waterfalls, and the craggy peaks. Discover the "undiscovered" beaches. Boogey board at Makapuu. Ride a horse at Turtle Bay. Watch the surfers at the Pipeline. Or sample a little fresh pineapple juice. Have fun! Get wet! This is Hawaii. It's an adventure!

This euphemistic but accurate overview of Oahu emphasizes Oahu's natural environment and ocean recreational and sporting activities. Sending someone off to "boogie board at Makapuu" and "to surf the world's biggest waves" can also be an invitation to trouble for those uninitiated in the intricacies of big surf, swift undercurrents, and rip tides. It does not help that the ocean environment is stunningly beautiful, entrancing, and, for some, the fulfillment of, perhaps, a sociocultural primeval memory and desire to frolic in paradise.

Oahu's deep harbors, geographic location, and equable society and climate have also made it a prime military site. The military's presence, however, brings a host of people and ocean safety problems, with a special psychological artifact that must be "confronted."

Both average visitors and average military personnel and their dependents are basically ignorant of ocean conditions in general, and probably have not even considered complex, specific aquatic conditions. The average tourist, inexperienced in the ocean environment, is on the island for a matter of days and seeks a peak enjoyment experience. Military personnel and their families are on Oahu for several years. Most are young and trained to be aggressive, to attack. This aggression translates into some interesting situations on the beach. Imagine such a "life-taker and heartbreaker" is beached, watching a young local kid gliding easily and effort-lessly in the beautiful, blue big waves at Sandy Beach. The soldier does not realize that the kid has been body surfing for several years, knows local conditions and, that notwithstanding, can still get hurt.

At any given time in Hawaii 10% of the *de facto* population (about 110,000 people) is comprised of visitors or military personnel and their dependents. Yet, over the years, about half of the deaths by drowning and near-drowning incidents have involved this visitor/military segment of the population, which is similarly signifi-cantly overrepresented in rescue and preventative incidents.

Local folks are becoming less and less ocean oriented. Oahu continues to move toward the status of an "international" city, like Paris, New York, and London. There is less emphasis on an agriculture-based economy. Oahu's plantation days are long gone. The tourism and military industrial complex is still influential, but it seems to have entered a consolidation, slight growth phase. Oahu is on the brink of a movement to high technology, providing service to service-type industries. Locals spend less time in the ocean and more time working and pursuing other endeavors. There is a "beach crowd." Oahu's estimated guarded beach attendance was more than 17 million in 1995, but the dependence on the ocean, the intimate familiarity with the ocean environment, and the allotment of significant time to ocean activities have diminished. There are few, if any, organized youth programs of rudimentary swimming instruction in Hawaii, but there is also no apparent decrease in major rescues and preventative actions by lifeguards or, as they are known in Hawaii, water safety officers.

BRICKS AND MORTAR — A SYSTEMATIC APPROACH

In the mid-1980s, senior management of the Water Safety Division met with the Hawaii Medical Association's Emergency Medical Services (EMS) program and faculty of the University of Hawaii's Graduate School of Public Health and Depart-ment of Geography. The result of this meeting was an internal decision at Water Safety to set up a system of ocean safety services, comprised of 15 components; advanced strategic, tactical, and media planning processes; and legislative interaction.

A SYSTEM

Simply stated, a system is a complex whole. A fully integrated, cohesive network of components was designed to provide a comprehensive aquatic safety program for the island of Oahu. This program includes lifeguard services at 19 city and county beach parks, patrol and rescue activities, injury prevention, public education programs, and emergency response to medical cases in the beach environment.

Components of this system include personnel, personnel training, communications, transportation, facilities, coordination with emergency medical and critical care services, coordination with and use of available public safety agencies, promotion of consumer participation, standardized recordkeeping, consumer information and education, independent review and evaluation, disaster linkage, mutual aid agreements, and other components necessary to system operation — particularly planning and legislative interaction.

Personnel An ongoing inventory of the numbers, types, and levels of different ocean safety personnel has been determined and is maintained. It was determined whether personnel were sufficient to provide for system needs. All affected city departments are routinely contacted to determine planning, operational, and budgeting factors impacting service delivery. Work loads are monitored to ensure that this inventory of service personnel is completed and annually updated.

Based on inventory of available personnel, it has been determined how many people must be trained and retrained to serve the needs of the system.

In certain instances, formulae were used to determine the numbers of personnel required. Work was performed to establish formulary to determine numbers of personnel to be trained. Using a civil service model, for example, to determine the number of personnel needed to staff a single shift, eight-hour-per day lifeguard unit, the equation factors in actual sick leave, vacation leave, and other considerations.

Personnel Training After the number of personnel for the system was determined, professional, command-rank staff oversaw performance training functions. Initially, we worked with the staff responsible for training of all public safety personnel: fire, police, and other public safety officers.

We assisted in negotiating the ability of these personnel to participate in at least a 51-hour emergency medical services "first responder" emergency medical care course. Initially, courses with our personnel intermingled with other public safety officers were often "competitive" with other training being provided. This was especially true with municipal police and fire personnel. We were virtually outnumbered as there are thousands of such personnel. Lifeguards who required training and retraining numbered in the hundreds at the time.

Eventually, the "first responder" training was institutionalized in the community college system of the University of Hawaii, but, first, discretely designed courses were developed for the particular needs of each public safety agency and separately offered to each. Areas of course emphasis were discrete to the potential worst case scenario and milieu confronting each personnel category. Our ocean safety personnel deals with a mix of respiratory-related, cardiac, and minor medical emergencies, in contrast to the predominately severe respiratory, cardiac, and major medical emergencies firefighters might see and severe traumatic injuries and wounds that might present to police officers.

The pre-hospitalization EMS system in Hawaii is based on a medical model. Besides logistics benefits, concentration of the medically related first responder training at the community colleges seems to work to ensure that there is a concentration of medical training expertise in a collegial atmosphere. In this setting, instructor intramural interaction, deliberation, and discussion ensures maintenance of first-rate basic life support training. Instructional personnel consult with medical and health authorities to ensure course content is context sensitive and appropriate. In addition to being educators, these personnel, in most instances, have professional nursing or paramedical credentials.

An interesting offshoot of training was the establishment of first responder equipment specific to the needs of our personnel in the early 1980s. This resulted from a review of the level and type of training to be provided. With our professional staff, the instructional staff of the then-EMS program, and its medical consultants, we helped put together a recommended emergency equipment listing for ocean safety first responders. Determining the training needs led to equipment specification. For example, we assumed that our personnel would be confronted with certain types of emergencies, for which they would have to be taught basic life support care measures. To accommodate these care requirements we considered alternatives. For example, we knew we would see respiratory problems. We then determined artificial respiration means had to be efficient and effective for the beach environment, so we added to our equipment list the ever-popular bag-valve-mask and oropharyngeal airways. A hospital respirator, to use an extreme example, was not added for obvious reasons, i.e., complexity and lack of suitability to the environment.

Related ancillary administrative support systems were similarly affected. For example, training assisted in helping us in the design and refinement of our beach and ocean incident reporting system's emergency medical sections. Teaching patient history and treatment involves instructional content on documentation. We designed our forms to include such documentation.

Presently all lifeguard personnel are recertified in cardiopulmonary resuscitation, Emergency Medical Services First Responder, and ocean lifesaving skills during the fiscal year. Physical performance testing is conducted in all districts to ensure the level of physical fitness the job of ocean lifeguard requires.

Ongoing in-service training activities for all full-time personnel include advanced techniques utilizing rescue craft and updates on patient airway management and resuscitation techniques.

Communications   We have been involved in establishing, enhancing, and monitoring the continuing operation of emergency communications systems on Oahu. We have worked with communications consultants, engineers, and other executives in ensuring the continued operation and enhancement of our communications system. We assisted in writing the grant for the initial $100,000 Federal funding that was used to implement a tactical radio communications system for Oahu's ocean life-guards that was obtained by the former EMS program.

Transportation   We initially attended and monitored numerous meetings and participated in the deliberations of what was then Chapter 48, Public Health Rules and Regulations on ambulances, ambulance equipment, ambulance personnel, and ambulance training. These are the state administrative rules that determine the minimum standards used to regulate the staffing, equipment carried, etc. on emergency medical and transfer vehicles providing basic and advanced life support services. We were also involved with the development and enhancement of the Military Assistance to Safety and Traffic Program and its transfer protocols, which involved the 25th Infantry Division, 25th Medical Battalion of the United States Army. This program is involved with the helicopter evacuation of patients in emergency circumstances from remote, rural areas on Oahu to facilities in town.

Facilities   We initially worked with all acute primary care hospital and freestanding emergency care facilities to ensure proper interface and the coordination of their emergency medical and critical care services with our system. Subsequently, we have monitored interagency meetings conducted under the auspices of our State Department of Health and its Statewide EMS Advisory which address this area.

Coordination With and Use of Other Available Public Safety Agencies   We have successfully moved our service, Oahu's only provider of ocean safety and lifeguard services, from the status of a recreational accessory to a fully functioning public safety service.

We routinely interact with all other principal public safety agencies providing services on Oahu, including the civilian and military fire, police, lifeguard, civil defense, mass casualty, and disaster relief agencies and establishments. We worked with these agencies in many ways with the object of bringing to bear the fullest feasible resources to ensure the public's safety in a harmonious and effective fashion.

For example, we worked with the fire department on Oahu to establish, develop, monitor, and evaluate a co-response system. Fire companies in the vicinity of an emergency incident more contemporaneously than ambulance units were (and still are) dispatched to the scene to render first responder-type emergency medical care or basic life support until an ambulance or other medical authority arrived at the scene to render more advanced care.

We have participated in major studies to determine whether the emergency ambulance service on Oahu and our agency should be incorporated as divisions or other administrative entities within the Honolulu Fire Department. We have also worked with the fire department to articulate its hazardous material response team prototype and rescue services.

Interaction with the police department has determined appropriate response mechanisms. Line police sergeants in the field were/are to be responsible for crowd coordination; our personnel provide first responder emergency medical care until disposition to more qualified personnel or transaction termination.

Promotion of Consumer Participation   This component is designed to ensure that consumers are involved within our system. We have addressed this concern by including consumers in board membership of the Hawaiian Lifeguard Association and our Junior Lifeguard Program.

Standard Recordkeeping   We developed a basic incident form that contains minimum, consistent data sets and "first responder" victim care information. We worked with our city's Department of Data Systems and our consultants in developing an incident report form and computerized systems. This included data set design, forms design, report listing design, development of an ad hoc and standing report generation system, related documentation, and materials used by coders and completers of the forms.

We also have worked with others who wished to link and communicate with us — the various data systems in the EMS system, medical researchers, state and county officials, and emergency-related facilities that were computerizing their systems.

Consumer Information and Education   We established and continued to implement a public information and education program. We strive to inform and educate the public on lifeguard services and ocean safety issues: what they are and how to access and use our services.

We routinely prepare the media and broadcast plan for the year, what safety or system messages to be broadcast or publicized, and when. For example, in summer, we emphasize general water safety, specifically for children who are out of school. In winter we raise consciousness of big surf conditions on Oahu's North Shore. In this connection, we have prepared public service messages and asked for related stories in the television and print news. We have appeared on the free public service broadcasts that all commercial and cable outlet stations are required to provide.

We arrange for speakers and act as spokespersons on ocean safety and related services or related topical material. We write or edit news releases, public service broadcast announcements, editorial requests, scan sheets, talking points outlines, and movie and television scripts. We work with professional public relations and advertising agencies on electronic and print media and other collateral.

We consult with others on their media strategies, materials, and outlet selection, e.g., the Hawaii Poison Center, the United States Lifesaving Association, the Honolulu Fire Department, the Hawaii Medical Association, the Hawaii Chapter of the American Academy of Pediatrics, and others. We have worked directly with the State Department of Health on its health education activities, particularly injury prevention and EMS-related matters. We also work with other state agencies on their public education materials. For example, we worked with the health education curriculum component of the State Department of Education to revise its health instructional educational materials to include ocean safety-related topics: use of emergency numbers, use of emergency facilities, ocean safety, general safety, the role of lifeguards and emergency personnel, etc.

We work a great deal with the visitor industry, its representative associations, organizations and agencies, and media outlets to develop materials for distribution to or use by visitors to Hawaii. Much of the work was to encourage the visitor industry to publicize emergency-related information not only to visitors, but also to persons involved in the industry. We also consulted or worked with others throughout the United States and some foreign countries on their education programs.

Independent Review and Evaluation   We evaluate the program periodically to determine if we are achieving the program objectives, to determine areas of possible improvement, and to determine whether fiscal and accounting practices are appropriate. We also work with system evaluators and consultants in conducting research to determine incident outcomes. We have worked specifically with our professional consultants to determine the type of case we were to track, research, design, and ensure appropriate access to and transfer of data. We also review and comment on prepared documents and directly participate in preparing reports, publications, and documents by other individuals and agencies.

Disaster Linkage   This component was concerned with whether the overall disaster system would be responsive in disaster circumstances. We worked with other agencies on protocols in disaster circumstances and remain involved with reviewing all state and county disaster plans.

Mutual Aid Agreements   This component was concerned with ensuring that the many disparate agencies involved would aid each other. We worked with all agencies to ensure that they would fully cooperate with each other in emergencies, critical care, mass casualty, and disaster circumstances. The co-response system described earlier is a good example of this.

Planning   The need for advance and ongoing master planning at strategic, budgeting, operational, and tactical levels is becoming increasingly apparent to us. We were the first division in our department to generate an overall strategic plan.

Our strategic plan is our overall action plan and policy *approach* to achieve our system objectives. Budgeting is planning, per se, and is particularly important in the present time of diminishing resources. We take into consideration not only our principal sources of funding but potential resources to tap for concrete assistance. Operational and tactical planning is an articulation and phasing of the steps and critical events necessary to meet specific, usually short-term, objectives.

We anticipate engaging in more pronounced, particular media planning. As noted earlier, we are trying to provide service to three discrete, identifiable groups — local residents, visitors, and military personnel and their dependents — and a most significant, vulnerable subset of each, children and youth. Each of these groups has specific informational needs and can be reached in different ways and by different forms of information dissemination and educational means.

Legislation   We find ourselves increasingly involved with ocean safety-related issues in local legislative bodies. In 1996, for example, we worked on state legislation to establish a public land liability immunity law, the purpose of which is to provide state and county governments with immunity from liability for injuries caused by a natural condition of any unimproved public land.

We have extensive experience with the state legislature, the Honolulu City Council, and the Federal Congress and have worked on various major, technical pieces of budget, finance, health, and safety-related legislation.

"OPS"

THE DIVISION

Staffing   The Water Safety Division provides ocean lifeguard, public safety rescue services at 18 beach parks on Oahu under the jurisdiction of the City and County of Honolulu. In 1995, the division was staffed by 91 full-time water safety officers (lifeguards). Full-time staff is augmented by 90–100 part-time, contract hire lifeguards who work on weekends, holidays, and during staff leaves.

Leadership   The division is headed by a water safety administrator and key administrative, secretarial, and clerical support personnel. In 1995, of the 91 full-time water safety officer positions, 7 were water safety captains, who serve as operations, district, and training supervisors, and 9 were lieutenants who function as links between beach personnel and the division's administration.

Districts   The Island of Oahu, which is primarily the City and County of Honolulu, is divided into four ocean safety districts:

District I — Honolulu (The South Shore): The area between Pearl Harbor and Hanauma Bay

District II — Windward (The East Shore): The area between Hanauma Bay and Kahuku Point

District III — North Shore: The area between Kahuku Point and Ka'ena Point

District IV — Leeward (The West Shore): The area between Ka'ena Point and Pearl Harbor

Significant Statistics   Water safety officers performed approximately 1,100 rescues at guarded beaches in 1994. They covered beachfronts with an estimated beach attendance, in 1994, of 17.5 million persons. Accident prevention is a key aspect of professional lifeguarding. In 1995, for example, divisional officers took 226,922 preventative actions.

International Recognition   The division's staff and services have been nationally and internationally recognized for their excellence. Many of the professional personnel are world-class athletes and water persons. The division's services have been cited as a "national model of excellence" for providing a fully integrated, cohesive network of components designed to provide ocean safety, accident, and drowning prevention services.

Innovative Techniques   Divisional staff are international leaders in technical developments associated with rescue and ocean accident prevention services.

USE OF THE PERSONAL WATERCRAFT AND RESCUE SLED

The personal watercraft has been used as an effective ocean rescue vehicle on Oahu and the other islands of Hawaii for several years. This apparatus has numerous advantages: speed, maneuverability, stability, quick launch from a variety of sites, and ability to operate in nearly all types of surf conditions. Despire a few maintenance- and environment-related disadvantages, maintenance is easy and fuel efficiency is considerable. Other than over-aeration in the ocean creating poor throttle response, the apparatus just "takes a licking and keeps on ticking."

To date in Hawaii, the Yamaha Waverunner® III is still the craft of choice for in-the-surf rescue work. The hull design allows for sufficient maneuverability, "surf-ability," and speed to cope with the very challenging surf conditions in Hawaii. Its 650cc motor (approximately 50HP) provides the power necessary to transport the craft operator (driver), crew person, and one or more victims to safety under the most demanding of conditions. We hope to acquire newer models with more power as they become available. The power should provide an added margin of safety by making available more low-end power, and consequently, improved "hole-shot" acceleration.

Despite its positive attributes, the craft alone is not a fully practical piece of rescue equipment in the surf environment. The success in applying this new technology to surf lifesaving techniques lies in the invention of the rescue sled. Prototyped by water safety captain Brian Keaulana and water safety officer Terry Ahue, the sled was a natural outgrowth of their "cutting-edge" experimentation with the personal watercraft in ocean rescues.

The sled enables the victim to be placed safely on board at water level quickly, effectively, and efficiently. The craft operator is left free to concentrate on maneuvering the craft safely in and out of the surf zone. The craft's crew person, lying securely on the rescue sled, is responsible for getting the victim onto the sled and holding the victim securely there for the ride to shore.

The rescue sled is about 5 1/2 ft long, 4 in thick, and just less than the width of the watercraft. There are handles along the upper sides and front of the sled that the victim and crew member can hold. The sled is made of body board materials, adequately reinforced, generally with fiberglass, for strength. But the sled also has a soft skin to cushion any unintended hard contact with rescuers or victims during rescue efforts. An important detail is the precise manner in which the sled is attached behind the craft. This is significant because the maneuverability and performance of the craft and stability of the sled can be affected.

At least one rescue craft is deployed daily to each of the four ocean safety geographical districts. A rescue craft's immediate area of responsibility covers an average of ten miles of coastline — generally, the stretch connecting the guarded beaches of that district. Often these craft are called upon to perform rescues at remote unguarded beach areas, particularly in the North Shore and West Shore ocean safety districts, which extend their effective patrol range to some 40 miles of coastline.

Deployment of one rescue craft unit, seven days a week, requires three full-time positions, allowing for two personnel to be assigned to a unit per day. An estimation of expenses for the initial year of operation is as follows:

I. Personnel Costs
     Three operators at $30,000 per year —$90,000
     Indirect overhead cost —$45,000
II. Equipment Costs
     1. Mobile Equipment Costs
          One rescue craft (Waverunner® III) —$8,000
          One rescue sled —$1,800

One road trailer —$1,400
One Roleez® Beach Dolly —$400
One rescue patrol vehicle (4 × 4 Pickup) —$25,000
2. Rescue Equipment Costs:
One Motorola Saber® radio —$2,500
Radio harness and waterproof pouch —$100
Helmet (Gath®) with visor —$450
Uniforms and wetsuits —$1,000
Miscellaneous equipment (knives, ropes, fins, etc.) —$800

OCEAN AND BEACH SAFETY SIGNS

The beach signs, developed by the Hawaiian Lifeguard Association in cooperation with the division and used locally in Hawaii, have been adopted and emulated in other areas of the world. The author of this chapter was recently appointed to chair a committee of the United States Lifesaving Association responsible for recommending national standards for beach and ocean signage. Additionally, in his capacity as president of the Hawaiian Lifeguard Association, the author has opened communications with the American National Standards Institute (ANSI) on establishing relevant beach and ocean safety signage. We are currently requesting comments on improvements to ocean and beach safety signs.

Budget   The division has an annual budget of more than US$3 million.

Annual Report   To review the current Annual Report of the Water Safety Division, see Page 161.

WATER SAFETY OFFICERS (WSOs)

Division success is due to the knowledge, expertise, and courage of its staff on the beach.

Duties   In addition to other duties that may be assigned that relate to water safety work, the water safety officer (WSO):

- makes ocean rescues
- administers first responder emergency life support measures
- learns and enforces ordinances, rules and regulations governing beach activities and shore water usage
- renders first aid in cases of emergency

Officers at all times are expected to maintain a high standard of courtesy and professionalism in relationship to the public and other divisional staff. As a key member of Oahu's public safety team — the WSO is a specially commissioned police officer involved in mutual aid activities and implementation of aspects of local disaster plans. They warn the public of dangerous and/or unsafe beach and ocean conditions, i.e., high surf, strong current, tsunamis, and other National Weather Service and/or Civil Defense warning signals.

Qualifications   The following are the necessary basic qualifications for a water safety officer. There are five civil service classes of WSO, with specific experience requirements for each level:

I. Necessary Requirements
    1. Must be 18 years old
    2. A valid Hawaii driver's license (Type 3 — Operator's)
    3. A high school diploma or responsible work experience that demonstrates the ability to perform the essential functions of the job
    4. A current American Heart Association or American Red Cross Cardio-Pulmonary Resuscitation (CPR) Certificate
    5. One of the following: A current Red Cross Standard First Aid Multimedia, a current Standard First Aid and Personal Safety, or a current First Responder Certificate that meets U.S. Department of Transportation guidelines
    6. A current U.S. Lifesaving Association Ocean Lifeguard Certificate or a Red Cross Lifeguard Training Certificate

II. Performance Requirements (Pass/Fail Examination — Must Pass to Qualify)
    1. 1000 × 1000 × 1000 Yards — Run/Swim/Run — Under 25 Minutes
    2. 500 Yards — Swim — Under 10 Minutes
    3. 400 Yards — Rescue Board Paddle — Under 4 Minutes
    4. 100 × 100 × 100 — Run/Swim/Run — Under 3 Minutes

Officers must meet recertification requirements in cardiopulmonary resuscitation, emergency medical services First Responder and ocean lifesaving, as well as undergo physical performance testing annually.

Training   The water safety officer participates in in-service training programs to maintain good physical condition, learn new first aid and rescue methods and techniques, and use new equipment such as personal watercraft, rescue boats, and the all-terrain vehicle.

Equipment   The water safety officer may operate rescue boats, personal watercraft (wave runners or jet skis), and emergency medical equipment such as resuscitators, radios, all-terrain vehicles, trucks, and cars.

Working Conditions   Officers may be exposed to various weather conditions for prolonged periods; hazards when effecting a rescue; high surf and strong currents; and the possibility of physical harm while monitoring beach regulations. The officer may have to perform duties unassisted.

Junior Lifeguard Program

Program Background   Hawaii is internationally renowned for the natural beauty of its magnificent beaches and surrounding ocean waters. Many have yet to realize that this magnificence is replete with dangers. Few realize the gravity and extent to which these dangers exist, especially for local children and youth.

Tens of millions visit Hawaii's beaches annually. With more than half of Hawaii's resident population under 18 years of age, one may surmise that a very high proportion of those beach visitors are youth. According to State of Hawaii Department of Health injury surveillance data, drowning is the second-ranking cause of childhood unintentional injury in the state. Injury data associated with Hawaiian ocean and beaches is even more glaring: Hawaii ranks second in the United States for such accidental injury data.

There is no organized state program to instruct large numbers of children in safe ocean practices, including swimming. Other than recreational facilities such as the "Y," there are few, if any, places in Hawaii where one can acquire basic ocean and water safety skills. Ocean skills and swimming are acquired naturally. Friends, parents, and beach acquaintances can teach, but often the individual is self-taught.

There is no routine instruction of children on ocean water or beach hazards in Hawaii's educational system. In fact, the health education instructional curriculum for basic instruction in general personal safety per se is taught only when it is not in conflict with the base curriculum of the schools. There are few, if any, public courses on ocean water safety other than those provided on an incidental basis by groups like the American Red Cross. These courses are intended as basic courses and may or may not be modified by the instructor to include local Hawaiian conditions.

What swimming and ocean-safety skills our children acquire, if any, are acquired in a haphazard, disorganized fashion, which explains our high injury rates.

Recognizing the safety and survival needs of youth, the Water Safety Division, in close cooperation and coordination with the Hawaiian Lifeguard Association, believes that it is imperative to establish an ongoing educational program for them. Other areas in the world have established fairly progressive junior lifeguard programs with great success. Participants in these programs seem to be those children and adolescents who are naturally inclined to recreate in an ocean and beach setting. Other than personally benefiting from such a program, if properly groomed as leaders, these youth can serve as role models and leaders among their peer group.

Program Purpose   The purpose of the Junior Lifeguard Program is to increase the self-confidence, physical conditioning, and ocean awareness of program participants by introducing them to water safety, first aid, and surf-rescue techniques.

Instructors   Course instructors are veteran beach lifeguards. Guest lecturers include ocean aquatic experts and champions in sports such as surfing, body boarding, and body surfing. All course instructors are required to have, at a minimum, current certifications in the State of Hawaii's "First Responder" emergency medical services course; Basic Cardiac Life Support; Standard First Aid; and United States Lifesaving Association Open Water Lifesaving Instructors' Certification Course.

During the summer of 1995, program coordinators were Water Safety Captain Kendall Rust and Acting Lieutenant Mark Cunningham, senior lifeguards who have been instrumental in establishing and conducting prototypes of the Junior Lifeguard Program in Hawaii. Captain Rust is a national champion in rescue racing and an all-around competitive ocean waterman. He is currently captain of the Training Division of the Water Safety Division of the Department of Parks and Recreation in Honolulu. Acting Lieutenant Cunningham is a veteran North Shore lifeguard and a world-class body surfing champion.

Classes   As many as 32 classes can be provided throughout Oahu when full funding is available. Currently, there are four lifeguard districts on Oahu: Waikiki-Ala Moana, the North Shore, Leeward Oahu, and Windward Oahu. Each of these districts has one module of eight junior lifeguard classes, each of which is five days in duration and accommodates at least 12 students per class. Class size has averaged about 15 students.

Admission Requirements   Participants must be 13–17 years old. They must possess a basic swimming ability with the capability of swimming 500 yds in less than ten minutes. Prospects should have passed a general physical examination within six months prior to application to take the course. Applicants must be able to dead lift 50 lbs.

Instruction and Syllabus   Instructional methodologies employed include didactic classroom instruction and lectures, skills training, and enhancement. A typical course day consists of instruction in the following:

Physical training — includes warm-up, stretching, running on the beach, and swimming.

Ocean Skills Training — Daily instruction alternates between paddling rescue boards, using surf boards, body boards and rescue apparatus, rescue tube, personal ("wave runner") rescue watercraft, performing water entries and exits, skin diving, surf swimming, body surfing, and skill topics, including surf awareness and safety.

Classroom Skills Training — Personal care topics are taught such as skin cancer awareness, eye safety, and maintaining a healthy lifestyle through appropriate diet, physical conditioning, etc. Lifesaving techniques and procedures are introduced through victim detection and first-aid instruction. This instructional component includes beach condition assessment, ocean current and surf condition detection, safety awareness, and marine life identification.

Competitive Training — Competitive lifeguard techniques, strategies, skills and sportsmanship are introduced through physical training with a competitive emphasis.

Certification   Students receive a certificate of course completion.

Costs   In 1996, the cost of the program — to run 32 classes — was estimated at $93,000. It should be noted that it was anticipated that certain of the costs would be offset by donations and *kokua,* i.e., in-kind contributions.

Appendix 1

WATER SAFETY DIVISION

The Water Safety Division provides a comprehensive aquatic safety program for the island of Oahu. This program includes lifeguard services at 19 city and county beach parks, patrol and rescue activities, injury prevention, public education, and emergency response to medical cases in the beach environment.

PERSONNEL

The division has a full-time staff of 97, including:

1 — Water Safety Administrator
1 — Administrative Assistant, SR-22
1 — Secretary I, SR-14
1 — Operations Chief, WSO V, SR-23
6 — Lifeguard Captains, WSO IV, SR-21
9 — Lifeguard Lieutenants, WSO III, SR-19
78 — Beach Lifeguards, WSO I/II, SR-15/17

The full-time staff is augmented by 90 part-time lifeguards employed on an hourly basis.

OPERATIONS

Organizationally, the island is divided into four geographic districts: Honolulu, East Oahu, North Shore, and Leeward. Each district is coordinated by a captain and two lieutenants who are responsible for scheduling and general supervision of beach lifeguards. Each district utilizes specialized rescue equipment including jet skis and all-terrain vehicles to respond to cases requiring lifeguard assistance in both guarded and unguarded areas.

The Water Safety Division continues to function as an essential component of the City and County of Honolulu's public safety team, and works closely with the Honolulu Fire Department, Honolulu Police Department, and the Emergency Ambulance Services Division of the City Health Department.

TRAINING

All lifeguard personnel were recertified in cardiopulmonary resuscitation, Emergency Medical Services First Responder, and ocean lifesaving skills during the fiscal year. Physical performance testing was conducted in all districts to ensure the level of physical fitness required by the job of the ocean lifeguard.

In-service training activities for all full-time personnel included advanced techniques utilizing rescue craft and updates on patient airway management and resuscitation techniques.

Program Highlights

Public Education and Prevention efforts continued to inform visitors and residents about water safety issues through the various media. The Junior Lifeguard Program was held at Ala Moana and Ehukai Beach Parks. Approximately 200 children were taught ocean safety.

Statistical Activities Report

Attendance figures are based on daily estimates made by lifeguards. All other figures are based on actual cases, incidents, and responses (Table 1).

TABLE 1
Department of Parks and Recreation
Water Safety Division Statistical Activities Report
July 1, 1994–June 30, 1995

Beach Area	Estimated Attendance	Violation	Prevent. Action	First Aid Minor	Public Contact	Rescue	Resuscitation	Drown
Ala Moana	1,205,001	295	8,584	2,415	40,101	62	2	0
Waikiki	6,751,943	64	17,135	13,829	45,976	140	4	1
Hanauma	2,242,576	21	29,760	15,220	55,695	214	7	1
Sandy	559,979	35	42,868	3,995	49,098	238	2	0
Makapu'u	314,184	140	22,935	19,174	30,535	79	0	0
Bellows	115,045	116	2,348	963	3,205	23	0	0
Kailua	1,011,088	0	3,481	1,250	11,469	9	1	0
Kualoa	215,628	0	1,784	430	3,327	4	0	0
Waimanalo	273,503	1	3,891	3,259	9,490	9	0	0
Sunset	581,789	0	6,027	217	11,456	33	0	0
'Ehukai	315,541	9	5,659	655	11,226	46	0	0
Ke Waena	165,209	22	4,832	615	10,558	14	0	0
Waimea	720,708	28	8,882	1,108	11,039	118	0	1
Alii	282,257	0	6,227	844	8,463	23	0	0
Nanakuli	646,745	386	17,890	1,706	22,838	60	0	0
Ma'ili	493,845	4	11,272	1,383	14,093	31	1	0
Pokai Bay	717,140	113	11,380	1,527	20,368	8	0	0
Makaha	616,910	32	12,029	1,447	17,290	11	0	0
Keauwaula	332,704	1	9,938	807	12,169	18	0	0
TOTAL	17,561,795	1,267	226,922	70,844	388,306	1,140	17	3

10 Drowning Intervention: An Army Corps of Engineers Perspective

Brad Keshlear

HISTORICAL PERSPECTIVE

The Army Corps of Engineers is the second-ranking provider of outdoor recreation opportunities among the seven major Federal land-managing agencies. In 1995, the Corps registered more than 385 million visits, which accounted for 30% of all recreation/tourism occurring on Federal lands. The Corps manages lakes in 43 states and more than 7 million surface acres of water and 4.5 million acres of land.

The land base of Corps lakes is relatively small compared to the Federal recreation land base (less than 2%), but the use is high (30% of Federal recreation) (Figure 1), because:

a. Many Corps lakes are located close to large cities. About 80% of Corps lakes are within 50 miles of major metropolitan areas.
b. In many parts of the country, Corps lakes are the only recreational resources within many miles.
c. Water always has been a focal point for outdoor recreation, and water is a principal feature at Corps lakes. The Corps is the largest provider of water-based recreational opportunities in the United States.

The U.S. Army Corps of Engineers has been in existence far longer than any of the other Federal land-management agencies. Early Corps missions were military in nature. The civil works mission of the Corps began in 1824 with the passage of the first Rivers and Harbors Act, when Congress provided the first appropriations for work in navigable waters. The Corps protected Yellowstone and Yosemite National Parks until the National Park Service was created in 1916. Flood control activities were added to Corps responsibilities in the 1920s and 1930s. Reservoir development expanded the scope of public service of the Corps. The development of Corps lakes nationwide for a variety of purposes attracted so many visitors that Congress passed the Flood Control Act (1944), which gave the Corps specific authority to provide public outdoor recreation facilities at its lakes.

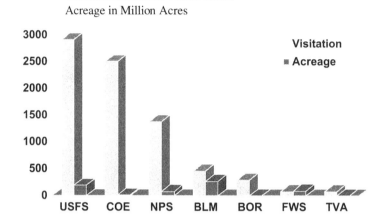

FIGURE 1   Federal Land Management Agency visitation and total acreage.

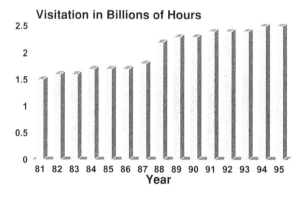

FIGURE 2   Visitation at Corps lakes.

RECREATION AT CORPS LAKES

Development of Corps lakes during the 1940s and 1950s occurred typically in rural settings. Suburban sprawl was in its infancy. Continued national growth, with its attendant increase in disposable income and leisure time, resulted in increased public use and pressures on these resources. Improved roads and automobiles quickly followed, and the cities grew out to meet and surround the once rural lakes. Visitation at Corps lakes continued to grow. By the mid-1970s, visitation to Corps lakes reached nearly 500 million visitor hours of use. Within the next ten years visitor hours had grown to 1.5 billion. By 1995, visitor hours totaled 2.5 billion. Approximately 10% of the United States population visits a Corps lake at least once each year (Figure 2).

ECONOMIC IMPACT OF RECREATION

As one of the nation's largest providers of outdoor recreation, the Corps of Engineers plays an important role in the U.S. tourism industry. Recent studies by the Corps indicate that significant economic activity is generated by recreational opportunities provided at Corps lakes. Visitors to Corps lakes in 1994 spent more than $12 billion for such nondurable goods and services as food, fuel, bait, restaurant meals, and lodging. This trip spending generated an estimated $20 billion in employee income and over 600,000 full- and part-time jobs for local economies. Total effects represent 4% of U.S. jobs, 4% of employee income, and one in 200 jobs in the United States.

RECREATION AT CORPS LAKES TODAY

Recreation is a major use for virtually all Corps lakes today. The Corps manages 4,382 recreation areas on 461 lakes in 43 states. Corps lakes cover 11,897,449 acres and have 40,647 miles of shoreline. Recreation facilities include:

- Campsites: 94,106
- Picnic sites: 55,141
- Boat dock slips: 177,154
- Boat launch lanes: 7,241
- Swimming beaches: 1,000

In 1995, visitation to Corps lakes totaled 2.5 billion visitor hours. Approximately 58% of this visitation (1.4 billion visitor hours) is attributable to water-contact recreational activities, such as swimming, wading, boating, water skiing, and fishing.

WATER-RELATED RECREATION FATALITIES

As visitation began increasing in the 1970s, the recreation-related public fatalities associated with water-based recreation also increased. During the early 1970s, 400–500 people drowned each year while engaged in recreational activities on Corps lakes. Recreational boating and fishing activities were expanding at phenomenal rates. The United States was entering its first "environmental awareness era" and outdoor recreational activities were the "in thing." Camping, hiking, fishing, boating, picnicking, and swimming became common activities for most Americans, many of whom were unfamiliar with the outdoors and the hazards related to recreational activities on and in large bodies of water.

Many of the Corps lakes built during the 1940s and 1950s were not designed with recreation in mind. They were built mainly for flood control, water supply, navigation, and power production. Recreation was a "supplemental" benefit and did not receive high priority status or resources.

As public recreational demand increased, recreational facilities like boat ramps, campgrounds, and picnic areas were added. Most were very primitive in nature and had very few amenities associated with them. Swimming and wading activities began to occur along stretches of unimproved shoreline. There were steep drop-offs, underwater tree snags, and other kinds of underwater obstacles and hazards. Properly designed and constructed swimming areas were virtually nonexistent.

Because of the increasing recreational use and the extremely high incidence of drowning, the Corps began to look carefully at managing its lakes for recreational use. Professional personnel, highly educated and trained in parks and recreation management, were hired. As these managers began taking control of Corps recreation programs, they were faced with the monumental task of retrofitting the Corps lakes to accommodate the large recreational use they were already receiving. This required establishing specific design standards and criteria for recreation areas and their associated facilities, such as boat ramps, swimming beaches, campgrounds, picnic areas, rest rooms, shower houses, roads, trails, etc.

ESTABLISHING DESIGN STANDARDS AND CRITERIA

The process of establishing design standards and criteria in an agency mostly geared toward massive civil and military construction projects was a challenging task. The exceptionally high quality of Corps of Engineers design standards were unrivaled anywhere in the world. Establishing specific design standards for recreational facilities was a lengthy and expensive task. Once the design criteria and standards were established, the process of obtaining funds to construct, operate, and maintain the facilities could begin.

In the interim, lakes operated independently in their attempts to accommodate the ever-increasing recreational use. Some lakes were able to begin establishing high quality recreational facilities, while others lagged behind. There was very little consistency in the types of recreational facilities that began springing up on Corps lakes. Some facilities were state of the art, while others were very primitive.

Initial recreation and design criteria for recreational facilities issued by the Corps in 1971 included very basic guidance for development of recreation facilities. Detailed guidance on specific recreation facilities such as swimming beaches, campgrounds, and picnic areas was very minimal, but even this basic guidance was better than none.

The importance of this design criteria and guidance cannot be overstated. This guidance provided on-site managers with the necessary tools needed to provide recreational facilities that were designed with the users' health and safety as primary considerations. More detailed design criteria and standards were established during the 1980s, which greatly enhanced the Corps ability to provide some of the highest quality outdoor recreation facilities found anywhere in the United States.

I focus on these design criteria and standards since they are among the primary bases for the dramatic reduction in drownings that resulted at Corps lakes when they were implemented (Figures 3 and 4).

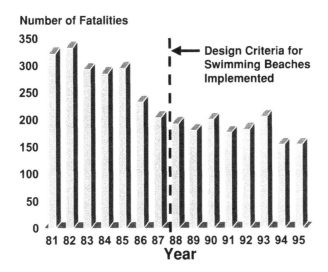

FIGURE 3   Number of persons drowned at Corps lakes, 1981–1995.

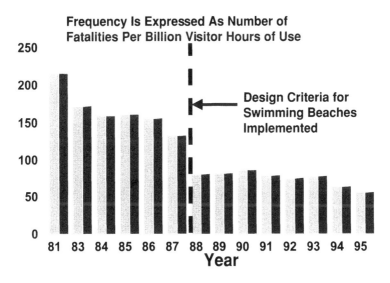

FIGURE 4   Fatality frequency rates, 1981–1995.

POLICY PROHIBITS THE USE OF LIFEGUARDS

The Corps of Engineers has a longstanding policy that prohibits the use of lifeguards at swimming beaches it manages. The basis of this policy is simply liability. While many disagree with this policy, all attempts to allow the use of lifeguards at Corps swimming beaches have failed. With this in mind, the design criteria for swimming beaches becomes of paramount importance.

Lifeguards are allowed and encouraged on beaches not directly managed by the Corps.

DESIGN CRITERIA FOR SWIMMING BEACHES

The design criteria for Corps of Engineers swimming beaches can be found in Engineer Manual (EM-1110-1-400), Recreation Planning and Design Criteria, July 31, 1987. The following highlights are the basis of the criteria:

A. *General*   The primary priorities in the design of a beach are:
   (1) Safety of the user
   (2) Effects the physical features of the site will have on the beach
   (3) Future operation and maintenance considerations
B. *Site Selection*   Site selection considerations include:
   (1) *Existing or projected visitation*   User patterns are determined from visitation records, area use observations, and user survey data sources. For new beaches, visitation trends at the lake or other locations are used to establish sizing requirements for the beach.
   (2) *Accessibility*   Beaches are only developed where vehicle entrances are feasible and where such entrances can be controlled or separated from other area uses. Access to a beach in a multi-use area cannot interfere with other uses, create safety hazards, or adversely impact the area.
   (3) *Slope Gradients*   The slope of the land, both above and below the water line, is one of the determining factors in the selection of a good beach site. Slopes in the underwater portion of beaches should ideally range from 2 to 5%, the most desirable slope being as flat as possible to disperse use. Beach bottoms are designed to eliminate sudden changes in grade or drop-offs in the 0–5 foot depth. Pre- and post-impoundment studies are performed to ensure acceptability of gradients. Daily, seasonal, and yearly water level fluctuations due to irrigation, flood control, evaporation, power generation, or other factors are considered in beach design to ensure optimum utilization. A detailed inspection of the underwater portion of the beach is accomplished each year just prior to opening to the public. The inspection includes the necessary detail to reveal sinkholes, depressions, or dangerous drift material, and corrective actions are then taken prior to opening of the beach. Inspection records are maintained on file.
   (4) *Soil composition and stability*   Sites are selected which offer a proper base for a sand beach. Beaches are not located in areas where extensive siltation occurs or is expected to occur.
   (5) *Water Characteristics*
       (a) Water quality at all beach locations must be acceptable for swimming. Prior to detailed design, water quality sampling data is collected, analyzed, and coordinated with appropriate state agencies.

(b) Beaches are located where adequate water circulation is present to assure continued acceptable water quality. Barriers and coves generally offer the best protection against wind and wave action; however, dead-water coves are avoided. Adequate circulation is also necessary to remove surface debris that may deposit on the beach.

(6) *Health Considerations*   Swimming beaches are planned to provide protection from boats, fuel spillage, sewage, industrial outfalls, and boat wakes. Beaches are sighted to ensure maximum southern exposure where possible. However, in non-Corps areas where lifeguards are provided, western exposure is avoided if possible so as to reduce afternoon glare to the lifeguards. Beaches are located upstream from boat ramps, marinas, etc. in order to minimize or avoid effects of fuel spills. Beaches are not located where concentrations of waterfowl exist.

(7) *Surface drainage*   During the planning and design of swimming beaches, special emphasis is given to surface drainage.

(a) Surface runoff must not be allowed to drain across the beach area; therefore, the runoff from any area upland of the beach must be diverted. Methods of diversion include grassed swales, terracing, inlets, landscaped walls, etc. Methods of diversion should complement the beach development and minimize impact to the site. If possible, outfall of diversion is located downstream of the swimming beach.

(b) Runoff from parking areas is controlled and diverted to an outfall away from the beach area.

(c) Runoff from commercial agricultural activities in the watershed is considered when site locating the beach.

C. *Design Criteria*   Figure 5 depicts a concept layout for a swimming area.

(1) *Buffer Zones*   Beaches, including turf sunbathing areas, are separated from parking areas with an adequate grass buffer. Trees are left in the turf areas adjacent to sand beaches. When surface runoff is anticipated to be heavy, diversion contouring or ditches are designed to carry runoff water away from the beach turf area and swimming area. Placement of picnicking facilities in the buffer area is only done if absolutely necessary. When such facilities are designed into the beach area, they are located so as not to interfere with the primary purpose of the beach.

(2) *Design Carrying Capacities*   Beach sizing is based on the assumption that approximately 60% of the total numbers of beach users will be on the beach at one time with 30% in the water and 10% elsewhere. As a rule-of-thumb a turnover factor of three is used for design purposes. Ideally, 50 sq ft of sand and turf and 30 sq ft of swimming area, inside a buoyed safety zone, is provided for each person. Beach capacities will vary according to the attendance, supervision, size of beach, anticipated usage, and type of beach experience desired.

■ Concept Design

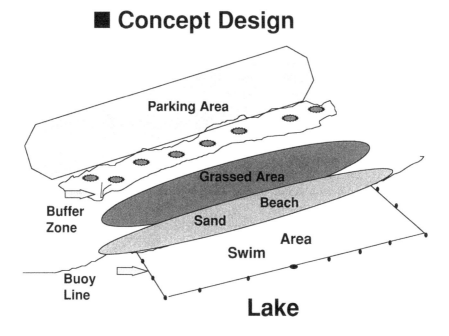

FIGURE 5   Concept layout for a swimming area.

(3) *Vertical Limits*   The uppermost limits of graded areas are based on an analysis of daily, seasonal, or yearly water level fluctuations. The lower limits are 6 vertical ft below the normal summer pool elevation. Deviations from this minimum limit must be fully justified. The beach and adjacent underwater areas are graded on a constant slope. Underwater slopes extend at least 10 horizontal ft beyond the lowest placement of buoy lines.

(4) *Beach Site Preparation*

    (a) *Beach construction prior to water impoundment*   The area is first cleared of all trees, shrubs, and manmade objects. The area is then stripped to a minimum depth of six inches. All depressions and holes are filled with suitable material and compacted. Grading operations are performed to establish the 2–5% slope. Two ft of sand is then placed on a prepared stone base to a uniform thickness to reduce turbidity. A layer of nonwoven filter fabric is placed on the base prior to sand placement.

(b) *Beach construction with water impounded*   A detailed survey and inspection are performed. Grading requirements are then established based on the survey. All trees and stumps within the beach area are removed. Holes and depressions are filled with granular materials such as sand, gravel, or crushed stone. Special efforts are taken to ensure that all holes are properly filled.

(5) *Sand*   A minimum depth of 2 ft of sand is applied on all above-water beach areas.

(6) *Diving Platforms and Swim Floats*   Diving platforms, rafts, floats, or similar facilities are not permitted in Corps-managed areas.

(7) *Facilities for the disabled*   Where practical, a paved walkway at least 4 ft wide with metal handrail is integrated into the beach area to aid disabled persons in gaining access to the swimming area.

(8) *Buoys and Markers*
   (a) The limits of the swimming area are marked off by buoy lines or foam-filled floated pipe lines. The PVC pipe buoy is preferred in beach areas that experience heavy traffic. Larger beaches may be sectionalized so that one or two sections can be used on slack days and additional sections utilized as needed during heavy use hours or days. International, orange-colored floats are used every 15 ft on buoy lines or at all angles when PVC pipe is used.
   (b) Ideally, buoy lines used to mark the limit of the swimming area are placed in water not more than 5 ft deep. However, at lakes where water level fluctuations occur, this would locate the buoy line in shallow water which would critically limit the usefulness of the swimming area. In such cases, buoy lines are placed in relation to the mean water level. In lakes where significant water level fluctuations occur, buoy lines are designed so they can be adjusted as necessary.
   (c) A minimum of two warning marked buoys or floating signs indicating the "boats keep out" symbol (diamond shape and international orange) are spaced at a maximum of 200-ft intervals and are located to provide adequate warnings to vessels approaching the swimming area from various locations. The buoys are located 100–300 ft from the swimming area buoy lines.

(9) *Additional Safety Measures*
   (a) Lifesaving devices consisting of life jugs, a ring buoy and line, and one 10- to 12-ft pole, are located every 200 ft along the beach. Depth gauge poles are placed at regular intervals along buoy lines. First-aid stations are provided, where conditions permit.
   (b) Bulletin boards or signs, prominently placed where swimmers can readily see them before entering the area, are provided to post emergency telephone numbers, safety messages, and other information.

WATER SAFETY CAMPAIGN AND NATIONAL FOCUS GROUP

The Corps supports an aggressive water safety campaign. A national focus group, comprised of employees from all levels within the organization that specialize in water safety, coordinate the development of an annual water safety campaign. The group obtains input from Corps lakes across the country concerning the previous years' water-related accidents and fatalities in order to identify trends and target areas where water-safety initiatives should be focused.

Based on this evaluation, specific water-safety issues are identified and high-quality posters, coloring books, book covers, safety pamphlets, and radio and TV public service announcements are produced and distributed to each Corps lake for use in promoting water safety.

Many of the items included in this campaign are targeted at young school-age children. The Corps is committed to devoting resources for water-safety education at the earliest age possible, since this is where the most impressionable impact can be made, and the greatest long-range impacts will result in fewer water-related accidents and fatalities.

DATA COLLECTION AND ANALYSIS

Accurate data collection and analysis of recreation-related, water-based accidents and fatalities is an important tool for correcting design and program deficiencies or weaknesses.

In 1991 the Corps of Engineers and the Centers for Disease Control (CDC) conducted a cooperative study effort to obtain data about drownings on Corps lakes. The study included drownings on Corps lakes between 1986 and 1990. The data collected during this effort has been invaluable in evaluating and guiding the Corps water-safety initiatives. The data revealed the following information:

A. Between 1986 and 1990 there were 1,107 recreation-related fatalities on Corps lakes.
B. Male/Female
   89% of the victims were male.
   11% of the victims were female.
C. Activity
   Swimming/Wading: 44%
   Boating: 23%
   Fishing: 6%
   Other Recreation: 14%
D. Alcohol- or Drug-Related
   Yes = 37%
   No = 63%
E. Minority/Non-Minority Victims
   Minority = 35%
   Non-Minority = 65%
   (This information is significant, since only 12% of the visitors to Corps lakes are minorities.)

F. Was the victim alone at the time the mishap occurred?
77% of the victims **were not alone** at the time of mishap.
G. **40%** of the fatalities occurred **inside a developed recreation area**.
H. **80%** of the swimming/wading fatalities occurred **outside a designated swimming area.**
I. Age
The average age of victims was 29 years old.
52% of the victims were between the ages of 11 and 30.

CONCLUSION

As a result of drowning interventions implemented by the U.S. Army Corps of Engineers, the number of recreation-related drownings at Corps lakes was reduced by 54% and the frequency of drowning was reduced by 73% between 1981 and 1995. This was accomplished during the same period that visitation increased by 66%. The primary initiatives that affected these reductions were the implementation of design standards (criteria) for swimming beaches and an aggressive water safety program implemented at all management levels within the Corps.

With continued emphasis on these drowning interventions, together with accurate data collection and trends analysis, the Corps intends to achieve additional reductions in the number and frequency of recreation-related drownings that occur needlessly each year.

Additional partnering efforts among Federal, state, and local entities, combined with the efforts of private industry, will greatly enhance the Corps ability to make positive impacts on reducing the number of recreation-related accidents and drownings in the United States.

11 Drowning Intervention and Prevention: A U.S. Coast Guard Perspective

Bruce Schmidt

It was a beautiful day for boating on an Arkansas river. The weather was clear, water conditions were calm, winds were light, and visibility was good. The air temperature was 90°F. A family of nine embarked on a fishing outing. The passengers loaded their fishing gear, ice chests, motor, and three-gallon gas tank into a lightweight, 14-ft, flat-bottom boat. The capacity label on the boat indicated a maximum load of three persons at 150 lbs each with motor and gear totaling 600 lbs. The heaviest passengers sat in the front of the boat on this outing. Shortly after pushing off from the riverbank, the boat began to take on water rapidly. When the passengers realized they were in trouble, they looked for their life jackets. Unfortunately, no life jackets were on board. Seven of the nine family members — ages 40, 32, 10, 7, 4, 2, and 1 — drowned that day.

What happened that beautiful summer day to turn an enjoyable boating outing into a tragedy? From the outset, family members put themselves at considerable risk by overloading their small boat — by more than 300 lbs — with passengers and gear. To make matters worse, no personal flotation devices (PFDs or life jackets) were on board the boat, and some of the boat's flotation was missing. All seven drownings could have been prevented that day if the family had not overloaded the boat and had worn life jackets prior to leaving shore. This chapter will focus on intervention and prevention efforts of Coast Guard and state officials to avoid this type of incident. The scope of the drowning problem will be defined through the discussion of recreational boating accident statistics, Coast Guard and state intervention efforts, and preventive measures boaters should employ to minimize risk of drowning in a boating accident.

RECREATIONAL BOATING ACCIDENT STATISTICS

Over 78 million people participate in recreational boating at least once during the year.[1] Water skiing, fishing, hunting, cruising, and sailing are all popular activities of recreational boaters. Although boating is an enjoyable recreational pursuit, over 800 recreational boating fatalities are reported annually to the U.S. Coast Guard.[2]

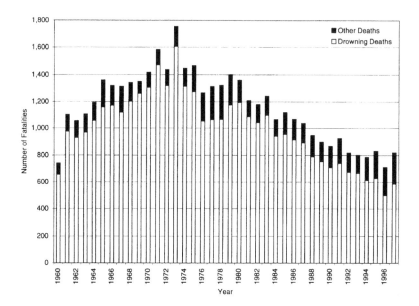

FIGURE 1   Recreational boating accident fatalities, 1960–1997.

TABLE 1
**Recreational Boating Accident Drownings
and Other Deaths, 1960–1997**

Years	Number of Drownings	Other Fatalities	Total Fatalities	Percent
1960–1969	10,499	1,374	11,873	88%
1970–1979	12,640	1,760	14,400	88%
1980–1989	9,658	1,452	11,110	87%
1990–1997	5,113	1,433	6,546	78%
Totals:	37,910	6,019	43,929	

Approximately eight out of ten of these boating fatalities are drownings. Figure 1 shows the total number of recreational boating fatalities and the number of drownings from 1960–1997.

Boating accident data in Table 1 reveals that over the past three decades and for available data in the 1990s, the percentage of drownings compared to total boating fatalities is decreasing.

Explanations for this downward trend include the implementation of recreational boat manufacturing standards and the wearing of life jackets. Basic and level flotation standards have contributed significantly to helping individuals stay afloat in the aquatic environment. These standards require a boat to float so people in the water have a platform to cling to which improves their chances for survival. Intervention efforts in keeping the boat afloat are not enough to prevent recreational boating

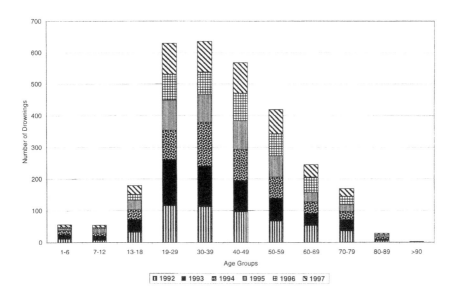

FIGURE 2 Preventable drownings, 1992–1997. A preventable drowning is defined as a reported boating accident drowning victim where a life jacket was not known to have been used or worn by the person who drowned.

accident victims from drowning. All recreational boaters need to wear their life jackets to assist them in staying afloat. The Coast Guard estimates that at least 500 drownings a year can be prevented if boaters wear their life jackets. Figure 2 shows the number of drownings who did not wear life jackets by age group, 1992–1997.

The vast majority of drownings occur on recreational boats under 16 ft in length. Over 95% of all numbered recreational boats in the United States are under 26 ft in length.[3] Chapter 123 of Title 46, United States Code requires each undocumented vessel equipped with propulsion machinery to be numbered in the state in which it is principally operated. Figure 3 shows the percentage breakdown of numbered boats reported in 1997 by the following length categories: less than 16 ft, 16–26 ft, and greater than 26 ft in length.

Boats less than 20 ft in length have an increased risk of becoming unstable in the aquatic environment when overloaded with passengers and gear. To prevent overloaded situations from occurring, boaters need to read and obey the capacity label located inside their boat. As of August 1, 1980, recreational boat manufacturers were required to install in all boats less than 20 ft in length a capacity label showing the maximum number of persons and weight the boat can safely hold. Figure 4 presents the number of drownings by boat length, 1982–1997.

Capsizing, swamping, and falls overboard are types of accidents contributing to the greatest number of drownings each year. Figure 5 shows a capsizing which is the overturning of a vessel where the bottom of the boat is uppermost; a capsized sailboat, however, lies on its side.

Mechanically Propelled Boats

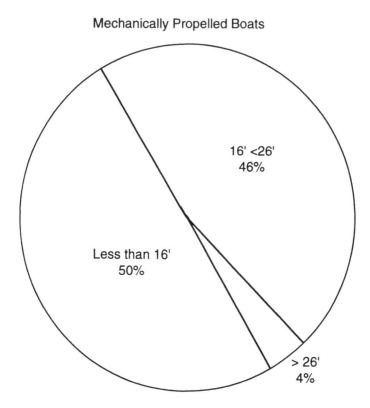

16' <26'
46%

Less than 16'
50%

> 26'
4%

FIGURE 3   Recreational boat lengths, 1997.

Figure 6 shows a swamping. A swamping is when a boat fills with water, particularly over the sides, but retains sufficient buoyancy to remain on the water's surface.

These accidents are caused by overloading a boat, improper weight distribution, movement of passengers or gear, or passengers who lean over the edge of a boat. Based on reported accidents, your risk of dying in a boating accident is greatest if your boat capsizes, swamps, or sinks, and you fall overboard.

Recreational boats can float because they displace a weight of water that is equal to their own weight. Boats stay on top of the water because they are designed to sink into the water only far enough to displace their own weight of water. The heavier the boat, the farther it sinks into the water before it floats. This means that the less weight you add to a boat, the higher it will float in the water. The stability of a boat depends upon its underwater shape and its centers of gravity and buoyancy. A boat's center of gravity is the center of its total mass.[4] An object is stable when its center of gravity is over its base (inside the boat) and unstable when it is over a point outside the base (leaning near the edge of the boat). The higher the center of gravity, the less stable the boat. Piling things in a boat or standing in a boat raises its center of gravity and reduces its stability. The lower the center of gravity of a boat, the

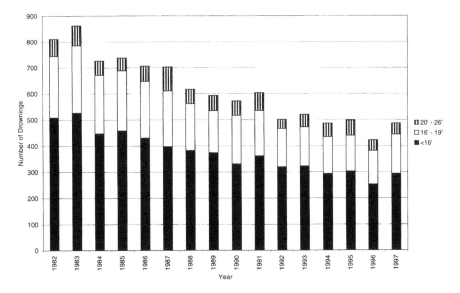

FIGURE 4   Drownings by boat length, 1982–1997.

more stable it is. The center of gravity of a boat varies with its load and where you place it. Another consideration in the stability of a boat is buoyancy. The buoyant force on a boat is equal to the weight of the water it displaces.[5] The center of buoyancy is the center of the mass of the water the boat displaces. The center of buoyancy varies as a boat heels to one side or the other. In an unloaded boat, the centers of gravity and buoyancy are in a vertical line, and the boat is in a stable condition. Boaters who are properly centered and seated low in a boat do not seriously disrupt the natural stability of the boat. If a boater stands up and reaches too far to the side, the center of gravity may move outside the boat and increase the risk of a swamping or capsizing incident. Once you sit in a small boat, stay seated, and do not lean over the side. When you enter a small boat, or if you need to move about, maintain three points of contact by holding onto both sides of the boat while keeping at least one foot on the deck. This keeps the center of gravity of the boat as low and as nearly centered as possible, which helps maintain the stability of the boat. If the elevated center of gravity moves off center, which occurs if a person stands and leans to one side, the boat may capsize. If your boat capsizes or swamps, stay with it and climb on top of it, if possible, so you are out of the water and in sight of others. The colder the water, the more urgent it is that you get out of it. Do not attempt to swim to shore because it is difficult to judge distances when you are in the water. The distance to shore may be farther than you think.

BOATING ACTIVITIES

Recreational boating drownings are reported most often when boaters are cruising, drifting, or fishing. An estimated 25% of recreational boaters fish and some hunt.[6] Sportsmen stand up to fish, to shoot their guns, to start their engines, to

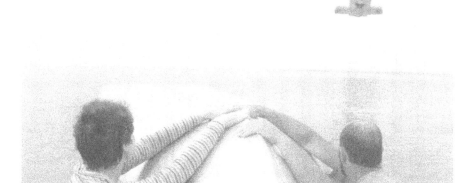

FIGURE 5 Capsizing.

exchange positions in the boat, or, in many instances, to raise anchor in boats 14 ft or less in length. Boats under 16 ft in length are safe but can become unstable under some circumstances. Hunters often overload their boats and neglect to make weather checks for the latest water and wind conditions. Regardless of the size of your boat, load it according to the weather. When the weather is rough, a boater needs more freeboard (height distance between the water and top side of the boat) to avoid swamping. A boat loaded properly in favorable weather conditions may not be safe in an approaching storm. Never exceed your boat's capacity in calm weather and reduce its load if the weather deteriorates. Hunting seasons are usually periods of changing weather, and the changes may be sudden and violent. If a boat is over-loaded, it may swamp in adverse weather or water conditions. Sportsmen who hunt or fish should never walk around or make sudden movements in a small boat. If you absolutely have to move, keep as low as possible and hold onto both sides of the boat — if you can — while keeping one foot on the deck, avoid drinking alcoholic beverages, wear your life jacket under all conditions, get a weather report before you launch, keep alert for changing conditions, and load your boat with current and anticipated weather conditions in mind.

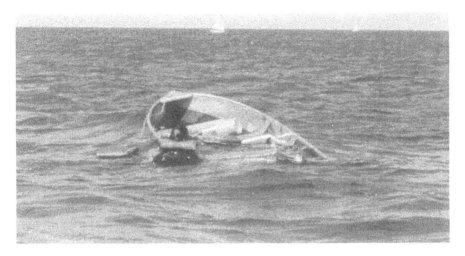

FIGURE 6 Swamping.

TABLE 2
Types of Boating Accidents, 1997

Type of Boating Accident	Drowning Deaths	Other Deaths	Total Fatalities
Capsizing	207	38	245
Collision with Fixed Object	24	32	56
Collision with Floating Object	11	2	13
Collision with Vessel	10	70	80
Fall in Boat	4	2	6
Falls Overboard	214	29	243
Fire/Explosion (Other than Fuel)	0	2	2
Flooding/Swamping	40	2	42
Grounding	4	11	15
Not Reported	9	2	11
Other	36	24	60
Skier Mishap	0	8	8
Struck by Boat	0	8	8
Struck by Motor/Propeller	0	1	1
Sinking	23	0	23
Struck Submerged Object	4	2	6
Totals:	586	233	819

Based on accident statistics, most boating fatalities occur on rivers or lakes when the weather is clear and the conditions are ideal for boating. Figure 7 shows the number of reported drownings for different types of known water conditions.

People need to respect the aquatic environment and stay alert because nearly 80% of recreational boating accidents are caused by operator-controllable factors

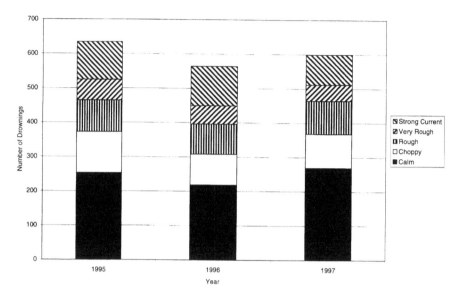

FIGURE 7   Drownings by known water condition, 1995–1997. Note: Accident report data may indicate strong current was involved with any one of the other types of water conditions.

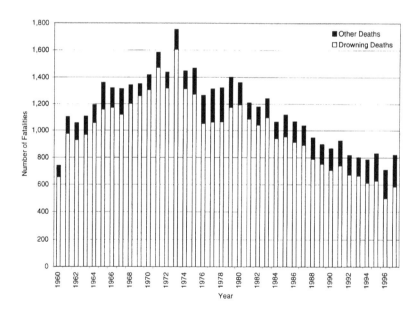

FIGURE 8   Drownings by water temperature, 1997.

(operator inattention or carelessness) rather than physical or environmental factors (boat, environmental conditions).

Most boating fatalities occur in waters 70–74°F. Figure 8 shows most boaters who drowned were reported in waters 50–79°F.

TABLE 3
Recreational Boating Drownings by Month*, 1997

Month	Number of Accidents	Number of Drownings
January	118	19
February	134	24
March	330	44
April	391	62
May	1,020	89
June	1,434	95
July	1,991	76
August	1,489	55
September	571	38
October	282	32
November	158	29
December	93	23

* When month was reported.

When waters are below 60°F, hypothermia can set in quickly. Table 3 shows that a greater percentage of the vessels involved in accidents during the fall and winter months result in drownings.

One third of all numbered recreational boats in United States are located in states that border the Great Lakes. Boaters in these states are more likely to experience the effects of hypothermia than boaters in warmer regions of the country.

HYPOTHERMIA

Hypothermia is a major killer in aquatic mishaps and occurs most rapidly in cold water, but it may occur in waters at 80°F. Hypothermia occurs more rapidly when you are wet than when you are dry and even faster when you are in water because water conducts heat away from your body. The 50–50 rule emphasizes the rapidity with which hypothermia can occur.[7] Using the 50–50 rule, a boater has a 50–50 chance to swim 50 yds in water at 50°F and a 50-year-old person only has a 50–50 chance of surviving for 50 minutes in waters at 50°F. Boaters who find themselves in water at or below 60°F should immediately get into the Heat Escape Lessening Position (HELP), keep on all clothing, and wear a life jacket. HELP is a position where a person makes his or her body as compact as possible to conserve heat. You do this by bringing your legs up toward your chest while keeping your arms folded. This position retains body heat and will help you survive until rescued. Remember to keep your head out of the water because the greatest source of heat loss from a person's body is the head. If two to three people are in the water, they should huddle together to conserve heat. The type of clothing a person wears makes a difference for surviving in the cold water. Air trapped in the clothing helps insulate a person against the cold water. Wool clothing retains a higher degree of its insulating properties when wet than most other fabrics. Synthetic clothing offers no protection against heat loss. When individuals try to

TABLE 4
Approximate Median Lethal Exposure Times

	Time in Hours		
Water Temp (°F)	Floating with a Life Jacket	Treading Water	Swimming
35	1.75	1.25	.75
45	2.50	1.75	1.00
55	3.50	3.00	2.00
65	7.75	5.75	4.50
70	18.00	13.00	10.00

swim, they rapidly lose any warmed air trapped in their clothing. Wearing your life jacket traps warmed water between it and your body and helps you stay afloat with a minimal expenditure of energy. When a person fails to wear a life jacket, they expend a significant amount of energy treading water to survive. A person expending energy in cold water looses a significant amount of body heat which increases the onset of hypothermia. Tests show the average rate of heat loss of a person treading water is approximately 34% faster than for that same person wearing a life jacket.[8] Table 4 gives the approximate survival times in water of various temperatures.[9]

A typical life vest has superb insulation qualities. A properly fitted life jacket will help retain the body heat of a person who remains still in the water, which significantly improves their chances of survival. A person attempting to swim for shore wearing a jacket will lose body heat rapidly. Studies show that the average person swimming in a life jacket cools 35% faster than a person remaining still.[10]

LIFE JACKETS

Whether you refer to them as life jackets, life vests, or personal flotation devices (PFDs), they are designed to (1) keep your head above water and in a position which permits proper breathing; (2) provide buoyancy to keep you afloat; and (3) save your life. The Coast Guard considers wearing a life jacket at all times to be the primary factor in ensuring survival after a boating accident. Most fatal boating accidents involve people who suddenly and unexpectedly find themselves in the water without life jackets. Unfortunately, most fatal boating accidents involve people who have life jackets on board their boats but are not wearing them. When a small boat capsizes, life jackets are often trapped under the boat's seats, are inaccessible, and, subsequently, not worn.

HISTORY OF LIFE JACKETS

In the earliest years of development, the "life preserver" resembled an empty barrel of wood planks used by Norwegian seamen, as seen in Figure 9.

Life jackets have been saving lives since 1852, the year Congress passed the first legislative requirement that commercial vessels carry a wearable life preserver

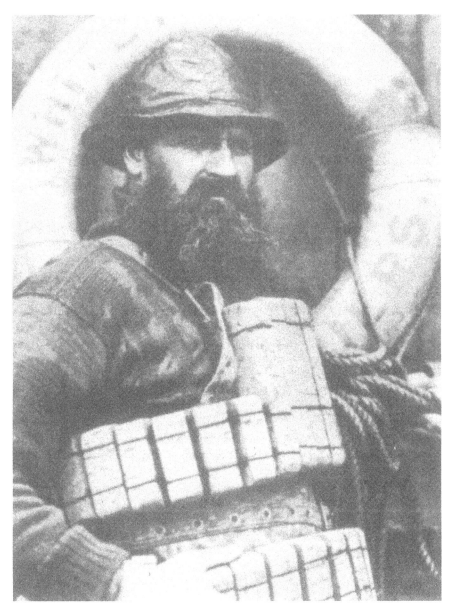

FIGURE 9   An early life preserver.

designed to be worn or secured to the body or have hand holds so a person could hold on to it securely in the water. With passage of the Motorboat Act of 1940, the U.S. Coast Guard began to address drowning prevention efforts for recreational boaters in its consideration of life preserver carriage. The Coast Guard recommended life preservers be designed to support a recreational boater for a shorter length of time than for a commercial vessel passenger and to reduce the bulk of the jacket to improve comfort and wear. During World War II, development and testing of life jackets were conducted to determine the effectiveness of buoyant materials such as kapok, balsa wood, cork, and air (inflatable life jackets). In 1964, the Coast Guard developed a standard for flotation devices that offered minimum restriction while providing for the needs of recreational boaters. As a result, life jackets were manufactured using new materials such as closed cell foam. These jackets were not as bulky as older styles, and they were more attractive and colorful. In 1985, the Coast Guard proposed and adopted extensive requirements for approving inflatable life jackets and additional requirements concerning their carriage on recreational boats. Continuing technological advances make inflatable life jackets more reliable, lighter, and easier to maintain.

TYPES OF LIFE JACKETS

Today's life jacket, the product of considerable research and development, offers boaters greater wear, comfort, and style. There are many different types of life jackets in sizes for everyone. The Type I Offshore life jacket, as seen in Figure 10, is designed to keep people afloat for an extended period of time in rough, open water and provides more protection to wearers than any other type of jacket. These jackets are recommended for boaters who cruise far offshore where a delayed rescue is probable. The jacket will turn an unconscious person in the water face up and gives an adult a minimum of 22 lbs of buoyancy and a child 11 lbs of buoyancy. They are bulkier and less comfortable than other types and only come in two sizes, one for children and one for adults.

The Type II Near-Shore buoyant vest, shown in Figure 11, comes in several sizes for adults and children. This vest is used in calm inland water where the likelihood of rapid rescue is great. It will turn an unconscious person in the water from a facedown position to a vertical or slightly backward position. It is less bulky than a Type I jacket and gives an adult a minimum of 15.5 lbs of buoyancy, a child 11 lbs, and a small child and infant 7 lbs.

The Type III life jacket or Marine Buoyant Device, also known as a flotation aid, shown in Figure 12, is considered the most comfortable type of life jacket. Type III life jackets come in several styles for different boating activities and sports. They are designed for use in calm water where rescue is likely to be quick. Their minimum buoyancy is 15.5 lbs, and they will not generally turn an unconscious person face up. They are usually worn for water skiing, fishing, or other activities where freedom of movement is a priority. Type IIIs are also available as flotation coats, which are useful in cold weather.

The Type IV device is thrown to a person in the water. Examples of these devices are boat cushions, ring buoys, and horseshoe buoys. They are not designed to be worn and must be supplemented by a wearable life jacket. They are also not to be used for small children, nonswimmers, or unconscious people. A Type V life jacket, shown in Figure 13, can either be a "special use device" or a hybrid. Special use devices include board sailing vests, deck suits, and work vests. They are designed and approved for only the special uses or conditions indicated on their labels and do not meet legal requirements for general use on board recreational boats.

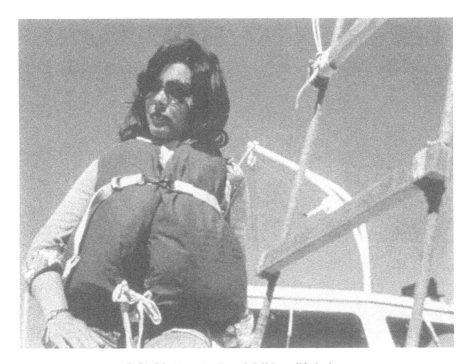

FIGURE 10   The Type I Offshore life jacket.

Hybrid life jackets are inflatable devices with some built-in buoyancy provided by plastic foam or kapok. They can be inflated orally or by cylinders of compressed gas to give additional buoyancy. In some hybrids, the gas used to inflate the life jacket is released manually by the wearer and in others, it is released automatically when the life jacket is immersed in water. The inherent buoyancy of a hybrid may be insufficient to float a person unless it is inflated. Because of its limited buoyancy when deflated, a hybrid is recommended for use by a nonswimmer only if is worn with enough inflation to float the wearer. To satisfy the legal carriage requirement, hybrids manufactured before February 8, 1995 must be worn whenever a boat is underway and the wearer is not below deck or in an enclosed space. Hybrids cost more than other life jackets but are more comfortable than Type I, II, or III life jackets. The Coast Guard has determined that improved, more comfortable, and less costly hybrids can save lives since they will be purchased and used more frequently. For these reasons, a Federal regulation, effective February 8, 1995, increased both the deflated and inflated buoyancies of hybrids and made them available in a greater variety of sizes and types.

On April 29, 1996, the U.S. Coast Guard approved inflatable life jackets for use by adult recreational boaters. Inflatable life jackets are gaining wider acceptance as more adults recognize their comfort and good fit. The Coast Guard anticipates boaters will wear inflatable life jackets more often than currently approved inherently buoyant life jackets (I, II, or III) and make a significant contribution to preventing the loss of life on the nation's waterways. An inflatable life jacket must be inflated either

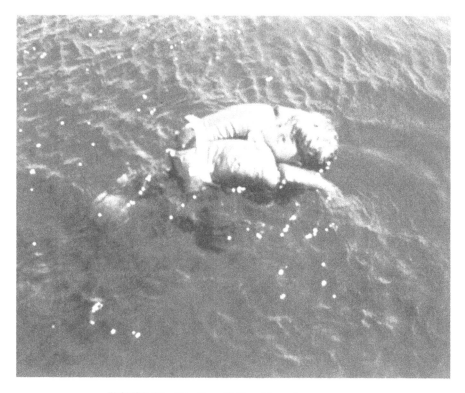

FIGURE 11   The Type II Near-Shore buoyant vest.

automatically, orally, or manually to become buoyant. An automatic system inflates when the device becomes immersed in the water without any action by the user. The manual system is activated when the wearer pulls a lanyard which inflates the device with a carbon dioxide cartridge. The manual system is considered a primary system because it is generally the simplest to maintain and less susceptible to unwanted or inadvertent inflation. The third means of inflating the device is an oral inflation system where the user blows air into the device through a tube. Oral inflation is considered a backup system because the user may panic in a drowning situation and be unable to inflate the device. Inflatable life jackets are approved only for adults and are not recommended for anyone who cannot swim.

Regardless of type, all life jackets must meet the following requirements: (1) Coast Guard approval, with a label and approval number attached; (2) all straps, buckles, zippers, and stitching must be intact, and the fabric should also be in good condition; (3) any devices with rips or tears must be replaced; (4) jackets must be readily accessible to occupants of the vessel; and (5) jackets may not be stored in sealed packages or in a locked storage area.

A Coast Guard-approved life jacket must show the manufacturer's name and approval number. Most are marked as Type I, II, III, IV, or V.

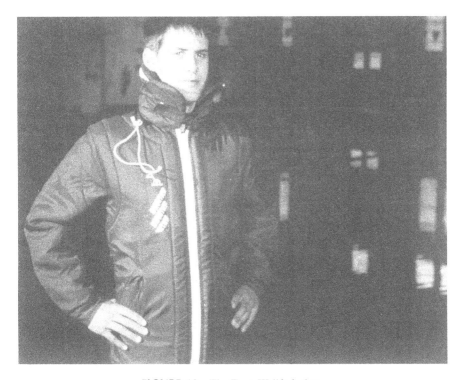

FIGURE 12   The Type III life jacket.

FEDERAL REQUIREMENTS FOR LIFE JACKETS

As of May 1, 1995 Federal regulations require the carriage of at least one wearable life jacket (Type I, II, or III) or hybrid for each person on board your recreational boat. If your boat is 16 ft or more in length and is not a canoe or a kayak, you must also have at least one Type IV on board. These requirements apply to all recreational boats that are propelled or controlled by machinery, sails, oars, paddles, poles, or another boat. A water skier being towed is considered to be on board the boat when judging compliance with legal requirements. Forty-three states mandate the wearing of life jackets. A common requirement among the states is that children under age 12 must wear a life jacket while on board a boat. Other states mandate their use when water skiing or operating a personal watercraft.

MAINTENANCE OF LIFE JACKETS

Proper maintenance of life jackets is critical for ensuring effective use for many boating seasons. After each outing, dry jackets thoroughly and store them in a dry, well-ventilated area. For inflatable life jackets, make sure the carbon dioxide cartridge is replaced after each use and thus fully operational for the next boating outing. Avoid throwing life jackets because they contain buoyant material

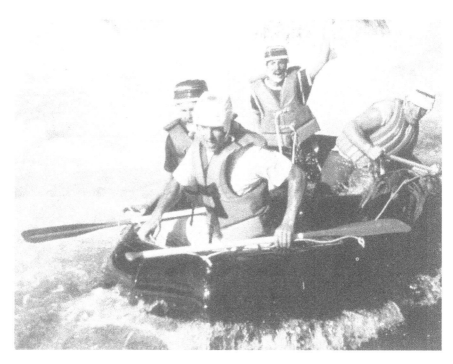

FIGURE 13   The Type V life jacket.

such as kapok or fibrous glass enclosed in plastic bags. These bags can rupture if damaged and render the jacket unserviceable. Every few months, check to see if air leaks out of your jacket by squeezing it. If air can leak out, water can leak in, and your jacket will not be safe to use. Avoid exposing your life jacket to direct sunlight because the covers of some life jackets are made of nylon or polyester, which may weaken due to extended exposure to sunlight. Ripped and badly faded fabric are indications that the covering of your life jacket is deteriorating. A test to determine the strength of your covering is to pinch the fabric between your thumbs and forefingers and attempt to tear the fabric. If the fabric can be torn, the life jacket should be destroyed and discarded. Compare the colors in protected places to those exposed to the sun. If colors have faded, the materials have been weakened. With normal use, a fabric covered life jacket should ordinarily last several boating seasons. Depending on the care and use of the life jacket, there is potential for buoyancy loss. Each life jacket should be checked at the beginning of the boating season to ensure that it can still provide adequate flotation for the wearer. You can do this by putting on the device, adjusting it properly, and gradually walking into the water until it completely supports the wearer. If the device floats the person out of the water and feels comfortable, the device is still usable. Wearing a life jacket does not ensure a boater is risk free from drowning. Water temperature and conditions, any injury rendering the boater unconscious while in the water, alcohol or drug impairment, and improperly fitted or maintained life jackets are factors that influence survival in the aquatic environment.

TABLE 5
State Requirements for Life Jackets

PERSONAL FLOTATION DEVICES

State	Mandate Wearing PFDs	Circumstances and Age Requirements
Alabama	Yes	Within 800 ft below a hydroelectric dam or navigational lock. All occupants.
Alaska	Yes	Under 13 while water skiing or on open deck
American Samoa	Yes	All on board while boat is underway.
Arizona	Yes	Children 12 and under when vessel is underway
Arkansas	Yes	Ages 12 and under; except within enclosed area while not under way
California	Yes	Under 7 years of age on vessels more than 26 feet, unless in an enclosed cabin.
Colorado	Yes	PWC operators and passengers. Waterskiers and persons on aquaplanes, surfboards and similar devices when towed behind a boat. All persons aboard outfitter's vessels.
Connecticut	Yes	Under 12; Between Oct. 1 and May 30th all people in canoes, PWC riders and skiers.
Delaware	Yes	All PWC operators and children under 12
District of Columbia	Yes	When the operator of a vessel is under 18, all others under 18 must wear PFDs.
Florida	Yes	Children under 6 on vessels 26 feet while underway, all PWC operators, skiers.
Georgia	Yes	PWC operators and passengers; skiers; in designated "hazardous area". Below age 10 in moving vessel, except when enclosed in cabin.
Guam	No	None
Hawaii	No	None
Idaho	No	None
Illinois	Yes	PWC only (current). Children under 13 effective 1/1/98.
Indiana	Yes	PWC Only
Iowa	Yes	Skiers or others being towed.
Kansas	Yes	PWC; 12 and under
Kentucky	Yes	Everyone on PWCs.
Louisiana	Yes	Children under 12 on vessels less than 26 feet.
Maine	Yes	10 years old and under
Maryland	No	None
Massachusetts	Yes	Persons being towed, PWC users, canoeists/kayakers (mid-September - mid-May). 12 years of age
Michigan	Yes	PWC operators, riders & skiers. Under 6.
Minnesota	Yes	All persons on PWCs
Mississippi	Yes	12 yrs or younger in boats under 26 ft and when boats are underway
Missouri	Yes	PWC operators and passengers; under age 7
Montana	Yes	Under 12 when vessel is in motion
N. Mariana Islands	No	None
Nebraska	Yes	Under 12
Nevada	Yes	Water skiers and PWC
New Hampshire	Yes	Any child 5 years or under; PWC operators and persons being towed.
New Jersey	Yes	All PWC operators and riders
New Mexico	Yes	n/a
New York	Yes	Under 12 years of age on a boat less than 65 feet unless inside an enclosed cabin.
North Carolina	Yes	Only on PWC
North Dakota	Yes	Everyone 10 years or younger, on boats less than 27 ft while in operation
Ohio	Yes	Children less than 10 on boats less than 18 ft; all PWC operators and passengers; skiers
Oklahoma	Yes	Skiers, PWC passengers / operators; under 13 when vessel is underway
Oregon	No	None
Pennsylvania	Yes	PWC, skiers, sailboards, children 12 years of age and under.
Puerto Rico	No	Children under 12
Rhode Island	Yes	On PWC's; under 10 on class A vessels underway.
South Carolina	Yes	All PWC operators and riders; under 12 on class A
South Dakota	No	None
Tennessee	Yes	Below dams in the areas marked and all PWC riders; 12 and under
Texas	Yes	Children 13 and under; PWC operators
Utah	Yes	PWC, Children 12 or less & all boaters on rivers.
Vermont	Yes	Under age 12 while under way & on an open deck
Virgin Islands	Yes	Operation of PWC / skiing
Virginia	Yes	Operating a PWC; 14 and under
Washington	Yes	Water skiers and all persons on PWCs
West Virginia	No*	All persons on PWCs
Wisconsin	Yes	On PWCs
Wyoming	No	None

RECREATIONAL BOAT FLOTATION STANDARDS

BASIC FLOTATION

When a boat capsizes, floods, or swamps, boaters are often caught by surprise and unable to put on their life jackets to save themselves. The basic flotation standard is a Federal regulation that helps boaters stay afloat by having part of the boat stay afloat. The basic flotation standard, effective August 1, 1973, requires any structural part of a swamped boat to float in any position while supporting the passengers clinging to the boat with water approximately at the neck level.[12] Basic flotation applies to all monohull inboard and inboard/outdrive powered boats less than 20 ft in length, except canoes, kayaks, and inflatable boats.[13] The problem with basic flotation is when boats are swamped, they have a tendency to capsize and float with their bow high in the air. This situation makes it difficult for survivors to hang onto and remain with the boat and almost impossible for them to right the boat and climb on board. The Coast Guard observed that people had great difficulty hanging onto an overturned boat. The tendency was to give up in the face of overwhelming odds against survival. Accident victims felt the boat provided insufficient security. As a result, they overestimated their swimming ability and swam for shore only to drown en route. When people are immersed in cold water, the shock and psychological effects of possibly drowning impairs their judgment and increases psychological deterioration. Faced with this situation, the Coast Guard analyzed reports and statistical data about fatalities from boats capsizing, flooding, sinking, or striking floating objects. A team of accident analysts and naval architects established a probability of how many lives could be saved with an improved flotation regulation. Their results showed that a large percentage of deaths would not have occurred if the boats involved in the accidents had been equipped with level flotation.

LEVEL FLOTATION

The level flotation standard is a regulation that has saved countless lives and addressed the drowning problem in recreational boating. This standard, which went into effect August 1, 1978, applies to all monohull outboard powered boats less than 20 ft in length, except sailboats, canoes, kayaks, and inflatable boats. Level flotation has enabled passengers to remain on board a swamped boat in a sitting position where they are warmer, less subject to panic, and less in danger of drowning while providing a large target for rescue groups to locate. The Coast Guard estimates that 210 lives would have been saved in 1975 had all boats been equipped with level flotation. Prior to passage of this regulation, Coast Guard research indicated almost half of the deaths caused by capsizing, swamping, and sinking could have been prevented by requiring boats to have enough buoyance to float level when swamped with the passengers seated inside, as shown in Figure 14.

When a boat capsizes, the tendency to panic is severe and the flooded stability of the boat can either aggravate or lessen that tendency. The accident victims need to feel secure when their boat is flooded to discourage any attempt to swim for shore. Boaters have a better chance of surviving in a boat equipped with level

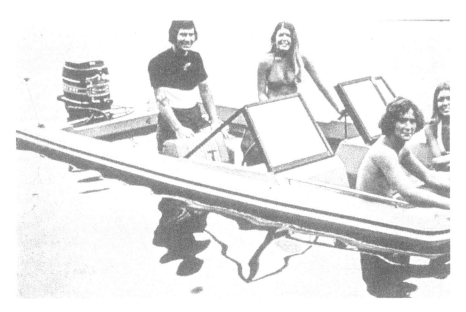

FIGURE 14   Boat equipped with level flotation.

flotation for a number of reasons. Boats equipped with level flotation swamp slowly and remain upright during the maneuver, as opposed to boats equipped with basic flotation that tend to capsize when swamped. In boats equipped with basic flotation, life jackets are often stored in areas where they could be trapped if the boat capsizes, making the life jackets inaccessible to boaters in danger of drowning. A study of recreational boating accidents prior to the implementation of the level flotation standard revealed that approximately 56% of the fatalities had access to a life jacket but failed to use it.[14] A boat equipped with level flotation offers the benefit of floating level and remaining upright when swamped. As a result, life jackets will be accessible and are more likely to be used properly. Since passengers are able to remain inside the boat during swamping, this will help save boaters who cannot swim, who are panic stricken, or who are physically impaired by age, weight, or heart disease.

As discussed earlier, prolonged exposure to cold water quickly leads to hypothermia where the body loses heat faster than it can produce it. The interval between the onset of hypothermia symptoms and collapse might be only one hour, between collapse and death, two hours. Level flotation allows a person to remain within a partially submerged boat with the upper part of the body out of the water. As a result, chances of survival are greater. In cases where the power head of the motor has not been damaged by immersion in the water, passengers can empty (bail) water from the boat, start the motor, and return safely under their own power. In summary, benefits of level flotation include the following: boats will float level when swamped providing a safe platform for occupants until rescue; boaters are more likely to stay with the boat which improves their chances of rescue; boaters can remain in the swamped boat with approximately 50% of their bodies out of the water, reducing the risk of hypothermia; the power head of the outboard motor will remain out of the water when the boat is swamped and can be restarted, allowing occupants to

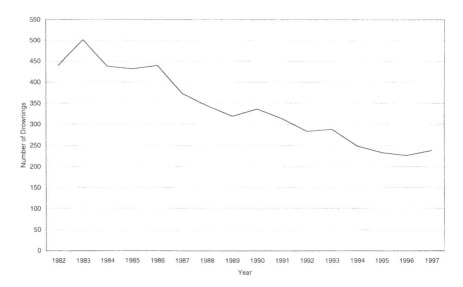

FIGURE 15   Drownings on open motorboats less than 20 ft in length, 1982–1997.

return home; and the boat is stable enough to allow passengers to climb back on board the boat without tipping it over.

Figure 15, which presents accident statistics involving open motorboats less than 20 ft in length powered by outboard motors, shows the direct benefits of level flotation. From 1982 to 1997, the number of drownings reported on boats in compliance with the regulation shows a downward trend.

Level flotation has proven to be one of the most beneficial boat construction standards ever developed and implemented for reducing the number of boating drownings.

ALCOHOL AND BOATING

Recreational boating can be a very strenuous activity due to the glare of the sun, vibration of the boat motor, pounding waves, and rocking motion of the boat. These conditions can affect a boater's equilibrium to the point the individual may exhibit signs of alcohol impairment just by boating over the course of a day. A boater's physiological response to the conditions in the aquatic environment are exacerbated by the effects of alcohol. Alcohol use is a major contributing factor in recreational boating casualties. Appointing a designated skipper to assume responsibility of the boat is not a good idea. Passengers who consume alcohol place themselves at considerable risk of personal injury or death. Boating accident reports reveal that passengers who drink are at risk of either falling in or out of the boat. Alcohol impairs judgment. Individuals lack the ability or skill to save themselves after taking any unnecessary risks. When people drink, their ability to measure distance is impaired at .035, their behavior and emotions are affected from .03 to .05, judgment and risk-taking are affected from .04 to .07, and balance and coordination are impaired from .06 to .10. In fact, a boat operator with a blood alcohol concentration above .10 is over ten times as likely to be killed in a boating accident than a sober boat operator.[15] When people under the influence of alcohol unexpectedly fall into the water, they are disoriented, tend to panic, hyperventilate, and attempt to push up on the water to save themselves. This behavior is a characteristic response a sober individual may exhibit when drowning. Being under the influence of alcohol further exacerbates this classic drowning response and greatly diminishes a person's chance of surviving. Alcohol impairs ability to operate a vessel safely in the same way that it impairs ability to drive a car safely. Other factors that add to the intensity of impairment when on the water include the motion of the boat and dehydration. Your balance deteriorates when you consume alcohol, and, when you combine this with the rocking of a boat, your chances of falling overboard increase. When you drink alcohol on a boat, the sunlight and heat cause you to perspire, which removes water but leaves the alcohol in your body. This causes impairment to occur more quickly. In a study of boating fatalities in four states, 51% of the people who died had a blood alcohol content of .04 or more, and a blood alcohol content of .10 or more was found in 30% of the fatalities.[16] All states have operating under the influence laws. Blood intoxication levels range from .08 to .10. Most states use .10 as the legal limit, but an increasing number of states have adopted .08 intoxication levels to be consistent with their motor vehicle law levels. When boaters operate a vessel in states where implied consent is the law, they agree to submit to a Operating Under the Influence (OUI) test at the request of a law enforcement officer. Implied consent is the law in 37 states. In 45 states, refusal to take an intoxication test can be used against a boater for criminal prosecution. Table 6 shows the state intervention efforts in enforcing OUI laws for recreational boaters.[17]

SWIMMING ABILITY

Results from the American Red Cross National Boater Survey show that approximately 96% of boat-owning households possess some degree of swimming ability.[18] Even though swimming ability is considered the key skill for surviving in the aquatic environment, many of the reported drowning victims in boating accidents could swim. Boaters with swimming ability can become disoriented by the sudden plunge into cold water, hit their heads on the boat as they fall in the water and be rendered unconscious, or be weighted down by their wet clothes. More than 80% of people who lose their lives in boating accidents drown, although most of them are "swimmers." Granted, a person who knows how to swim is at less risk of dying in the aquatic environment than a nonswimmer, but knowing how to swim does not guarantee survival.

TABLE 6
State Operating Under the Influence (OUI) Laws

OPERATING UNDER THE INFLUENCE

State	Vessel OUI Laws	Blood Alcohol Concentration Intoxication Level	Implied Consent Law For Watercraft	Refusal of Test Can Be Used Against Boater
Alabama	Yes	0.10	No	Yes
Alaska	Yes	0.10	Yes	Yes
American Samoa	Yes	0.10	No	No
Arizona	Yes	0.10	Yes	Yes
Arkansas	Yes	0.10	Yes	Yes
California	Yes	0.08	Yes	Yes
Colorado	Yes	0.10	Yes	Yes
Connecticut	Yes	0.10	No	Yes
Delaware	Yes	0.10	Yes	Yes
District of Columbia	Yes	0.10	Yes	Yes
Florida	Yes	0.08	Yes	Yes
Georgia	Yes	0.08	Yes	Yes
Guam	Yes	0.08	No	No
Hawaii	Yes	0.08	Yes	Yes
Idaho	Yes	0.08	Yes	Yes
Illinois	Yes	0.10/0.08*	Yes	Yes
Indiana	Yes	0.10	Yes	Yes
Iowa	Yes	None	No	No
Kansas	Yes	0.08	Yes	Yes
Kentucky	Yes	0.10	No	No
Louisiana	Yes	0.10 / 0.04*	Yes	Yes
Maine	Yes	0.08	Yes	Yes
Maryland	Yes	0.10	No	Yes
Massachusetts	Yes	0.08	Yes	No*
Michigan	Yes	0.10	Yes	Yes
Minnesota	Yes	0.10	Yes	Yes
Mississippi	Yes	0.10	Yes	Yes
Missouri	Yes	0.10	Yes	Yes
Montana	Yes	0.10	No	Yes
N. Mariana Islands	Yes	0.08	No	No
Nebraska	Yes	0.10	Yes	Yes
Nevada	Yes	0.10	Yes	Yes
New Hampshire	Yes	0.08	Yes	Yes
New Jersey	Yes	0.10	Yes	Yes
New Mexico	Yes	0.08	No	Yes
New York	Yes	0.10	Yes	Yes
North Carolina	Yes	0.08	No	Yes
North Dakota	Yes	0.10	Yes	Yes
Ohio	Yes	0.10	Yes	Yes
Oklahoma	Yes	0.10	Yes	Yes
Oregon	Yes	0.08	Yes	Yes
Pennsylvania	Yes	0.10	Yes	Yes
Puerto Rico	Yes	0.10	No	Yes
Rhode Island	Yes	0.10	Yes	Yes
South Carolina	Yes	0.10	Yes	Yes
South Dakota	Yes	0.10	No*	Yes
Tennessee	Yes	0.10	Yes	No
Texas	Yes	0.10	Yes	Yes
Utah	Yes	0.08	Yes	Yes
Vermont	Yes	0.08 / 0.02	Yes	Yes
Virgin Islands	Yes	0.10	Yes	Yes
Virginia	Yes	0.08	Yes	Yes
Washington	Yes	0.10	No	Yes
West Virginia	Yes	0.10	No	Yes
Wisconsin	Yes	0.10*	Yes	Yes
Wyoming	Yes	0.10	No	No

SUMMARY

Saving lives is the primary goal of the U.S. Coast Guard's Recreational Boating Safety Program. Over the years, we have worked with our partners in boating safety to lower the number of recreational boat drownings from an all-time high of 1604 in 1973 to 586 in 1997. The Coast Guard bases its drowning intervention and prevention efforts by analyzing: (1) Boating Accident Reports (BARs); (2) accident investigation reports; and (3) accident data and appropriate statistics. In this chapter, the scope of the drowning problem was defined by looking at statistics relevant to drowning victims. We found that smaller boats (less than 16 ft in length) are at risk of either capsizing and/or swamping when overloaded with passengers or gear. When passengers improperly distribute their weight by standing or moving around in an overloaded boat, their risk of falling overboard increases significantly. A passenger who does fall overboard usually is not wearing a life jacket and succumbs to the conditions in the aquatic environment.

From the analysis of boating accident statistics, boating safety regulations are created and implemented to help minimize a boater's risk of drowning. In this chapter, we discussed the benefits of (1) wearing your life jacket; (2) basic and level flotation standards for boats; (3) not drinking alcoholic beverages while you boat; and (4) swimming ability.

A life jacket is designed to (1) keep your head above water and in a position which permits proper breathing; (2) provide buoyancy to keep you afloat; and (3) save your life. The Coast Guard considers wearing life jackets at all times to be the primary factor in ensuring survival after a boating accident. Today's life jacket is the product of considerable research and development offering boaters greater comfort, fit, and style. There are many different types and sizes for everyone. As of May 1, 1995, Federal regulations require at least one wearable life jacket be carried for each person on board a boat. On April 29, 1996, the Coast Guard approved inflatable life jackets for use by adult recreational boaters. Inflatable life jackets are gaining wider acceptance as more adults recognize they are comfortable and fit well.

When a boat capsizes, floods, or swamps, boaters are often caught by surprise and unable to put on their life jackets if they are not already wearing them. The basic flotation standard, which went into effect on August 1, 1973, requires any structural part of a swamped boat to float in any position while supporting the passengers clinging to the boat with the water approximately at the next level. Basic flotation applies to all monohull inboard and inboard/outdrive powered boats less than 20 ft in length, except canoes, kayaks, and inflatable boats. A boat equipped with level flotation goes one step further by enabling the boat to float level and remain upright when swamped. Level flotation enables passengers to remain on board a swamped boat in a sitting position where they are warmer, less subject to panic, and in less danger of drowning. Level flotation, which went into effect on August 1, 1978, applies to all monohull outboard powered boats less than 20 ft in length, except canoes, sailboats, kayaks, and inflatable boats. It is a safety standard that has saved countless lives since its inception.

A boater's physiological response to the conditions in the aquatic environment are exacerbated by the effects of alcohol. Over the course of a day, individuals exposed to the sun, vibration of the boat motor, pounding waves, or rocking motion of the boat can be affected to the point where they exhibit signs of alcohol impairment while sober. If these same individuals consume alcohol and fall overboard, they usually are not wearing life jackets, become disoriented, panic, hyperventilate, push up on the water in an attempt to save themselves, go under the water, and drown. All states have operating under the influence laws with blood intoxication levels ranging from .08 to .10.

Although swimming ability is considered the key skill for surviving in the aquatic environment, many reported drowning victims in boating accidents could swim. Boaters with swimming ability can become disoriented by the sudden plunge into cold water, hit their heads on the boat as they fall into the water, and be rendered unconscious, or be weighted down by their wet clothes. Nevertheless, a person who knows how to swim is at less risk of drowning as a result of a boating accident than a nonswimmer.

The Coast Guard and its partners have accomplished a great deal since 1973, cutting the number of recreational boating drownings from 1604 to the most current figure of 586. In future, we will work with our partners to improve safety by informing the public of the benefits of wearing life jackets, operating boats in a safe manner, obeying the rules of the road, and taking safe boating courses. Every year, boating accident reports indicate that at least 500 drownings could have been prevented had boaters simply worn their life jackets.

REFERENCES AND NOTES

1. National Marine Manufacturers Association, *Boating 1997*, Chicago, IL, Revised 1997.
2. U.S. Coast Guard, U.S. Department of Transportation, Washington, D.C.: Current regulations (33 Code of Federal Regulations 173–174) require the operator of any vessel numbered or used for recreational purposes to file a Boating Accident Report (BAR) if the vessel is involved in an accident that results in: (a) loss of life; or (b) personal injury which requires medical treatment beyond first aid; or (c) damage to the vessel and other property exceeding $500.00; or (d) complete loss of the vessel. Boat operators are required to report their accidents to authorities in the State where the accident occurred, or directly to the Coast Guard if the accident occurred in Alaska. States with approved numbering systems furnish the Coast Guard with copies of Boating Accident Reports (BARs). The minimum reporting requirements are set by Federal regulation, but States are allowed to have stricter requirements. The recreational boating accident statistics in this chapter are derived from accident data abstracted from BARs that have been entered into the national BAR database for the years 1969–1997.
3. Report of Certificates of Number Issued to Boats — 1997 (33 CFR Parts 173–174).
4. Coast Guard Auxiliary National Board Inc., 1995, "Small Boat Stability," *Boating Skills and Seamanship,* Eleventh Edition.
5. Coast Guard Auxiliary National Board Inc., 1995, "Small Boat Stability," *Boating Skills and Seamanship,* Eleventh Edition.

6. Coast Guard Auxiliary National Board Inc., 1995, "The Rest of Our Story," *Boating Skills and Seamanship,* Eleventh Edition.
7. Coast Guard Auxiliary National Board Inc., 1995, "The Rest of Our Story," *Boating Skills and Seamanship,* Eleventh Edition.
8. Coast Guard Auxiliary National Board Inc., 1995, "The Rest of Our Story," *Boating Skills and Seamanship,* Eleventh Edition.
9. Coast Guard Auxiliary National Board Inc., 1995, "The Rest of Our Story," *Boating Skills and Seamanship,* Eleventh Edition.
10. Coast Guard Auxiliary National Board Inc., 1995, "The Rest of Our Story," *Boating Skills and Seamanship,* Eleventh Edition.
11. Noll, J. G. and Sarver, R., *Reference Guide to State Boating Laws*, Third Edition. Lexington, KY: Council of State Governments and National Association of State Boating Law Administrators, 1997.
12. Blanton, J. William, Granholm, E. Lars, and Lysle, Gray B.: U.S. Coast Guard, Department of Transportation, *Level Flotation Research to Regulation.*
13. Blanton, J. William, Granholm, E. Lars, and Lysle, Gray B.: U.S. Coast Guard, Department of Transportation, *Level Flotation Research to Regulation.*
14. Blanton, J. William, Granholm, E. Lars, and Lysle, Gray B.: U.S. Coast Guard, Department of Transportation, *Level Flotation Research to Regulation.*
15. Disario, Robert, Mengert, Peter, and Susman, E. Donald, *A Study of the Relationship Between the Risk of Fatality and Blood Alcohol Concentration of Recreational Boat Operators.* U.S. Department of Transportation, Research and Special Programs Administration, John A. Volpe National Transportation Systems Center. Cambridge, MA, May 1992.
16. U.S. Coast Guard, U.S. Department of Transportation, *Boating Statistics 1994*, U.S. Government Printing Office, Washington, DC, September 1995.
17. Noll, J. G. and Sarver, R., *Reference Guide to State Boating Laws*, Third Edition. Lexington, KY: Council of State Governments and National Association of State Boating Law Administrators, 1997.
18. U.S. Coast Guard, U.S. Department of Transportation, American Red Cross National Boating Survey, *A Study of Recreational Boats, Boaters, and Accidents in the United States,* Grant Agreement #1801.82, 1991.

12 Scientific Facts Show Heimlich Maneuver Best Method for Drowning Resuscitation

Henry J. Heimlich and Eric G. Spletzer

The Heimlich Institute has reviewed all available studies on the treatment of drowning from 1933 to 1995, a total of more than 400 scientific papers. The scientific data provided in this chapter proves that the Heimlich Maneuver is the best method for saving drowning victims. Not one scientific study showed mouth-to-mouth is effective for oxygenating drowning victims, without first draining water from the lungs. The Heimlich Maneuver is the only method that removes water from the lungs without instrumentation. The scientific facts concerning drowning and resuscitation are presented below, and references to medical journals and other sources in which the studies appear are provided so that readers may examine them in full to determine how to treat drowning victims.

WATER FILLS THE AIRWAYS IN 85–90% OF DROWNING VICTIMS

Joseph Ornato, past chairman of the American Heart Association (AHA) Committee on Special Resuscitation (drowning), reported in the *Journal of the American Medical Association*: "In humans, breath holding is frequently followed by laryngospasm of variable duration. Asphyxia eventually causes the glottis to relax and permits the lungs to fill with water in most, not all, humans who succumb to drowning. Ten percent to 15% of drowning victims maintain tight laryngospasm until death and do not aspirate at all."[1]

Jerome H. Modell, an advisor on drowning to the American Heart Association and the American Red Cross (ARC), reported in the *New England Journal of Medicine*, "Drowning, which is defined as suffocation by submersion, especially in water, occurs without actual aspiration of water in only approximately 7 to 10 percent of victims, while approximately 90 percent aspirate fluid … active respiration, not passive flow of water, determines the volume of water aspirated." (Water will not enter the lungs of a cadaver; the water is inhaled by drowning persons, which fills the lungs with water.)[2]

Drs. Nicholas Manolios and Ian Mackie (former chairman of the World Life Saving Association Medical Advisory Committee) reported in a study of drowning in Australia over a period of ten years that "A predisposing medical condition (proved at a coroner's autopsy) that likely contributed to the drowning was noted in 11 of the 100 victims, all of whom were male. Of these 11 victims, seven had a myocardial infarction, two victims had suffered a fractured cervical spine, one victim had asthma and one victim had suffered a subarachnoid hemorrhage."[3] Those who die of other causes before inhaling water do not have water in their lungs. They are not drowning victims.

Anatomy textbooks show the volume of the adult tracheobronchial tree is 170 ml (one half cup); therefore, only one half cup of water totally fills and blocks the entire airway.

WATER IN THE LUNGS CAUSES DEATH

L. Quan, chairperson of the 1992 American Heart Association Drowning Committee, reported in the medical journal *Annals of Emergency Medicine*:

> Time is the critical factor. Animal and multiple human studies in the past decades have shown that four to five minutes of anoxia is the limit that the submersion victim can most likely survive with a reasonable likelihood of good neurological outcome. However, submersion victims may suffer additional hypoxic injury after retrieval from the water.[4]

This means water in the lungs even after the drowning victim is on shore is equivalent to the victim still being submersed underwater. These drowning victims suffer brain and heart damage from prolonged asphyxia even when out of the water. Water must be removed from the lungs as soon as possible to enable oxygenation.

Quan also found that "bystander cardiopulmonary resuscitation was not associated with improved outcome in this study (of near-drowned children), which differs from reports in studies of adults with ventricular fibrillation who were resuscitated by Medic I."[5] The Medic I study, conducted in the same area, found that bystander CPR doubled cardiac arrest victims' survival rate.[6] Bystander CPR doubled the survival of older victims with damaged hearts in cardiac arrest, but did not improve outcome in previously healthy near-drowned children, because heart attack patients do not have water in their airways.

A report from the Institute of Medicine, a branch of the National Academy of Sciences, referenced a study that found when 100% oxygen was given by positive pressure mechanical ventilation to animals with water-filled lungs, half of the animals died. This outcome would have been worse with CPR, because it is impossible to get oxygen into water-filled lungs with mouth-to-mouth. No test animals died when water was drained from the lungs before ventilation. This result proves that water in the lungs causes drowning deaths.[7]

A Patrick Institute study reported that in a series of unconscious, non-breathing, pulseless drowning victims, 87% survived when the Heimlich Maneuver (a drainage step) was performed, whereas only 27% survived when CPR was performed without the Heimlich Maneuver (no drainage).[8]

As stated previously, none of the more than 400 scientific papers reviewed on the treatment of drowning from 1933 to 1995 showed mouth-to-mouth is effective for reoxygenating drowning victims, without first draining water from the lungs.

DOCUMENTED LIFEGUARD RESCUES SHOW HIGH MORTALITY AFTER CPR IN CONTRAST TO HIGH RECOVERY RATE WITH THE HEIMLICH MANEUVER

Quan also reported in the medical journal *Pediatrics* the following from a ten-year study of pediatric drownings she conducted in the Seattle area:

"In spite of lifeguard staffing, public and semi-public swimming pools still represent a risk for school-aged children. The large case fatality rate of 42% for submersions in the presence of lifeguards seems high."[9]

Tragically, nearly half of the children died after being pulled out by the lifeguards who were present. Lifeguards in this study were not permitted to use the Heimlich Maneuver, only CPR (no drainage). A 42% death rate of drownings in the presence of lifeguards should have caused concern about the method the lifeguards were being taught.

Ellis & Associates is responsible for training and certifying the lifeguards at 950 water parks, including Disney World, and numerous city pools. These lifeguards oversaw 58 million persons admitted to the parks in 1996. Ellis adopted the Heimlich Maneuver as the first step in its resuscitation protocol on January 1, 1995, after conducting an extensive examination of scientific studies of drowning. Of the 80 drowning victims Ellis lifeguards saved in the following two years, only one victim needed CPR. CPR was required in only one case because the Heimlich Maneuver, by pushing up on the diaphragm, jump-starts breathing (reported by Ellis lifeguards on the television broadcast *Inside Edition*, July 25, 1997).

Many documented reports of drowning rescues by highly qualified professionals show that the Heimlich Maneuver successfully revived drowning victims after CPR failed. These rescuers describe how water gushes from the mouths of victims with application of the Heimlich Maneuver, after which the victims recover. Among rescuers who have saved drowning victims with the Heimlich Maneuver after CPR failed are Dr. Victor Esch, chief medical advisor to the Washington, DC, Fire Department; Terry Watkins, emergency medical technician and chief of the Destin, Florida, fire department; and Ron Watson, vice president of the U.S. Lifesaving Association and park director of Jacksonville, Florida. In an official sheriff's report to the mayor, Mr. Watson stated, "Before you try to provide oxygen to the victim, it makes sense to clear water from the lungs."[10,11]

Since 1995, The Heimlich Institute has received more reports of drowning victim saves with the Heimlich Maneuver than of choking victim saves.

THE HEIMLICH MANEUVER REMOVES WATER FROM THE LUNGS

Dr. Peter Safar is the AHA/ARC advisor who established mouth-to-mouth as the accepted choice for emergency ventilation. In dog drowning studies done at the University of Pittsburgh, he proved that four Heimlich Maneuvers expelled all the water from the lungs of drowning dogs. In contrast, with dogs intubated with an endotracheal tube and lying horizontal, Safar reported it took ten minutes to drain the same amount of water from the lungs of the dogs.[12] Brain damage occurs in five minutes.

Horizontal drainage is only possible through an inserted endotracheal tube; the Heimlich Maneuver removes water from the lungs without instrumentation. Ellis & Associates found that the water is expelled from the lungs in six to nine seconds with the Heimlich Maneuver.

CPR CAUSES COMPLICATIONS AND DEATH

American Heart Association Guidelines for 1992 state:

> Even properly performed chest compressions can cause rib fractures in some patients. Other complications may occur despite proper CPR technique, including fracture of the sternum, pneumothorax, hemothorax, lung contusions, lacerations of the liver and spleen, and fat emboli.[13]

Paaske and associates reported an autopsy series of 323 persons who died after receiving CPR. The chest thrusts were performed by physicians in 90% of the total cases, and 80% of them were performed in a hospital. Chest thrusts resulted in rib fractures in 44% of cases, 21% of which were bilateral, and in two thirds of the cases these fractures were significant factors in the subsequent deaths. There were 22% sternal fractures and 13% heart lesions. One liver lesion occurred in a 13-year-old child, and Paaske and associates report other series in which this injury occurred in up to 20% of the cases. In 17% of cases the various lesions resulting from the chest thrusts were sufficiently severe to be a contributory cause of death.[14]

THE HEIMLICH MANEUVER IS SAFE

As Surgeon General, Dr. C. Everett Koop made the following declaration:

> Millions of Americans have been taught to treat persons whose airways are obstructed by a foreign body by administering back blows, chest thrusts, and abdominal thrusts. Now they must be advised that these methods are hazardous, even lethal. A back slap can drive a foreign object even deeper into the throat. *Chest and abdominal thrusts*, because they refer to blows to unspecified locations on the body, *have resulted in cracked ribs and damaged spleens and livers, among other injuries* ... The best rescue technique in any choking situation is the Heimlich Maneuver ... The Heimlich Maneuver is safe, effective, and easily mastered by the average person. It can be performed on standing or seated victims and on persons who have fallen to the floor. It can be performed on children and even on oneself.[15]

Tens of thousands of rescuers, trained or lay persons, throughout the world have, over the past 20 years, used the Heimlich Maneuver to save lives. There are nine known published case reports of serious injuries following the Heimlich Maneuver. As Surgeon General Koop stated, some of these injuries are the result of the American Red Cross using the lethal term "abdominal thrust." An abdominal thrust is not a Heimlich Maneuver. The correct descriptive term for the Heimlich Maneuver is "subdiaphragmatic pressure."[11]

CPR CAUSES VOMITING IN MOST DROWNING VICTIMS

American Heart Association Guidelines for 1992 state:

> The major problem associated with rescue breathing is gastric distension ... Marked distension of the stomach may promote regurgitation and reduce lung volume by elevating the diaphragm.[13]

Mouth-to-mouth resuscitation blows air into the stomach, especially in drowning victims because the airway is blocked with water.

Drs. Manolios and Mackie describe vomiting as "the scourge of resuscitation." They found that vomiting and/or regurgitation occurred in 86% (25/29) of drowning victims following CPR. In 13 patients, vomitus was responsible for the extreme difficulty that was experienced in maintaining a clear airway.[3]

In contrast, Patrick's study of 1,364 choking and drowning victims showed less than 3% vomited after the Heimlich Maneuver was performed.[16]

THE DANGER OF CPR TO VICTIMS WITH CERVICAL FRACTURES

Drowning victims with suspected fractured cervical spine are treated by immobilization of the head and neck. The greatest danger for these patients is performing mouth-to-mouth on them because mouth-to-mouth is effective only when the head is tilted backward. It is backward or forward bending of the head that causes transection of the cervical spinal cord.

After immobilization with a neck brace, the safest method to use is the Heimlich Maneuver because it is performed nowhere near the head. Since the water is ejected from the mouth, it will not be inhaled again.

DROWNING AND THE ABCs OF RESUSCITATION

The ABCs of resuscitation are **A**irway, **B**reathing, and **C**irculation.[13] Some organizations' recommendations for drowning consist of B and C (omitting A), because they incorrectly assume that the airway is not blocked when filled with fluid.

Since 85–90% of drowning victims' lungs are filled with water,[1] and given the safety of the Heimlich Maneuver and its proven ability to expel blocking fluid, the Heimlich Maneuver should be the first step applied in drowning resuscitation to ensure the airway is clear. The Heimlich Maneuver should be performed until water no longer flows from the mouth, which usually occurs after two to four applications, over a period of four to six seconds.

The ABCs of CPR continue to be the sequence when the Heimlich Maneuver is used to resuscitate drowning victims:

(A) *Airway* must be cleared from the mouth to alveoli (Heimlich Maneuver).
(B) Rescue *Breathing* (mouth-to-mouth).
(C) *Circulation* (chest compressions).

CONCLUSIONS

The scientific facts concerning drowning and resuscitation, including published case reports, prove that drowning victims die when their lungs fill with water. Air cannot get into water-filled lungs. The Heimlich Maneuver removes the water from the lungs in four to six seconds. Pressing upward on the diaphragm jump-starts breathing. Many drowning victims have been saved by rescuers performing the Heimlich Maneuver, even after CPR failed. The Heimlich Maneuver should be the first step in resuscitating a drowning victim, followed by CPR, if necessary.

More importantly, however, you now know the scientific facts. When faced with a drowning victim, you can make an informed decision. Can you in good conscience not use the procedure you know is the best lifesaving technique?

Furthermore, the American Academy of Pediatrics reports that most drownings of children take place in residential swimming pools where the first person on the scene is a parent or neighbor. There are 250 million Americans not trained in CPR, but who know how to perform the Heimlich Maneuver for choking victims or who can learn the Heimlich Maneuver in one minute. When the public knows that same Heimlich Maneuver saves drowning victims, 1,000 lives — mostly those of children — will be saved every year.

save a DROWNING victim
HEIMLICH MANEUVER®
You can't get air into the lungs until you get the water out!

STANDING IN A POOL OR SHALLOW WATER
Buoyancy Of Water Lightens Victim's Weight

1. Stand behind the victim and wrap your arms around victim's waist.

2. Make a fist and place the thumb side of your fist against the victim's abdomen, below the rib cage and above the navel.

3. Grasp your fist with your other hand and press into the victim's abdomen with a quick upward thrust.

4. Repeat until water no longer flows from mouth.

VICTIM LYING ON GROUND

1. Place victim on back. Turn face to one side to allow water to drain from mouth.

2. Facing victim, kneel astride victim's hips.

3. With one of your hands on top of the other, place the heel of your bottom hand on the abdomen below the rib cage and above the navel.

4. Use your body weight to press into the victim's abdomen with a quick upward thrust. Repeat until water no longer flows from mouth.

If the Victim has not recovered, proceed with CPR. The Victim should see a physician immediately after rescue.

REFERENCES

1. Ornato, J. P., 1986, "The resuscitation of near-drowning victims," *JAMA* 256: 75–77.
2. Modell, J. H., 1993, "Drowning," *New Eng. J. Med.* 328: 253–256.
3. Manolios, N. and Mackie, I., 1988, "Drowning and near-drowning on Australian beaches patrolled by life-savers: A 10-year study, 1973–1983," *Med. J. Aust.* 148:165–171.
4. Quan, L., 1993, "Drowning issues in resuscitation," *Ann. Emerg. Med.* 22: 366–369.
5. Quan, L., Wentz, K. R., Gore, E. J., and Copass, M. K., 1990, "Outcome and predictors of outcome in submersion victims receiving prehospital care in King County, Washington," *Pediatrics* 86: 586–593.
6. Thompson, R. G., Hallstrom, A. P., and Cobb, L. A., 1979, "Bystander-initiated cardiopulmonary resuscitation in the management of ventricular fibrillation," *Ann. Int. Med.* 90: 737–740.
7. Tütüncü, A. S., Faithfull, N. S., and Lachmann, B., 1993, "Comparison of ventilatory support with intratracheal perfluorocarbon administration and conventional mechanical ventilation in animals with acute respiratory failure," *Am. Rev. Resp. Dis.* 148: 785–792.
8. Patrick, E. A., 1995, "Resuscitation (Patrick-Heimlich method and other techniques): Pitfalls and other medicolegal/forensic scientific considerations," *Legal Med.* 77–115.
9. Quan, L., Gore, E. J., Wentz, K., Allen, J., and Novack, A. H., 1989, "Ten-year study of pediatric drownings and near-drownings in King County, Washington: Lessons in injury prevention," *Pediatrics* 83: 1035–1040.
10. Heimlich, H. J., Autumn 1996, "The Heimlich maneuver saves drowning victims," *Certified Pool Operator.*
11. Heimlich, H. J., 1975, "A life-saving maneuver to prevent food-choking," *JAMA* 234: 398–401.
12. Werner, J. Z., Safar, P., Bircher, N. G., Stezoski, W., Scanlon, M., and Stewart, R. D., 1982, "No improvement in pulmonary status by gravity drainage or abdominal thrusts after sea water near drowning in dogs," *Anesthesiology* 57 (Suppl. 3A): A81.
13. Emergency Cardiac Care Committee and Subcommittees, American Heart Association, 1992, "Guidelines for cardiopulmonary resuscitation and emergency cardiac care, II: Adult basic life support," *JAMA* 268: 2184–2198.
14. Paaske, F., Hart Hansen, J. P., Koudahl, G., and Olsen, J., 1968, "Complications of closed-chest cardiac massage in a forensic autopsy material," *Dan. Med. Bull.* 15: 225–230.
15. Koop, C. E., 1985, "The Heimlich Maneuver," *Pub. Health Rep.* 100: 557.
16. Patrick, E. A., 1980, "Choking: A questionnaire to find the most effective treatment," *Emergency* 12(7): 59–64.

13 Water Safety Measures for Hotels and Resorts

John R. Fletemeyer

The objective of this chapter is to recommend water safety standards for hotels and resorts that offer water recreational opportunities to their guests.

INTRODUCTION

A concept commonly known as "premises liability" makes hotel and resort owners, management, and staff responsible for keeping their premises safe. For establishments with swimming pools, ocean beaches, and/or lakefront premises, liability takes on an added significance because water represents an alien environment with many hidden and inherent hazards. In most cases, these hazards have the potential to cause serious injury (even death) if action is not taken to eliminate the hazard. When it is not practical to eliminate the hazards, appropriate warnings must be provided to guests. Failure to do so not only exposes guests to possible injuries but also exposes hotels and resorts to potentially devastating litigation.

In addition to premises liability, some states hold hotels and resorts to a higher duty because of their special relationship with their guests. This is called "innkeeper" or "common carrier" duty. The rationale for this higher standard of duty is that guests depend on proprietors to keep the premises safe; therefore, it is the responsibility of the hotel or resort to inspect its premises for safety hazards and then institute appropriate safety procedures and warnings.

While hotels and resorts bear the primary responsibility for maintaining their premises at an acceptable industry level for guests, this responsibility is not theirs alone. Guests must act "reasonably" in regard to their personal safety and to the safety of their immediate families. In some cases, this responsibility may extend to a small group, e.g., a scoutmaster charged with the responsibility of his troop.

If a guest fails to act reasonably when confronted with a known hazard, he or she may be held totally or partially accountable for whatever injury ensues or for the injury to an individual for whom he or she is responsible (Figure 1). For example, if a father leaves his son unattended at the pool where the boy fails to heed a "Danger No Diving" sign and consequently suffers a spinal injury, the father may be held responsible for his son's injury. In many cases involving water-related injuries, the courts have ruled according to the concept of "shared responsibility" where the hotel and the injured party were held jointly accountable for the injury as determined by a percentage.

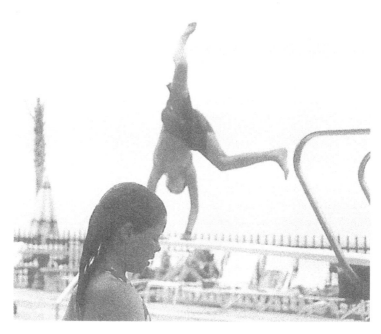

FIGURE 1   Boy doing a handstand off the diving board. Such behavior may lead to serious injury, and it is unlikely that a hotel would be held accountable because it is something a "reasonable" person would not do on a diving board.

An example is the above incident involving the father and his son. The court may find the father 75% liable for leaving his son by the pool and the hotel 25% liable for not providing an appropriate "No Diving" warning. Civil damages would then be awarded accordingly.

HOTEL AND RESORT WATER SAFETY PROGRAMS

Any hotel or resort that provides aquatic recreational opportunities has a duty to provide guests with a comprehensive water safety program. Such a program must include carefully identifying the type of guests staying on the premises, conducting a professional safety audit that attempts to identify all inherent dangers and risks associated with the aquatic facility, performing and documenting periodic safety inspections of the premises, and providing appropriate training to management and staff. When developing a safety program, the following considerations should be taken into account:

- What types of aquatic environments are located on the premises (pools, lakefront, beach, etc.)?
- What kinds of water recreational opportunities are offered to guests (wind surfing, kayaking, springboard diving, etc.)?
- What types of hazards are present, including those that can be eliminated and those that cannot be eliminated but require warnings?
- What are the local, state, and federal laws that relate to aquatic safety?
- What are the industry standards that govern aquatic safety?

IDENTIFYING GUEST DEMOGRAPHICS

The first step management must take when developing an aquatic safety program for its hotel or resort is to identify the demographic makeup of the clientele. This is necessary because in some cases when ethnically and/or geographically diverse groups use the premises different responses and considerations may be required to ensure their safety. For example, a hotel located in South Florida that attracts a large number of French-Canadian guests must provide written warnings in both French and English. Failure to take demographic considerations into account may potentially be regarded as negligent by the courts, especially in those states where hotels and resorts are held to a "higher level of duty."

The following real-life example helps us to better understand this consideration. In recent years a relatively large number of ocean drownings occurred when tourists were caught in rip currents — strong and temporary currents that run from the shore directly out to sea. A study conducted by the author (Fletemeyer, 1994) of the Panama City bathing population revealed that the majority of bathers using the beach were from inland states. Consequently, most of the bathers had little or no experience swimming in the ocean and were unfamiliar with the many inherent hazards present in this aquatic environment. The study indicated that most bathers were unaware of what to do when caught in a rip current. Based on the results of this study, it was recommended that a comprehensive public education program be conducted targeting out-of-state bathers and aiming to inform them about local marine hazards known to impact beach safety.

INSPECTING FOR HAZARDS

The second responsibility of management is to conduct a comprehensive safety audit of the premises. In most cases, it is unlikely that management will have the necessary background and expertise required to conduct a professional audit. Consequently, a risk-prevention expert with an aquatics background should be consulted to conduct this audit. If the safety audit reveals any unreasonable risks or safety hazards, it is incumbent upon management to take immediate action to either eliminate the risk or, if this is not possible, to provide appropriate warnings (Figure 2). Failure to respond in this manner places the hotel at a high level of liability exposure.

A safety audit should be accompanied by a written report and a formal meeting with management to discuss problems and suggest possible solutions. Audits

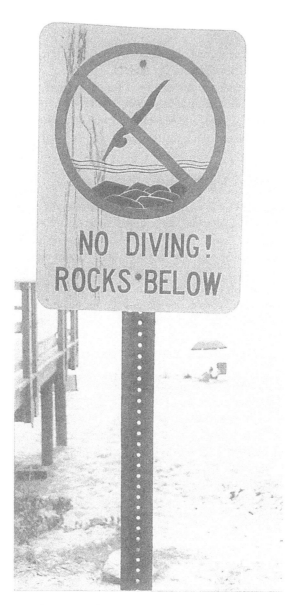

FIGURE 2   A resort takes appropriate measures to warn guests about a hazardous area with submerged rocks.

should never be considered a one-time task, because water environments, especially those associated with beaches and lakes, change constantly and must be periodically inspected.

Whenever possible, hazards identified in the audit should be eliminated. Removing a diving board from a pool is perhaps the best example of eliminating a hazard. Diving board-related injuries have been responsible for more litigation than any

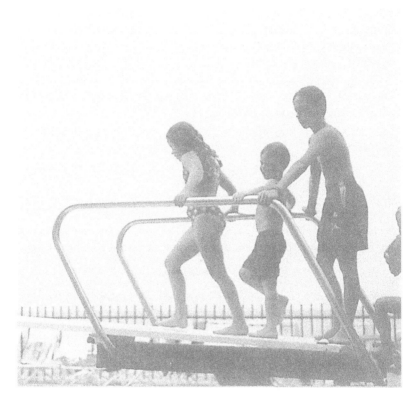

FIGURE 3 Diving board-related injuries are perhaps best prevented by removing the board.

other hazard in a pool environment (Figure 3). When it is not feasible to remove a hazard, appropriate warnings must be provided.

A monthly safety audit usually will be sufficient, but in some cases it may be necessary to conduct daily audits. Such daily audits tend to be less formal than a monthly audit and are sometimes called "safety inspections" to avoid confusion with the more formal safety audit. Safety inspections generally are conducted by a trained member of the hotel or resort staff, who attempts to identify risks and hazards known to materialize or occur over a period of time. Some examples of these appear in Table 1. Like the monthly audit, records should be maintained in a log in the event documentation is needed in defense litigation involving the injury of a guest.

RECORDKEEPING

Accurate recordkeeping should be considered a key element in any water safety program. Missing or sloppily maintained records have the potential of impacting a defense in a litigation proceeding. Accurate, well-maintained records and logs, on the other hand, may have the opposite effect. Records should be regularly inspected by management and should contain the following information:

- Results of the monthly audit, including management responses to problems
- Training of staff, including initial training and recurrent training. It is recommended that an evaluation instrument (test) of some kind be designed for each program
- Daily log record, including such information as water quality results in the case of pools, and water, current, and weather conditions in the case of lakes and the ocean
- Incident reports noting injuries to guests, first-aid administration, and rule violations
- Miscellaneous information, including the names of the on-duty staff and any other factors that might impact safety

---

TABLE 1
Inventory of some hazards that may occur over a relatively short time.

Pool	Ocean Beach
Broken glass	Broken glass and various kinds of debris
Vandalized or missing warning sign	Vandalized or missing warning sign
Loose electrical wire	Hypodermic needles
Loose or broken tile	Fish hooks
Loose hand rail	Rip currents
Broken gate latch	Underwater rock or debris
Misplaced shepherd's hook	Feeding fish
	Man-o-war
Detached depth marker or lane line	Jellyfish
	High energy waves
Missing drainage gate	Beach scraps
Slippery pool deck	Surfing or boat activity in designated bathing area

---

ESTABLISHING RULES

Pools and other water environments where recreational activities are conducted must have an established set of rules for the guest to follow (Figure 4). There are two general types of rules: safety rules and general purpose rules. An example of the latter would be to place used towels in a nearby hamper.

In many states rules governing commercial pools are determined by code or law. For example, in Florida, the Department of Health and Human Rehabilitation Services (HRS) defines a number of rules dealing with safety, bathing load, water chemistry, and pool construction. National organizations such as the United States Lifesaving Association (USLA) and the YMCA help to set guidelines for rules involving the ocean and other open-water environments.

Once hotel or resort management has identified the appropriate rules for its facility, they should be posted at all access points, using a method that makes them clearly visible. Rules partially hidden by a tree branch or a building structure provide

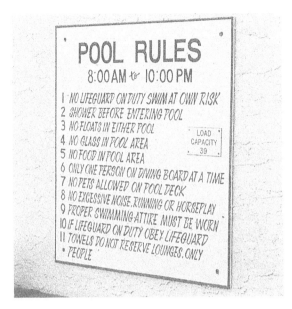

FIGURE 4   An example of general rules and safety rules. Since these rules do not include some basic safety precautions, such as "no diving headfirst" and "no alcoholic beverages," they are not adequate for the premises.

excellent ammunition for litigators. Posting pool rules is facilitated by national vendors who sell signs with standard rules.

Certain pool rules, if not followed by guests, become life threatening and sometimes merit special warnings. A rule prohibiting diving headfirst into shallow water, for example, may require a separate sign that meets American National Standards Institute (ANSI) guidelines.

One particular hazard requiring a rule and strict enforcement that is frequently ignored by hotels and reports involves consumption of alcohol on the pool deck or on the beach. Regarding the beach, some qualification is needed, because, in some cases, although a hotel or resort may be located in an area designated as beachfront, the actual sand may be owned and controlled by a public entity. In Florida, for example, the area between the water and the mean high-tide line is owned and controlled by the state. It should be noted that the rule prohibiting the consumption of alcohol is well justified because statistics reveal that a relatively high percentage of drownings involve victims who had been drinking previously.

SAFETY EQUIPMENT

Every hotel and resort is required to have some basic safety equipment. In some cases, this is mandated by the state while in others, it is mandated by industry-accepted standards. All pools, regardless of size, must have a shepherd's hook located within visual range of all parts of the pool deck. Pools must also have a ring buoy or throw buoy attached to 3/8-inch polypropylene line that is at least 50% longer

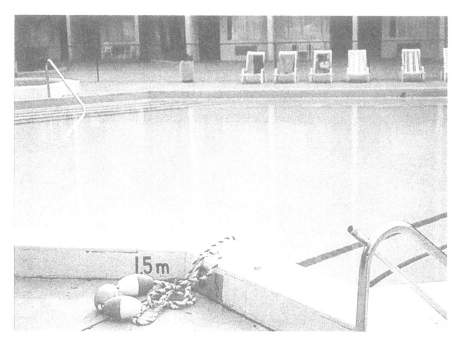

FIGURE 5 The purpose of a daily safety inspection is to identify problems that could lead to injury of a guest. Here a detached deep water/shallow water buoy line could lead to drowning.

than the length of the pool. In the case of lakes and beaches, a line 200 ft long should be attached to a throw bag. Beyond this length, throw bags are usually not very effective.

Another important equipment item is a floating pool line that marks the location where the shallow end of the pool meets the deep part. Usually this line has a number of small buoys strung through it to increase its visibility and buoyancy. It is important to permanently secure the line to both sides of the pool so bathers cannot detach the line. It is not uncommon for a bather intent on swimming laps to remove the pool line (Figure 5). It is incumbent upon management to make frequent inspections of the line to ensure that it is secure.

A dedicated emergency telephone line should be located in close proximity to the pool, beach, or lake. Figure 6 shows a dedicated emergency phone located on the beach next to a popular Florida resort and hotel. Clear instructions should be posted regarding how to use the phone in the event of emergency. The phone should be checked daily by a staff member and the operational status noted in a log book.

All hotels and resorts should have a well-stocked first-aid kit on the premises. Deciding what to include in the kit may be confusing; however, ready-stocked kits are available. Depleted supplies should be replaced immediately (Figure 7).

Plastic can buoys or tube buoys are important equipment for hotels and resorts with open-water environments. These buoys should be strategically located on the

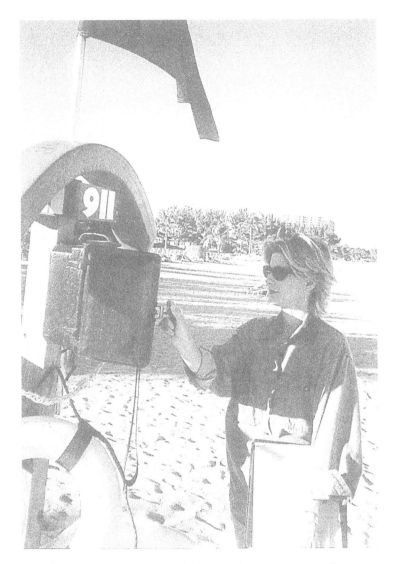

FIGURE 6 An example of a dedicated emergency phone line.

waterfront so they can be used by guests or staff in the event of emergency. It is necessary to periodically check buckles and straps attached to buoys because they often become frayed over time and must be replaced.

Other safety equipment may be used to further enhance a hotel or resort's water safety program. In areas where severe and frequent electrical storms occur, a lighting detector may be used to sound a warning for bathers to leave the water. Another safety item gaining in popularity and acceptance is a "CPR PROMPT." This device provides verbal instructions to a rescuer on how to administer CPR to a victim.

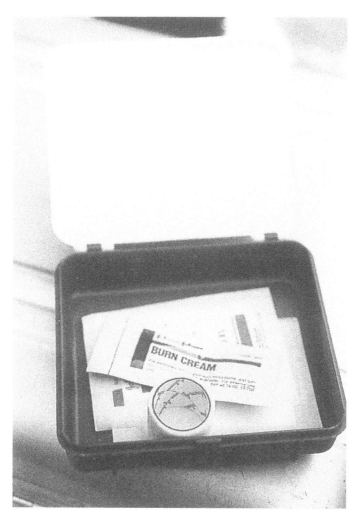

FIGURE 7   Inspection of a first-aid kit discloses a lack of essential items.

Because of the possibility of back or head injury, spinal boards equipped with cervical collars are recommended. Before this equipment is placed on the premises, staff members must be trained in its use. This usually requires training at the "Advanced" first-aid or "First Responder" level. Improper use of a spine board or placing the wrong size cervical collar on a victim could cause additional trauma.

WARNING SIGNS

A fundamental assumption about the use of warning signs is that once an individual is informed about the risks associated with a particular hazard, he or she will act responsibly. A review of the literature on this subject indicates little evidence to support this notion. Studies on the effectiveness of warning signs reveal that warning signs are often ignored for the following reasons:

- They are confusing or ambiguous.
- They are placed in inappropriate locations making them difficult to read.
- They are not obeyed because individuals may have motives for ignoring them.

Despite evidence that warning signs often are not heeded, they nevertheless represent an important element in any hotel or resort's water safety program. To increase the level of effectiveness of warning signs, they should be designed according to the guidelines set forth in the ANSI "Specifications for Accident Prevention Signs" (Z35.1-1973). The objective of this publication is to develop a standard format for constructing warning signs. For a warning sign to be effective, it must meet the following criteria:

- The message must be clearly received.
- The message must be comprehended.
- The message must be acted upon in an appropriate way.

When designing a warning sign for a water-related hazard, it is important to consider that guests who wear corrective lenses often leave them in their rooms before going to the pool or beach. Consequently, it is prudent to take this behavior into consideration and increase the size of the letters beyond ANSI requirements.

The fact that many guests are from different countries and cannot read or speak English significantly reduces the effectiveness of written warnings. A solution to this problem is to use nonverbal symbols to convey the warning. Usually a nonverbal warning consists of a particular symbol indicating a particular behavior and a circle with a slash running through it meaning "NO." An example of an international warning sign appears in Figure 8. This sign is commonly used on beaches to warn bathers of dangerous rip currents.

Despite the advantage of using nonverbal signs, Pepper (1989) previously reports in *Warning Signs, Why Do They Fail?* that quite often nonverbal warnings are not heeded because the symbols are too abstract, which makes them confusing. In various studies on this subject, the comprehension rate of nonverbal signs was 20–40% (Fletemeyer, unpublished).

For a variety of reasons, warning signs used to inform guests about particular water hazards are not always effective. Consequently, management must use other strategies in conjunction with signage to protect guests.

WARNING FLAGS

Another type of nonverbal warning hotels and resorts sometimes use is the flag warning (Figure 9). Evidence shows that perhaps as many as 74% of those who come to the beach rely on flags for information (Fletemeyer, 1994); however, as

DANGER
RIP
CURRENTS
No Swimming

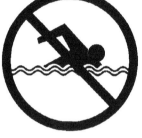

FIGURE 8   Example of international-type warning about rip currents.

is the case with sign warnings, there is little evidence that flags are effective. A paper that focused on developing effective warnings (Fletemeyer, 1995) noted that flag symbols require individuals to have previous knowledge about what the various colors represent. Without this prior knowledge, flags are useless, and, because there is no uniform code, warning flag information is often confusing (Figure 9).

An inspection of a number of Florida beaches using warning flag systems revealed that information posted about the meanings of flag colors was seldom consistent. On one beach, for example, a blue flag was posted to convey safe water conditions, while, on a neighboring beach, a green flag was flown to convey the same message about the water conditions. On yet another beach, yellow and red flags were flown at the same time (Figure 10); it is not known what this was meant to convey. To add to the confusion, flag systems used in different countries may have entirely different meanings and colors. For a flag system to be effective, a uniform standard must be adopted. The following uniform standard is recommended:

GREEN   Safe conditions prevail — No apparent safety hazards.

YELLOW   Caution — Unsafe hazards may be present. Experienced swimmers only.

RED   Danger — Life-threatening hazards exist. No swimming.

Another problem associated with a flag warning system relates to the fact that ocean conditions are constantly changing. For flags to be effective, they must be changed frequently to reflect existing ocean conditions.

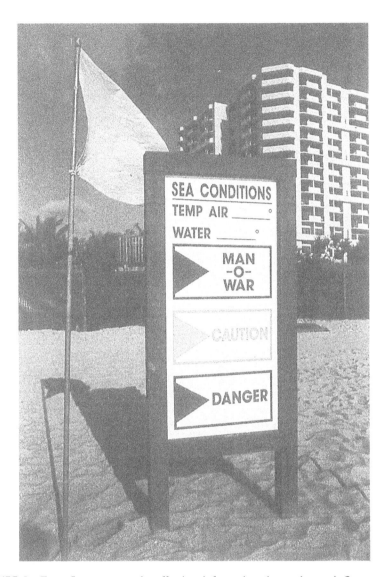

FIGURE 9   For a flag system to be effective, information about what each flag represents must be provided. This information often is confusing because there is no industry standard.

CONDITION BOARDS

Many hotels and resorts use condition boards to convey information about hazardous conditions (Figure 11). Condition boards have the advantage of presenting more accurate and detailed information about conditions. Like the flag system, they must be updated frequently to reflect changes. If they are not changed, a hotel or resort can be held accountable if the water conditions are implicated in injury to a guest.

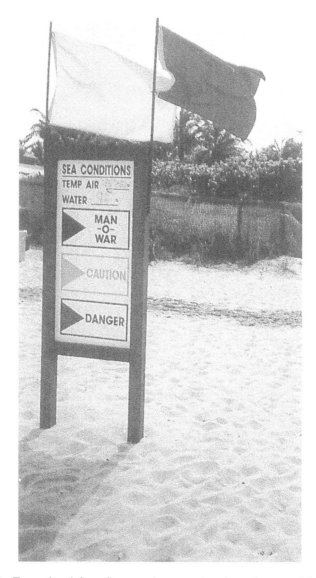

FIGURE 10   Two colored flags flown at the same time have the potential of sending a confusing message to bathers.

To remedy this potential problem, management must give staff a written directive detailing when a condition board should be changed. Any changes should be recorded in a daily log book.

A second problem with condition boards is that they are sometimes not easily seen by the public. Condition boards must always be strategically placed, and the public must be informed about their location. Failure to follow these guidelines may constitute negligence.

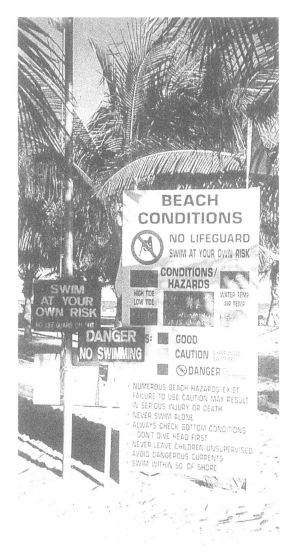

FIGURE 11 Example of a condition board that conveys information about rules and water conditions. For such boards to be effective, they must be updated frequently to reflect current water conditions.

INFORMATION BROCHURES

Information brochures are of value, provided that they are accurately and systematically distributed to guests. Perhaps the best time for distribution is during check-in time by the desk clerk. It is recommended that brochures contain the following information:

- Types of aquatic environments located on premises, i.e., beach, pools, lake, etc.
- Types of recreational opportunities being offered, i.e., scuba diving, sailing, windsurfing, kayaking, etc.
- A description of hazards that may be present
- Warning that there are **no** lifeguards on the premises and swimming is at your own risk
- Pool and/or beach rules including:
  — Never swim alone
  — Never leave children unattended
  — Never drink alcoholic beverages and swim
  — Never dive headfirst into shallow water
  — Never swim in rip currents
  — Never swim far from shore
- Methods of receiving information about the status of hazards, such as condition boards, telephone lines noting weather and beach conditions, flags, etc.
- Procedure for dealing with a water-related emergency, including how to contact help

If hotels regularly attract guests from foreign countries, information brochures written in different languages should be distributed accordingly.

TELEPHONE AND TV INFORMATION LINES

Another way of disseminating information about water safety is through a dedicated telephone information line and by an in-house closed circuit TV system. Local conditions can be recorded on the telephone system answering machine for guests to access.

Many large hotels and resorts have a special information channel that presents information about the premises, including rules and regulations.

LIFEGUARDS

Some large hotels and resorts have incorporated professional lifeguards into their safety programs. While scientific data regarding the benefit of lifeguards is meager, there is little doubt among professionals that lifeguards are responsible for preventing many serious injuries. In Chapter 10, Brad Keshlear notes that a significantly lower drowning rate occurs in areas with lifeguards versus areas without lifeguards.

Despite the increased level of safety that lifeguards provide, many hotels and resorts are reluctant to provide this service to their guests. There are two reasons for this. The first is economical. The second relates to the fact that liability exposure may increase if a lifeguard is present when a guest suffers a water-related injury

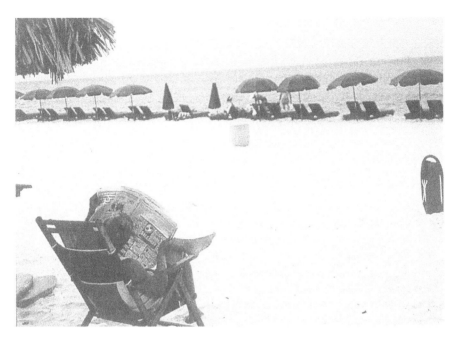

FIGURE 12   Lifeguards offer an enhanced level of water safety to guests at hotels and resorts; however, lifeguards who do not meet professional levels of conduct and behavior may expose the resort to liability. Here, a lifeguard reading a newspaper is guilty of a breach of conduct.

(Figure 12). Lifeguards also may create some logistical problems that a hotel or resort is ill-equipped to handle, including certification updates, scheduling, recurrent training, and equipment issues.

To date, there is no industry standard requiring lifeguards at hotels and resorts. In areas where injury and/or drowning rates are high, or in areas of unusual circumstances, it may be prudent to offer lifeguard services. In Panama City, for example, where there is a history of high annual drowning rates, a study (Fletemeyer, 1994) to determine if cultural factors contribute to the large number of drownings on this beach found that most bathers were from outside Panama City and from states without beaches. This study also found that bathers did not have an extensive swimming background. The conclusion was that these two variables were largely responsible for the high drowning rate on Panama City beaches. Another conclusion was that local beachfront hotels had a duty to provide lifeguards because of the lack of ocean experience and the poor swimming ability of the "typical" guests.

The Panama City study indicates it may be prudent for other hotels and resorts to provide lifeguards. Before such a determination can be made, however, professional assessments should be made at each resort and hotel to identify the characteristics of the guests and any particular water hazards located on the premises.

OPERATIONS MANUAL

An operations manual should be an essential element of a hotel or resort's water safety program. It can either stand alone as a separate document or be incorporated into an existing operations manual as a section or chapter. An operations manual should contain the following items:

- The stated objective of the manual
- A statement of the chain of command, including who is in charge and a description of personnel duties and responsibilities
- A list of subordinates, including a description of their responsibilities
- A description of a daily protocol, including designated work area and how daily inspections are to be conducted and recorded
- Policies and procedures regarding how and when to take breaks
- Policies and procedures regarding how to respond to an emergency
- Policies and procedures regarding when and how periodic safety audits are to be conducted and reported to management
- Policies and procedures regarding rules and how to enforce them
- Policies and procedures regarding who to contact in an emergency
- Policies and procedures regarding when a pool or beach is to be opened and closed for bathing and related recreational activities
- Policies and procedures determining the bathing load
- Policies and procedures regarding contact with and statements to the press following injury to a guest

Since writing a policies and procedures manual for a hotel or resort water safety program is a complicated process, it is recommended that a water safety expert be consulted to assist in this capacity.

CONCLUSION

All hotels and resorts that offer aquatic recreational opportunities to guests have a legal and moral responsibility for their safety. This responsibility begins with a risk management audit that attempts to define all potential hazards (permanent and temporary) on the premises. Once these hazards are identified, management must take steps to either eliminate the hazards, usually by removing them (e.g., removing a diving board), or provide appropriate warnings enabling guests to make a reasonable and informed decision to avoid the hazard.

Since water environments are dynamic, especially open-water environments such as lakes and oceans, additional safety audits may be necessary. In many cases, daily inspections by properly trained staff may be necessary.

In most cases, a water safety program consists of a number of elements designed to increase safety, which, when combined, must meet or even exceed a "standard" all hotels and resorts must strive to meet. Failure to achieve this standard exposes a hotel, its owners, management, and staff to the possibility of being sued if a guest is injured and negligence is proven.

No safety measure discussed in this chapter is intended to stand alone. Warning signs, for example, are essential, but not sufficient, to ensure the safety of guests. When signs are used in conjunction with other safety measures, they become crucial and essential elements of the safety process.

Since hotel and resort water safety program standards are constantly changing, it is critical that management remain current about changes within the industry. This can be accomplished by reading literature and attending seminars and water safety courses.

REFERENCES

Fletemeyer, J., 1994, *Panama Beach Safety Study.* Report prepared for Florida Beach Patrol Chiefs Association, pp. 1–7.
Pepper, P., 1989, *Warning Signs, Why Do They Fail?* National Safety Council Study.

14 Reflections on Lifeguard Surveillance Programs

Frank Pia

STATEMENT OF THE PROBLEM

Lifeguarding seems to be in a state of change. In the attempt to reduce drowning by training new lifeguards and retraining experienced lifeguards, new perspectives, ideas, terms, concepts, and training programs are constantly being proposed.

Public health officials, lifeguard training agencies, and experts in the field of lifeguarding agree that the recognition of drowning persons is a critical skill lifeguards must develop. Drownings occur in supervised areas because lifeguards lack this skill. Intrusions and distractions, the other two factors shown to be causal elements in these drownings, are presented in the article "The RID Factor as a Cause of Drowning."[1]

A New York State Health Department study on the causes of drownings while lifeguards were on duty noted instances when drowning persons displayed the behavior of the Instinctive Drowning Response; however, because of inadequate training, the lifeguards on duty did not recognize the signs of drowning. They dismissed the drowning person's behavior as "someone merely playing in the water."[2] A statement by the Service National des Sauveteurs (National Lifeguard Service) to a coroner's inquest in Montreal also noted the need to train lifeguards in distressed swimmer and drowning persons recognition skills and cited the role of the RID Factor in drownings.[3]

The aim of this chapter is to provide the reader with an understanding of contemporary water crisis recognition theory. This understanding is necessary because, in trying to establish patron surveillance programs, professionals often feel they are "drowning" in a flood of confusing terminology and behavioral descriptions. To help the reader evaluate patron surveillance programs, a historical review and critical analysis of the terms *distress, drowning,* and *behavior* vs. *trait-centered recognition concepts*[4] will be undertaken.

This historical method will provide an organizing scheme for student and professional alike since many of the current "big questions" about water crisis recognition training programs for lifeguards were asked decades ago. This method will help the reader to trace the evolution of this type of training over the past 40 years.

This chapter will not use the traditional lifeguarding term "victim" when referring to a distressed swimmer or a drowning person. Epidemiologists tell us this term carries a negative connotation. They recommend that the term be avoided when describing or referring to an injured person.

Different uses of the terms *distress* and *drowning* in lifeguard training textbooks have caused unclear references to the behavior that lifeguards should be trained to both recognize and react to. A critical training issue emerges when we frame recognition and rescue objectives for the lifeguard. If there is neither a theoretical difference (both terms mean the same thing) nor a behavioral difference (both behaviors are the same), then only a single term should be used and only one rescue technique taught. Since a dictionary helps systematize the way words or concepts are used in everyday life, this will be the starting point of the analysis.

The following excerpts are from the definition of the word *distress* in *Webster's New Ninth Collegiate Dictionary.*[5] Distress implies an external and often temporary cause of great physical or mental strain and stress, hence the attachment of the prefix *di* (double) to the root word *stress*, implying double stress. Other definitions include "to subject to great strain or difficulties or to cause to worry or to be troubled." The common themes that recur in the various definitions of *distress* are *physical* or *mental strain* or *trouble*.

Using the same dictionary to define *drowning*, a sharp distinction between *drowning* and *distress* emerges. The term *drown* is defined as "to become drowned." The behavioral definition "to suffocate by submersion especially in water" helps us by noting a crucial difference between the two terms. Research by the author has revealed that the actual or perceived feelings of suffocation in the water trigger universal unlearned behavior — the Instinctive Drowning Response — that life-guards must be trained to detect.[6]

In distress situations, the rescuer looks for an individual experiencing great physical or mental stress or strain in the water. In drowning situations, the lifeguard scans for an individual who is suffocating in the water.

If the differences between *distress* and *drowning* were merely semantic, we would not spend time debating trivial terminology. Underlying the terms *distress* and *drowning* is the primary question of lifeguards' scanning of bathing areas: What behavioral signs must the lifeguards identify?

REVIEW OF LITERATURE

The first published classification of the behavioral differences between *distress* and *drowning* were presented in the lifeguard training film *On Drowning.*[7] This 16mm documentary film, made at Orchard Beach, Bronx, New York, during the 1970 bathing season, recorded the movements of people drowning and being rescued. A detailed explanation of the differences between *distress* and *drowning* were presented in the 1974 article "Observations on the Drowning of Nonswimmers" in the YMCA publication *Journal of Physical Education.*[8]

Beginning in 1974, references to the original research regarding the difference between *distress* and *drowning* have been incorporated in the following lifeguard textbooks and manuals: *Alert*, the lifeguard training manual of the Royal Life-saving Society Canada[9]; *The Canadian Lifesaving Manual*, also from the Royal

Lifesaving Society Canada[10]; *Modern Concepts in Lifeguarding,* ALT International[11]; *Lifeguard Training,* The American National Red Cross[12]; *On the Guard II,* the YMCA Society of North America[13]; *Lifeguarding in the Waterparks*, Huint's definitive textbook on the subject[14]; *Lifeguarding Today,* The American National Red Cross[15]; and the U.S. Lifesaving Association's *Manual of Open Water Lifesaving.*[16] These textbooks point out that distressed individuals were not yet drowning and because of a swimming or floating skill were able to summon help by waving or calling out. Generally, these publications are in agreement that drowning persons are neither able to call out for help because they are suffocating in the water nor able to wave for help because, in their moments of peril, they lack a swimming or floating skill.

BEHAVIOR-CENTERED SURVEILLANCE

These concepts of *distress* and *drowning* are the foundations of bather-centered surveillance. The basic premise of behavior-centered surveillance is that a lifeguard's determination of a person's difficulty in the water must always be based on a person's behavior, not on physical characteristics such as age, weight, or ethnic or racial background. Implicit in this approach is the belief that scanning is a task that requires constant observation and evaluation of the behavior of all bathers.

The most efficient way for lifeguards to maintain surveillance over people at their facilities is to understand the behavior that indicates that a person is in distress or drowning and to evaluate a patron's movements against four target behaviors. The four target behaviors a lifeguard looks for while scanning a bathing area are breathing, arm and leg motions, body position, and movement in the water. The reader is encouraged to read Table 5-1 in *Lifeguarding Today* which compares the movements of swimmers, distressed swimmers, and both active and passive drowning persons.[17]

DISTRESS

Lifeguards can recognize distressed swimmers by the way they support themselves in the water and by their voluntary actions. Because of their swimming or floating skills, persons in distress have enough control of their arms and legs to keep their mouths above the surface of the water. Although distressed swimmers may use inefficient swimming strokes and might be unable to move to safety, they can continue breathing in a labored way and may call for help.

Another characteristic that differentiates distressed swimmers from drowning persons is that the distressed swimmers have voluntary control over their movements. Movements that attempt but fail to make any progress toward safety, trying to use another patron for support, and waving or calling out for help all signal the lifeguard — and often other patrons — that help is needed.

It has been documented that in times of acute stress the autonomic nervous system (ANS) causes an increase in pulse rate, breathing rate, and blood pressure. These phenomena generally cannot be observed by lifeguards while they are scanning a bathing area. It is only when ANS functions lead to observable voluntary behavior such as waving and calling out for help, the inability to swim or move to safety, or grabbing another patron, that the lifeguards react and initiate rescue procedures.

As conditions such as fatigue, becoming chilled, the progress of a sudden illness, or a rip current continue to affect distressed swimmers, they are less able to support themselves in the water. Distressed swimmers most often are found at surf or open-water beaches, and the USLA estimates that rip currents at surf beaches account for more than 80% of rescues at these locations.[18]

Anxiety increases as these conditions cause the person's mouth to come closer to the surface of the water. If distressed swimmers are not rescued, they begin to drown.

This description of distressed swimmers' behavior does not mean there is always a transition from *distress* to *drowning* behavior. On the contrary, data indicates that most drowning persons do not pass through the distress stage, but almost immediately go from a position of safety into Instinctive Drowning Response behavior.[19]

DROWNING BEHAVIOR

As mentioned earlier, an active drowning person struggles on the surface of the water in a highly predictable, patterned, and — to the trained eye — recognizable way. The Instinctive Drowning Response represents a person's attempts to avoid actual or perceived suffocation in the water. The key concept in understanding a drowning person's behavior is to keep in mind that suffocation in water triggers a constellation of ANS responses that lead to external, unlearned, instinctive drowning movements. Research has shown that this response is present whenever and wherever active drownings occur (pools, lakes, beaches, rivers, and water parks).

The reader must keep in mind that the drowning process starts at the point when persons are no longer able to keep their mouths above the surface of the water. The aspiration of water which leads to a wet or dry drowning occurs at a later point in the drowning process, so it is misleading to tell lifeguards that distress includes all behavior until the aspiration of water occurs, and that drowning includes all subsequent behavior.

CHARACTERISTICS OF THE INSTINCTIVE DROWNING RESPONSE

The following information describes the movements of the Instinctive Drowning Response, explains why certain behaviors occur or do not occur, and offers insights into what physiological processes prompt the drowning person's movements. The Instinctive Drowning Response is a group of signs that collectively indicate an active drowning is occurring and differentiate drowning from the distress.

The first characteristic of Instinctive Drowning Response is that persons who are drowning, except in very rare circumstances, are physiologically unable to call out for help. The respiratory system is designed for breathing; speech is the secondary or overlaid function.[20] This means the primary function — breathing — must be satisfied, before the secondary function — speech — occurs.

The second reason drowning persons cannot call out for help is their mouths alternately sink below and reappear above the surface of the water. The mouths of drowning persons are not above the surface of the water long enough for them to exhale, inhale, and call out for help.

When drowning persons' mouths are above the surface, they exhale and quickly inhale as their mouths begin to sink below the surface of the water. While their mouths are below the surface of the water, drowning persons generally keep their mouths tightly closed to avoid swallowing water.

The second characteristic of the Instinctive Drowning Response is that drowning persons cannot wave for help. Immediately after drowning persons begin gasping for air, they are instinctively forced to extend their arms laterally and begin to press down on the surface of the water with their arms and hands. This response, over which the drowning person has no voluntary control, renders them unable to wave for help.

The arm movements of drowning persons are intended to keep their heads above water so they can continue to breathe. By pressing down on the surface of the water, they lift their mouths out of the water to breathe.

The third characteristic of the Instinctive Drowning Response is that drowning persons cannot voluntarily control their arm movements. Physiologically, a drowning person who is struggling at the surface of the water cannot stop drowning to perform voluntary movements such as waving for help, moving toward a rescuer, or reaching out for a piece of rescue equipment. These actions require a swimming or floating skill, which, using the definition of the term *drowning*, drowning persons do not have.

When a drowning person grabs a rescuer, it is because the rescuer did not provide enough support to stop the Instinctive Drowning Response. Rather, the rescuer only provided the drowning person enough support to use either the rescuer or the rescue device as a base of support to grab the lifeguard. In such cases, lifeguards did not provide the drowning persons enough support to convince them they were no longer suffocating.

The fourth characteristic of the Instinctive Drowning Response is that the drowning person's body is perpendicular to the surface of the water and unable to move in a horizontal or diagonal direction. There is no evidence of a supporting kick.

The fifth characteristic of the Instinctive Drowning Response is that drowning persons struggle at the surface of the water 20–60 seconds. This data was obtained and validated over a 21-year period at Orchard Beach, Bronx, New York, where 40,000 rescues, an average of 2,000 per summer, occurred.

Observations at Orchard Beach also revealed that drowning persons were often surrounded by patrons who did not realize that a drowning was occurring nearby. It is imperative that new lifeguards be trained to recognize and rely upon the signs of drowning to begin their rescue procedure and not wait for patrons or more experienced lifeguards to tell them that a person is drowning.

Because manipulation of variables in my observational drowning studies at Orchard Beach were neither ethically nor morally possible, the only way to obtain this data was direct observation of drowning persons during rescues. This methodology followed the qualitative research methods noted by Patton[21] and others.

This behavior of drowning persons, originally studied at Orchard Beach in the 1950s and 1960s, and then written about in the 1970s, has been shown to exist in other areas. The confirmation for this conclusion is letters and telephone calls from lifeguards, parents, camp counselors, and park employees who noted that drowning person recognition concepts contained in *On Drowning,*[22] *Drowning: Facts & Myths,*[23] and *The Reasons People Drown*[24] enabled them to identify a drowning person who was surrounded by bathers who did not recognize the Instinctive Drowning Response.

Further validation of the existence of the Instinctive Drowning Response can be found in the Binghampton Tape,[25] a videotape that shows a firefighter being caught in a hydraulic at the base of a low-head dam. Although the firefighter was fully clothed, and alternatively pulled below and recirculated above the surface of the water, the Instinctive Drowning Response was observed as he struggled to stay afloat at the surface of the water.

Another piece of dramatic footage that illustrated the Instinctive Drowning Response was the rescue of an airline passenger that occurred in cold water near Dulles International Airport, in Washington, DC. The arm movements of the person being rescued clearly illustrated the presence of the Instinctive Drowning Response in cold water.[26]

The final support for the existence of Instinctive Drowning Response can be found in the instructional tape *In Too Deep.*[27] Using the documentary style of *On Drowning,* footage of near-drownings and rescues at Dorney Park was recorded.

Having defined behavior-centered surveillance and established the existence of the Instinctive Drowning Response and the characteristics that differentiate it from the behavior of distressed swimmers, the next section of this chapter will examine the ways *distress* and *drowning* are used in other lifeguard-training programs. In addition, trait-centered surveillance, the method of using external characteristics to predict people's behavior and then designate them as "high-risk guests" will be discussed.

In 1983, Ellis & Associates offered a new definition of the term *distress*. Two events — the expansion during the past few years of this program from the water park environment into pools and still water areas and the listing of 10 characteristics of distress — have led to confusion as to which water crisis recognition concepts lifeguard training agencies should use. The confusion is greatest when a lifeguard service has supervisors or staff members whose training backgrounds cause them to use different definitions of *distress* and *drowning*.

In the National Pool and Waterpark Lifeguard/CPR textbook, *distress* describes any individual "experiencing difficulty" in the water. People in distress are given characteristics, categorized as conscious or unconscious, and then found on the surface, just below the surface within arm's reach, or below the surface beyond arm's reach.[28]

The greatest source of confusion has been this organization's listing of certain Instinctive Drowning Response characteristics under the category of *distress*. This confusion is then compounded by including certain behaviors which persons may be experiencing but which are not observable to lifeguards.

NATIONAL POOL AND WATER PARK DISTRESS CRITERIA

The National Pool and Waterpark Lifeguard/CPR textbook notes one of the first indicators of distress in individuals is eyes wide open or tightly shut. For this characteristic to be useful to lifeguards scanning a bathing area, it must accompanied by other behavioral descriptors. Lifeguards cannot use this criteria if the persons being observed are turned away from the lifeguards or at a distance where lifeguards cannot, without binoculars, observe the persons' eyes.

Another characteristic of distress presented in this text is that the individual's body may be stiff or tense. It is extremely difficult, if not impossible, for a lifeguard to make this determination when most of a person's body is submerged in the water.

The third distress criteria cited is conscious victims who are in a diagonal or vertical position. This characteristic is consistent with the "a" distress indicator used by other agencies.

The fourth behavior of distressed persons is that "their arms flail up and down or reach and grab." While distressed swimmers may reach and grab for persons and objects, drowning persons, unless incorrectly supported by the rescuer, do not have the swimming or floating skills that enable them to perform these actions. It is incorrect to state that a drowning person is flailing in the water. Drowning persons use the surface of the water to press down upon to raise their mouths out of the water.

The fifth characteristic of distress is "their heads are back with their mouths gasping for air." Published research, which predated the NPWP program by more than a decade, clearly established that feelings of suffocation can sometimes cause this behavior, which is characteristic of drowning and not distress.

The sixth characteristic is that "no leg movement is evident." While this statement is true about drowning persons, distressed swimmers use their legs to support themselves while they wave for help or move toward shore or another swimmer.

The seventh characteristic states that "distressed persons are disorientated." For this characteristic to be useful to lifeguards scanning a bathing area, it must be accompanied by behavioral descriptors.

The next two characteristics of distress are that the persons are "unconscious in either a limp or rigid form" and there is "no body movement." These characteristics describe the behavior of someone suffocating in the water and should therefore be placed in the drowning category.

The tenth characteristic is that the "person may be trying to grasp an object to get support. This may be either a lane line, inner tube, or another guest." This behavior belongs with the distressed swimmer criteria cited earlier.

After listing ten characteristics of distress, the NPWP also notes a person in distress quickly can become a drowning victim who usually follows a pattern of reactions. Knowledge of the factors in the drowning process, specifically the

Five Stages of Drowning, and the difference between wet and dry drownings are thought to help lifeguards recognize a drowning.

Before examining the applicability of using the *Five Stages of Drowning* to teach recognition skills, it would be useful to review the animal research studies that led to the formulation of the five stages of drowning. In his article, *Water in the Lungs of Drowned Animals,* Peter Karpovich, M.D., described the drowning of rats, guinea pigs, and cats in a flat-walled aquarium that facilitated the accurate observation of all stages of drowning.[29] He notes that, while the behavior of these animals varied somewhat upon being submerged, he was able to divide the entire phenomenon into five stages. Lougheed, Janes, and Hall described the same five-stage process for dogs.[30] In his textbook, *The Pathophysiology and Treatment of Drowning and Near-Drowning,* Jerome Modell, M.D., reviewed these animal studies and noted there was no agreement upon the exact sequence of events during the drowning episode.[31]

A review of these studies shows the investigations reveal the progression of pathological processes that occur after aspiration of water in animal experiments; however, these studies cannot be used to extrapolate data about the surface struggle humans exhibit before submerging.

The five stages of drowning in the NPWP textbook are surprise, involuntary breath-holding, unconsciousness, hypoxic convulsions, and clinical death. The six characteristics of the first stage of drowning, surprise, closely resemble Instinctive Drowning Response behavior.

The use of the term *surprise* appears to have originated from animal studies in which water was introduced into the airway of animals to study the effects on the respiratory and circulatory systems of these unfortunate subjects. While it is under-standable that the animal was surprised, no research is cited that quantifies that amount of time to 10–20 seconds for either animals or humans.

It is the author's view that the correct sequence of the stages of drowning in humans is (1) Stage One: surprise or distress; (2) Stage Two: gasping for air; (3) Stage Three: the instinctive drowning response; (4) Stage Four: submersion; (5) Stage Five: unconsciousness; and (6) Stage Six: death. In passive drownings the sequence begins at Stage Four when the person's mouth is submerged in the water.

The first characteristic of *surprise* occurs when the person has recognized the danger and remains afraid for 10–20 seconds. Analysis of *On Drowning* shows that the feelings of surprise are replaced almost immediately, not after 10–20 seconds, by the gasping for air. The actual or perceived suffocation then triggers the Instinctive Drowning Response.

The second characteristic of the *surprise* stage is that the person's body is in a diagonal or vertical position. Here we have an example of criteria that are used in two classifications, *distress* and *drowning*. To be useful to lifeguards criteria must differ from one another.

The third characteristic of *surprise* in the drowning process is: "The person will probably not be kicking or using their legs." This finding is consistent with the research on the Instinctive Drowning Response.

The fourth characteristic describes the arm movements of the drowning person by noting that the arms will be moving at or near the surface of the water in random grasping or flapping movements.

The flapping or grasping movements this text describes as happening randomly are actually instinctive attempts by the drowning person to avoid suffocation. Analysis of the arm movements of drowning persons, which were first described in *On Drowning* (1970), shows these arm movements are designed to lift the mouths of drowning persons above the water to enable them to breathe, and they last as long as 60 seconds.

The fifth characteristic of *surprise* is that the persons' heads will be tilted back with the persons gasping for air. This description is generally accurate for the phase of the Instinctive Drowning Response during which persons' mouths are above the surface of the water.

The sixth characteristic notes that a person may or may not be making any sounds because a person who is drowning is too busy trying to get air to call for help. The physiological explanations provided earlier about the function of the respiratory system detail why the drowning person is rarely able to call out for help.

When these six characteristics are combined it is apparent that the heading *surprise* is not an accurate way to describe the behavior that is occurring. Rather, a term should be chosen which better reflects the three stages or processes which have occurred while the drowning person is attempting to avoid suffocation on the surface of the water: surprise/distress, gasping for air, and the Instinctive Drowning Response.

Stage Two of the drowning process, *involuntary breath-holding*, lasts 30–90 seconds. The victim is not breathing because his or her muscles have taken over the breathing process and are not under conscious control.

Since Stage One, *surprise*, which lasts 10–20 seconds, is followed by Stage Two, *involuntary breath-holding* which lasts 30–90 seconds, the inference can be made that involuntary breath-holding occurs at the end of Stage One and the beginning of Stage Two. The scenes in *On Drowning,* however, show that involuntary breath-holding does not occur within 30 seconds after the drowning person starts to struggle. While the persons' mouths are above the surface of the water, they will attempt to breathe. The breath-holding occurs after the person submerges, but certainly not while the drowning person is struggling on the surface of the water.

Further analysis reveals that voluntary breath-holding occurs in the distressed swimmer who is able to control his/her actions at the surface of the water. *Understanding Drowning*[32] depicts a little boy who is ill at ease holding his breath while a friend is looks on.

The last three stages — *unconsciousness*, *hypoxic convulsions*, and *clinical death* — present the physiological progress of a drowning. In the author's view, recognition of these stages would be simplified by using the new American National Red Cross' standard which calls for a lifeguard to respond to any person floating face down or remaining submerged for longer than 30 seconds.[33]

TRAIT-CENTERED SURVEILLANCE

The final section of this chapter will examine the appropriateness of using statistical data as the rationale for trait-centered surveillance. Trait-centered surveillance gives lifeguards a set of traits they must look for while scanning their zones. Persons possessing these traits or features are described as "high-risk guests" who need special attention.

Under this system, lifeguards are trained to look for certain characteristics such as age, gender, body weight, race, or ethnic background and then presumably watch individuals possessing these characteristics more closely than individuals not possessing these characteristics. The database that supports the approach of teaching trait-centered recognition concepts appears to come from statistical studies that show certain groups either drown or experience difficulty in the water more frequently than other groups.

The 1994 National Pool and Waterpark textbook lists ten types or groups of people who are "high-risk guests" at water parks. The reader is then encouraged to use this information by generalizing the findings and applying them to pools and waterfronts. The following is a summary of the individual classifications, an analysis of the criteria individually, and then an evaluation by the author of what he believes to be the deficiencies in using a trait-centered surveillance system.

The first type is "children ages 7–12." According to this publication, these children are at risk because they are smaller, not very strong, and have less skill in the water and less awareness of danger.

The second group is "minorities," which includes African-Americans, Hispanics, Asians, and others. The explanation for the "high-risk" designation is that these groups may have had less opportunity to gain aquatic experience.

While there can be no legitimate objection to targeting aquatic education programs, learn-to-swim campaigns, or other intervention strategies for "at risk" groups cited in sound epidemiologic research studies, we cannot, as aquatic professionals, single out a member of a group for special surveillance or swimming ability testing, based on anything but behavior. Besides drawing incorrect conclusions about an entire group of people, criteria that identify people as "high-risk guests" are absolutely useless when a lifeguard works at a facility that is used primarily by members of a group labeled "high-risk."

For example, attempting to apply "high-risk guest" criteria to teach drowning person recognition concepts to lifeguards at Orchard Beach, Bronx, New York, (where almost 90% of the population is African-American or Hispanic) illustrates the methodological weakness of this approach. While the data may show that African-Americans, for example, drown at statistically significantly higher rates than whites, misuse of the data occurs when all African-Americans are labeled "high-risk guests" who need special attention at swimming facilities. This approach causes resentment by minorities and reinforces racial stereotypes.

The third group is "parents with small children." The reason supplied for the "high-risk" designation is that the parents may lack sufficient swimming skills to support themselves and their children in the water.

The fourth group is "intoxicated guests." Here it is noted that even one drink can slow down reactions and the ability to control movement, balance, and judgment. Without using a Breathalyzer or drawing blood to obtain a blood-alcohol level, lifeguards have no reliable way of knowing a person is intoxicated except for his/her behavior. It is the behavior of individuals that indicates they are under the influence of alcohol.

The fifth group is "obese or overweight persons." The rationale for their designation as "high-risk guests" is that because fat is very buoyant, obese people have difficulty standing up if they lose their balance.

The sixth group is "guests wearing life jackets." The explanation given for this designation is that the life jacket may not fit properly, may not hold the person up, or the person, unaccustomed to the feeling of wearing a life jacket, may panic.

The seventh high-risk group is "the elderly." Elderly people may tire easily or have medical conditions that prevent them from having the strength or mobility of their younger years.

The eight group is "disabled guests." Here it is reasoned that disabled individuals may not be familiar with how the facility affects their abilities to move.

The ninth group is "guests wearing clothes." Clothes, it is noted, absorb water, become heavy, and make movement in the water more difficult. If a guest does not have a bathing suit, it may indicate a low swimming experience level.

The tenth group is "every guest." The rationale for this high-risk designation is that an unexpected aquatic accident can happen to anyone, regardless of swimming ability or experience.

This last high-risk designation, "every guest," provides the clearest example of the deficiency of the trait-centered surveillance. Unless there is, within the trait-centered surveillance system, a hierarchy of "high-risk guests" where one is presumably at greater risk of drowning than a member of another group, then the classification system, while useful for data collection and statistical analysis, is of little practical use to lifeguards while they scan their assigned zones.

Analysis of these ten categories prompts several other questions. First, when do lifeguards make the "high-risk" designation? Is it when the person walks into the facility, is out on the deck, or enters the water?

The next question is, once lifeguards have made the "high-risk" designation what do they do with the designation? Asking lifeguards to keep track of designations for what could potentially be hundreds of patrons is an unrealistic expectation.

Finally, the most important reason for not using trait-centered "high-risk guest" surveillance concepts is that they will interfere with the lifeguards' ability to quickly recognize distressed swimmers and drowning persons. The ten classifications listed will increase the number of variables for which lifeguards have to look from 4 behavior variables to 14 behavior/trait variables. Of the additional ten trait variables, only one — blood-alcohol level — has been shown to be significantly correlated with drowning.

CONCLUSION

It is clear from this discussion that public health and lifeguard training agencies must undertake two tasks. First, a uniform classification of *distress* and *drowning* terminology is needed to help lifeguards during scanning. The author proposes that, whichever classification is adopted by public health agencies that certify lifeguard training programs, the categorical classification be based on criteria that have defining features. The categorical approach to the classification of water crises will work best when all characteristics of the diagnostic classes of *distress* and *drowning* are mutually exclusive with clear descriptive boundaries between the definitions.

Second, the use of trait-centered surveillance and the depiction of people as "high-risk guests" who need special surveillance, has no place in modern lifeguarding. Just as the concepts of phrenology, the science of skull reading, and physiognomy, a system of using facial traits as clues to a person's inner personality, have been discredited by modern psychologists, so must the use of "high-risk guest" definitions be eliminated by today's lifeguards.

This article first was presented as a keynote address at the 1994 Reflections on Lifeguarding Conference sponsored by A.L.T. International and held at the University of Victoria, British Columbia, Copyright: Advanced Lifeguard Training International, Victoria, British Columbia. Used with permission.

REFERENCES

1. Pia, F., June 1984, "The RID Factor as a Cause of Drowning," *Parks & Recreation,* 52–67.
2. New York State Department of Public Health, *Drownings at Regulated Bathing Facilities in New York State, 1987–1990,* New York State Department of Health, Albany, NY.
3. Royal Lifesaving Society of Canada, October 1988, *Statement of the Royal Lifesaving Society of Canada for the Inquest of Coroner Roch Heoux,* Royal Lifesaving Society Canada, Montreal, PQ.
4. Pia, F., 1994, *Reflections on Lifeguarding,* Keynote Address, A.L.T. International, Victoria, BC, Canada
5. 1991, *Websters Ninth New Collegiate Dictionary.* Merriam-Webster, Springfield, MA.
6. Pia, F., 1971, *On Drowning,* 2nd revised edition, Water Safety Films, Inc., Larchmont, NY.
7. Pia, F., 1971, *On Drowning,* 2nd revised edition, Water Safety Films, Inc., Larchmont, NY.
8. Pia, F., 1974, "Observations on the Drowning of Nonswimmers," *Journal of Physical Education,* The YMCA Society of North America, Warsaw, IN.
9. Palm, J., Ed., 1978 and 1993, *Alert: Aquatic Supervision in Action,* The Royal Lifesaving Society of Canada, Toronto, ON.
10. Royal Lifesaving Society of Canada, 1995, *The Canadian Life Saving Manual,* Toronto, ON.
11. Anderson, S. and Kirchhof, C. W., Eds., *Modern Concepts in Lifeguarding,* 15th edition, ALT International, Victoria. BC, Canada.
12. The American National Red Cross, 1983, *Lifeguard Training,* The American National Red Cross, Washington, DC.
13. Forsten, D. and Murphy, M., Eds., 1994, *On the Guard II,* Second Edition, Human Kinetics, Champaign, IL.
14. Huint, R., 1990, *Lifeguarding in the Waterparks,* AquaLude, Inc., Montreal, PQ.
15. The American National Red Cross, 1994, *Lifeguarding Today,* The American National Red Cross, Washington, DC.
16. Brewster, B. C., 1995, *Manual of Open Water Lifesaving,* Brady, Englewood Cliffs, NJ.

17. The American National Red Cross, 1994, *Lifeguarding Today,* The American National Red Cross, Washington, DC.
18. Brewster, B. C., 1995, *Manual of Open Water Lifesaving,* Brady, Englewood Cliffs, NJ.
19. Pia, F., *On Drowning* and observational studies, Orchard, Beach, Bronx, NY.
20. Basis of speech.
21. Patton, M., 1990, *Qualitative Evaluation and Research Methods*, Sage Publications, Newbury Park, CA.
22. Pia, F., 1971, *On Drowning*, 2nd revised edition, Water Safety Films, Inc., Larchmont, NY.
23. Pia, F., 1976, *Drowning Facts & Myths*, Water Safety Films, Inc., Larchmont, NY.
24. Pia, F., 1988, *The Reasons People Drown*, L.S.A. Productions, Inc., Larchmont, NY.
25. Binghampton Tape: News footage.
26. Dulles Airport Rescue: News footage.
27. J. Ellis & Associates, 1990, *In Too Deep,* Houston, TX.
28. Ellis, J. and White, J., 1994, *National Pool and Waterpark/CPR Training*, Jones & Bartlett, Boston, MA.
29. Karpovich, P. V., 1933, "Water in the Lungs of Drowned Animals," *Arch. Path.,* 15: 828–833.
30. Lougheed, D. W., James, J. M., and Hall, G. E., 1939, "Physiological Studies in Experimental Asphyxia and Drowning," *Canadian Medical Association Journal*, 40: 423–428,
31. Modell, J., 1971, *The Pathophysiology and Treatment of Drowning and Near-Drowning*, Charles C. Thomas, Springfield, IL.
32. Huint, R., 1992, *Understanding Drowning,* AquaLude, Inc., Montreal, PQ.
33. The American National Red Cross, 1994, *Lifeguarding Today,* The American National Red Cross, Washington, DC.

15 Drowning in a Closed-Water Environment: Lessons That Can Be Learned

E. Louise Priest

The water recreation industry has taken a positive and aggressive stance on improvement of safety and reduction of accidents in aquatic facilities. Participation is increasing dramatically, and managers and owners take daily measures to improve patron safety and reduce the possibility of injuries. As the industry grows, most of the marketing is targeted at family participation, with "Lazy Rivers" and interactive play structures accounting for the majority of development. Injuries and accidents are carefully documented, and it is a rare park manager who cannot tell you where the "trouble spots" are in his or her facility. "Risk management" has become a common term in the recreation industry, as managers and other risk-management personnel analyze past occurrences and gain insight into the development of injury prevention. The management of risk is multifaceted, from the very simple act of stopping a young child from running to outmaneuvering the intentional thrill-seeking, risk-taking behavior of the average 18-year-old (Figure 1). In the constant attempt to manage risk while providing thrilling recreation, park managers and others have learned some specific things that help the process: better signage, electronic ride release signals, audio cues, and intensive in-service training, to mention several.[1]

National participation and detailed accident statistics relating to aquatics always have been difficult to access. Estimates are by definition inaccurate. For example, the National Sporting Goods Association estimates[2] that 61 million people participate in recreational swimming. Actual participation statistics of clients of Ellis & Associates (E&A)[3] show, however, in 1995 there were more than 40 million participants at E&A client facilities, mostly water parks. This indicates the estimate of 61 million is quite low.

The statistics and charts that follow are from the 1995 annual report of Jeff Ellis & Associates. The divisions listed refer to the size of the facility and/or the number of participants per year, with Division 1 being the largest. Since there were no drownings at these facilities in 1995, it should be remembered that the statistics discussed refer to *rescues*, not *drownings*. The rescues may or may not be immersion incidents, that is, the person may have gone underwater, but more likely would have been "in trouble" at the surface. In both cases the person was rescued and did *not* drown.

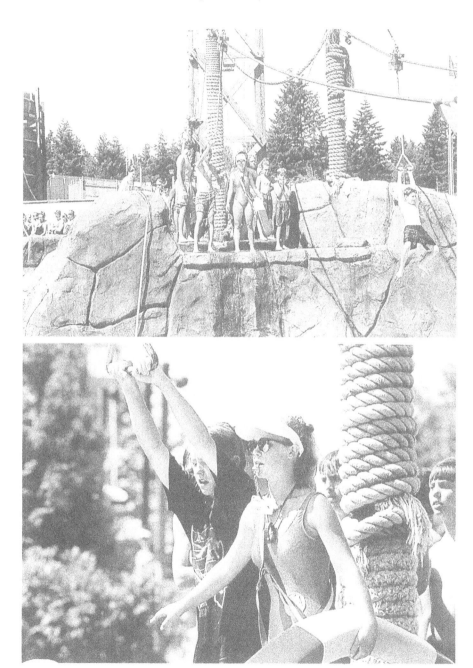

FIGURE 1a-b Managing risk-taking behavior.

IMMERSION INCIDENTS AND RESCUES

The fact that there were **60 million participants and *no drownings*** indicates that risk management has reached a high level at these facilities. Some background

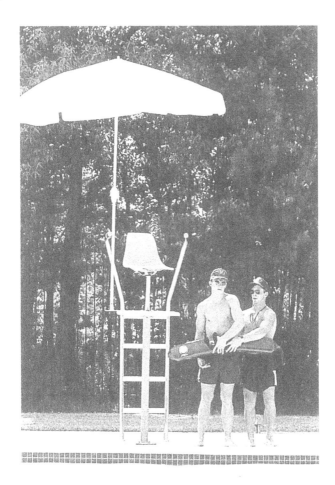

FIGURE 2   Training programs — lifeguard rotation.

information on policies and procedures will be provided here, for the benefit of those who are unfamiliar with E&A.

In the early 1980s, having observed a lifeguarding course specific to water parks was necessary, Jeff Ellis devised the National Pool & Waterpark Lifeguard Training course and created a total risk-management program for water parks. Drastically different from other lifeguarding courses at the time, with a philosophy of "use what works," the lifeguarding course — one component of the total program — was modified yearly, based upon input from the lifeguards themselves (Figure 2). The methods and program devised were of such quality and effectiveness that insurance companies were willing to insure those parks that adopted the program, and in less than ten years, 80% of the country's water parks were clients of E&A. In the early 1990s, a collaborative agreement with the National Safety Council and the National Recreation & Parks Association broadened the E&A base to include flat-water parks and facilities and the development of a learn-to-swim program.

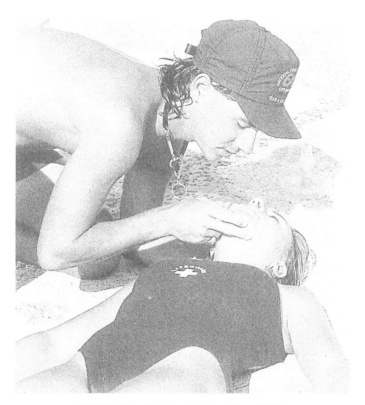

FIGURE 3a   Training in first aid and CPR.

Subsequent materials developed include safety training for water exercise instructors, a similar one for coaches, a safety awareness program for motel pool operators, and an adapted aquatics segment for the *Learn to Swim Instructor's Manual*. National Safety Council programs in CPR and first aid are used as components of the total training program (Figures 3a and 3b). The NPWLT program is currently used in 42 states, as well as in Canada, Mexico, China, Spain, Puerto Rico, and Hong Kong.

The dynamics of the firm are such that courses and materials can be modified yearly, enabling the organization to adopt new techniques and developments rapidly, and stay "on the cutting edge" of technical and medical information. In many instances, E&A sets the standard in the industry, as the nearly universal adoption of the E&A 10/20 response rule shows. Created by E&A, the 10/20 rule mandates observation of a distressed swimmer in 10 seconds and rescue contact in 20 seconds. This 10/20 response rule has been totally accepted as the standard of care lifeguards should provide. The unique features of the program devised include:

- an initial assessment of facility for safety practices and risk control
- training of staff in the NPWLT course

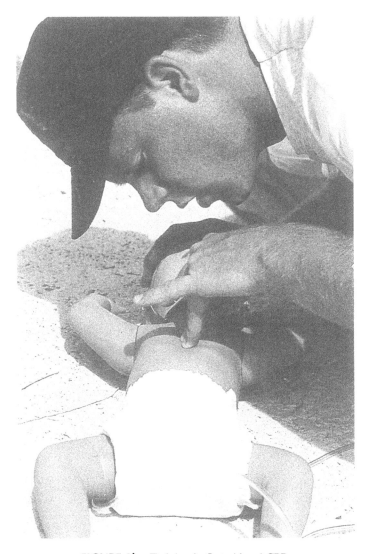

FIGURE 3b   Training in first aid and CPR.

- an agreement, signed by the trainee, to maintain fitness and skills at all times
- an agreement with facility management to maintain recommended risk management procedures
- unannounced audits of facility and staff, to ensure competence and maintenance of standards
- immediate counsel and help from E&A in the event of an aquatic incident[4]

The program incorporates many factors considered critical in recreation risk management, including the commitment of management, proactive risk policies, training and commitment of staff, and accountability (Figure 4).

pools, in particular, always have signs warning about the depth of the water, yet many of the people rescued there are nonswimmers. Of the 24,366 rescues made, 21,000, or 87%, were in five specific areas. Such data does not mean that the other six areas described should not be equally protected, but it does show the continued need for aggressive and proactive risk management in those areas (Figures 5 and 6).

RESCUES BY AGE

These charts do not contain many surprises. More than 75% of the rescues were of children 12 years of age or younger. The data does invoke the old question of parental supervision, since 24% of the children were only 6 years old or younger. It would be most interesting to know the location of the parents of these children. Unfortunately, that data is not available (Figures 7 and 8).

RESCUES BY SEX

While males still hold a small majority in the number of rescues, the division is almost equal. Boys 6–12 years of age are still more at risk than any other group (Figures 7 and 9).

RESCUES BY DEPTH OF WATER

Rescues by depth of water (Figures 10, 11, and 13) show, not unexpectedly, that most rescues are made in water 4–10 ft deep. The 23% made in 0–4 ft make a not unexpectedly close correlation with the 24% rescues in the 0–6 year age range shown in Figure 10. (Drownings by age and depth of water will be discussed later.)

ETHNIC BACKGROUND

Figures 12 and 13 show rescues by ethnic background. It may be more useful if we also knew the percentage of *participants* from various ethnic backgrounds. What these figures do show is that participation in aquatic recreation is certainly not limited to our white population, as was virtually the case in the past.

RESCUES BY DAY OF WEEK AND TIME OF DAY

The charts of rescues by day and time of day (Figures 14 and 15) reflect the fact that almost half the rescues were made on weekends, with almost equal distribution on weekdays, and almost 55% made between noon and 4 P.M.

Figures 16–18 deal with follow-up protocol and other data, and present an interesting picture of the handling of such incidents in E&A client facilities. The data, of course, could be extrapolated to apply in general terms to other facilities with well-trained staff and risk management policies. Figures 16–18 contain a myriad of facts worthy of study and comparison.

RESCUES BY AREA

CLIENT DIVISION		LAP/LANE POOL	REC POOL	CHILD POOL	DIVE WELL	ACTIVITY POOL	SLED RIDE	WAVE POOL	SLIDE POOL	LAZY RIVER	RAPIDS RIDE	LAKE-FRONT	OTHER	TOTAL
I	TOTAL	0	117	51	2,134	333	22	1,237	1,128	118	1,236	47	63	6,486
	AVG	0.0	7.3	3.2	133.4	20.8	1.4	77.3	70.5	7.4	77.3	2.9	3.9	405.4
II	TOTAL	4	46	37	788	1,624	6	1,153	830	18	21	0	32	4,559
	AVG	0.3	3.5	2.8	60.6	124.9	0.5	88.7	63.8	1.4	1.6	0.0	2.5	350.7
III	TOTAL	22	96	13	1,144	1,057	107	1,957	511	77	84	21	31	5,120
	AVG	0.9	3.8	0.5	45.8	42.3	4.3	78.3	20.4	3.1	3.4	0.8	1.2	204.8
IV	TOTAL	24	317	4	308	269	0	881	233	20	24	2	13	2,095
	AVG	1.0	13.8	0.2	13.4	11.7	0.0	38.3	10.1	0.9	1.0	0.1	0.6	91.1
V	TOTAL	127	740	74	404	126	0	0	661	25	0	115	48	2,320
	AVG	4.1	23.9	2.4	13.0	4.1	0.0	0.0	21.3	0.8	0.0	3.7	1.5	74.8
VI	TOTAL	71	545	89	393	125	0	17	344	442	0	34	24	2,084
	AVG	1.9	14.3	2.3	10.3	3.3	0.0	0.4	9.1	11.6	0.0	0.9	0.6	54.8
VII	TOTAL	81	282	26	252	46	0	132	263	9	0	0	8	1,099
	AVG	2.7	9.4	0.9	8.4	1.5	0.0	4.4	8.8	0.3	0.0	0.0	0.3	36.6
VIII	TOTAL	63	163	28	129	6	0	2	207	0	0	4	1	603
	AVG	1.2	3.2	0.5	2.5	0.1	0.0	0.0	4.1	0.0	0.0	0.1	0.0	11.8
ALL	TOTAL	392	2,306	322	5,552	3,586	135	5,379	4,177	709	1,365	223	220	24,366
	AVG	2	10	1	25	16	1	24	18	3	6	1	1	108

FIGURE 5   Printout of Jeff Ellis & Associates 1995 NPWL Activity Report showing rescues by area.

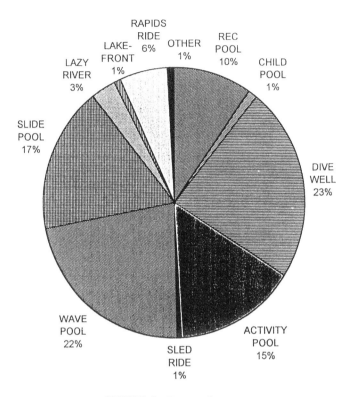

FIGURE 6   Rescues by area.

SUMMARY

The preceding data is from the 1995 annual report of Jeff Ellis & Associates.[5] It must be emphasized that the figures cited represent rescues, ***not drownings***. Rescues are delineated by area of the facility; age, sex and ethnic background of the rescued persons; the day of week and time of day of the rescues; and the follow-up protocol used. While these more than 24,000 persons were rescued, and fortunately did not drown, the circumstances of the incidents can certainly provide both victim and incident profiles, useful in future risk management. The fact that there were 60 million participants, no drownings, and more than 24,000 successful rescues certainly shows a high level of attentiveness and responsiveness in the lifeguards. Instructors, staff, and clients of E&A all have voiced the opinion that such performance is due to the training, audit procedures, and accountability demanded of E&A lifeguards and facilities.

DROWNINGS

The National Safety Council lists drowning as the third-leading cause of accidental death in children 1–4 years of age, and catalogs 529 yearly deaths in that age

RESCUES BY AGE

CLIENT DIVISION		0 - 6	7 - 12	13 - 19	20 - 30	31 - 45	46 - 60	60 +	UN-KNOWN	TOTAL
I	TOTAL	939	3,276	905	501	533	115	38	179	6,486
	AVG	58.7	204.8	56.6	31.3	33.3	7.2	2.4	11.2	405.4
II	TOTAL	945	2,418	584	265	212	49	13	73	4,559
	AVG	72.7	186.0	44.9	20.4	16.3	3.8	1.0	5.6	350.7
III	TOTAL	1,076	2,833	580	264	174	41	17	135	5,120
	AVG	43.0	113.3	23.2	10.6	7.0	1.6	0.7	5.4	204.8
IV	TOTAL	577	1,131	170	93	57	42	6	19	2,095
	AVG	25.1	49.2	7.4	4.0	2.5	1.8	0.3	0.8	91.1
V	TOTAL	847	1,181	114	36	23	8	7	104	2,320
	AVG	27.3	38.1	3.7	1.2	0.7	0.3	0.2	3.4	74.8
VI	TOTAL	757	968	144	78	76	16	10	35	2,084
	AVG	19.9	25.5	3.8	2.1	2.0	0.4	0.3	0.9	54.8
VII	TOTAL	467	481	61	27	21	3	4	35	1,099
	AVG	15.6	16.0	2.0	0.9	0.7	0.1	0.1	1.2	36.6
VIII	TOTAL	289	252	36	11	6	4	1	4	603
	AVG	5.7	4.9	0.7	0.2	0.1	0.1	0.0	0.1	11.8
ALL	TOTAL	5,897	12,540	2,594	1,275	1,102	278	96	584	24,366
	AVG	26	55	11	6	5	1	0	3	108

RESCUES BY SEX

	MALE	FEMALE	UN-KNOWN	TOTAL
TOTAL	3,248	3,022	216	6,486
AVG	203.0	188.9	13.5	405.4
TOTAL	2,339	2,166	54	4,559
AVG	179.9	166.6	4.2	350.7
TOTAL	2,574	2,449	97	5,120
AVG	103.0	98.0	3.9	204.8
TOTAL	1,151	938	6	2,095
AVG	50.0	40.8	0.3	91.1
TOTAL	1,369	835	116	2,320
AVG	44.2	26.9	3.7	74.8
TOTAL	1,079	963	42	2,084
AVG	28.4	25.3	1.1	54.8
TOTAL	643	446	10	1,099
AVG	21.4	14.9	0.3	36.6
TOTAL	340	262	1	603
AVG	6.7	5.1	0.0	11.8
TOTAL	12,743	11,081	542	24,366
AVG	56	49	2	108

FIGURE 7 Ellis & Associates 1995 NPWL Activity Reports showing rescues by age and by sex.

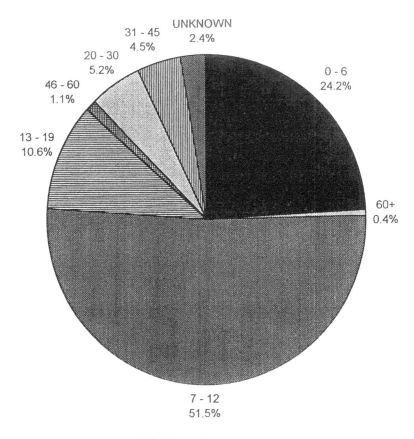

FIGURE 8   Rescues by age.

group in its latest *Accident Facts* book,[6] and a total of 3,524 drownings (all age groups). The Council does not tabulate drownings by type of facility, or any circumstances other than age, so the data really cannot be applied to a specific context such as "closed-water environment"; nevertheless, it is obvious that some of those drownings were in a closed-water environment and that some of them occurred when lifeguards were present. No system is perfect, and no system is free from human error, even where the safety record is excellent. It is difficult, if not impossible, to factually isolate causal factors. It is interesting, however, to find that everyone interviewed on the subject mentions three factors that they *believe* to be responsible: accountability demanded by the audit process, in-service training, and adherence to the 10/20 rule. Post-incident interviews[7] with the lifeguards certainly reinforce the accuracy of these perceptions. Excerpts from several interviews follow.

Mike   "In-service training is very necessary to keep on top of your skills, so you don't freeze in an emergency. I'd tell new guards 'Keep your zone. You can have fun on breaks, but it's all business when you're in the chair.'"

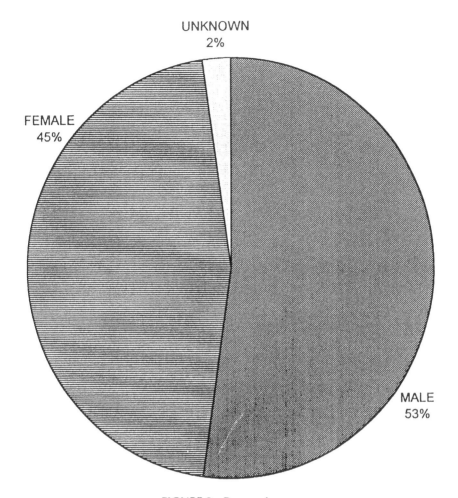

FIGURE 9   Rescues by sex.

Mark   "The training in the NPWL training program was more than adequate to prepare me to deal with this emergency. I would tell a lifeguard candidate that what we learned in training we need to know. We wouldn't be able to carry out a rescue without the skills we were taught. A lifeguard's job is not 'fun in the sun' at all. It is a very serious job."

Liz   "Don't goof around in in-service training. They are preparing you every week for what may happen. I'd tell a future lifeguard, don't think it's not going to happen to you, or that your pool is immune to injury. We had over 18 guards on staff, and something like this happened. It's just a matter of time. Be ready … be looking. Do your skills. Go to your in-service. Know when you get into your chair that you may have to pull someone out of the pool, and be ready and looking for it. You take this job knowing that this is the ultimate rescue. This is what it boils down to: It is possible

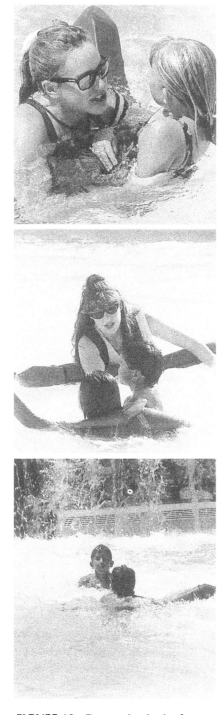

FIGURE 10 Rescues by depth of water.

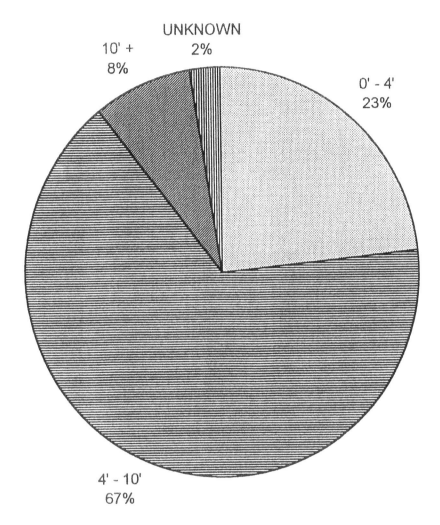

FIGURE 11   Rescues by depth of water.

that we may never eliminate drownings from aquatic recreation. There will always be some patrons who refuse to read or adhere to warning signs, and human error will remain with us. Experience does show, however, that training, retraining, and accountability go a long way toward eliminating these tragic incidents in our society."

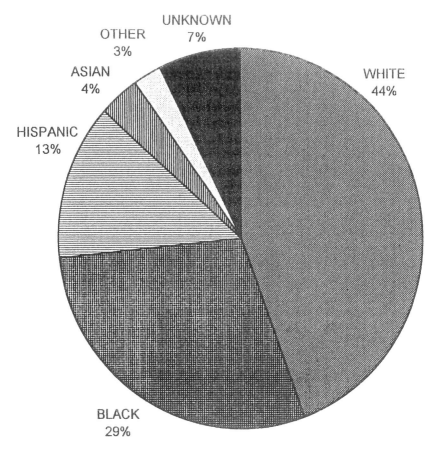

FIGURE 12   Rescues by ethnic background.

RESCUES BY ETHNIC BACKGROUND

CLIENT DIVISION		WHITE	BLACK	HISPANIC	ASIAN	OTHER	UN-KNOWN	TOTAL
I	TOTAL	2,254	2,422	914	295	230	371	6,486
	AVG	140.9	151.4	57.1	18.4	14.4	23.2	405.4
II	TOTAL	1,815	1,561	727	186	87	183	4,559
	AVG	139.6	120.1	55.9	14.3	6.7	14.1	350.7
III	TOTAL	2,368	1,385	720	237	145	265	5,120
	AVG	94.7	55.4	28.8	9.5	5.8	10.6	204.8
IV	TOTAL	1,250	314	181	39	23	288	2,095
	AVG	54.3	13.7	7.9	1.7	1.0	12.5	91.1
V	TOTAL	1,203	645	128	48	26	270	2,320
	AVG	38.8	20.8	4.1	1.5	0.8	8.7	74.8
VI	TOTAL	1,007	424	344	38	48	223	2,084
	AVG	26.5	11.2	9.1	1.0	1.3	5.9	54.8
VII	TOTAL	594	224	102	30	68	81	1,099
	AVG	19.8	7.5	3.4	1.0	2.3	2.7	36.6
VIII	TOTAL	307	120	93	9	14	60	603
	AVG	6.0	2.4	1.8	0.2	0.3	1.2	11.8
ALL	TOTAL	10,798	7,095	3,209	882	641	1,741	24,366
	AVG	48	31	14	4	3	8	108

RESCUES BY DEPTH OF WATER

CLIENT DIVISION		0' - 4'	4' - 10'	10' +	UN-KNOWN	TOTAL
I	TOTAL	1,340	4,392	525	229	6,486
	AVG	83.8	274.5	32.8	14.3	405.4
II	TOTAL	464	3,912	87	96	4,559
	AVG	35.7	300.9	6.7	7.4	350.7
III	TOTAL	1,202	3,763	66	89	5,120
	AVG	48.1	150.5	2.6	3.6	204.8
IV	TOTAL	564	1,317	178	36	2,095
	AVG	24.5	57.3	7.7	1.6	91.1
V	TOTAL	976	768	505	71	2,320
	AVG	31.5	24.8	16.3	2.3	74.8
VI	TOTAL	477	1,332	242	33	2,084
	AVG	12.6	35.1	6.4	0.9	54.8
VII	TOTAL	419	383	272	25	1,099
	AVG	14.0	12.8	9.1	0.8	36.6
VIII	TOTAL	257	197	145	4	603
	AVG	5.0	3.9	2.8	0.1	11.8
ALL	TOTAL	5,699	16,064	2,020	583	24,366
	AVG	25	71	9	3	108

FIGURE 13 Ellis & Associates 1995 NPWL Activity Reports showing rescues by ethnic background and by depth of water.

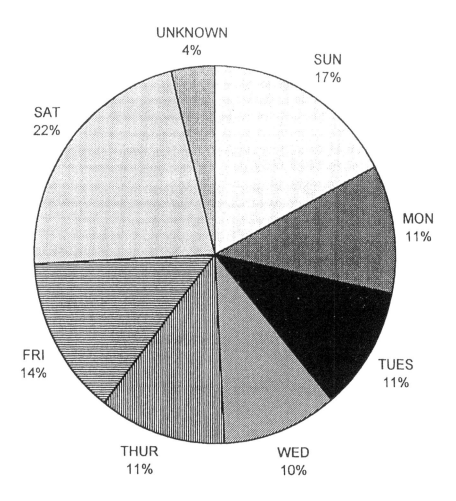

FIGURE 14   Rescues by day of week.

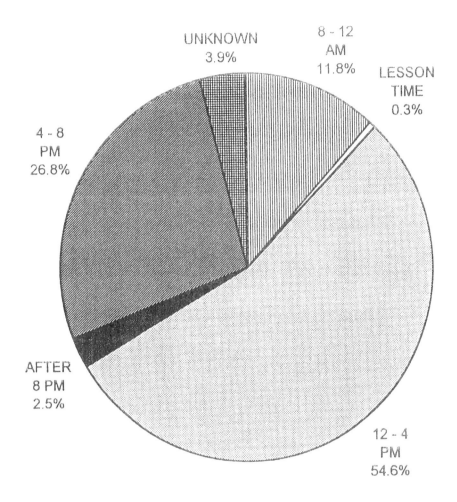

FIGURE 15   Rescues by time of day.

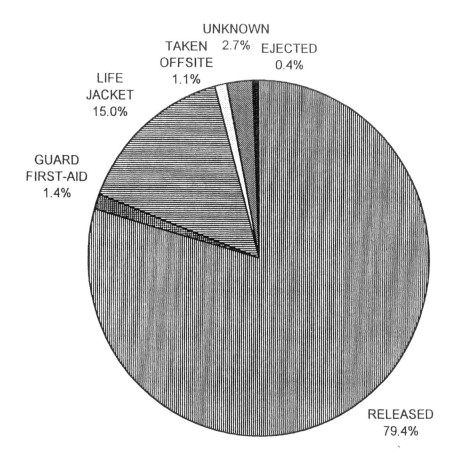

FIGURE 16   Rescues by follow-up protocol.

RESCUES BY FOLLOWUP PROTOCOL / OTHER DATA

CLIENT DIVISION		RELEASED	LIFE JACKET	GUARD FIRST-AID	TAKEN OFFSITE	EJECTED	UN-KNOWN	TOTAL	MULTIPLE VICTIMS	MULTIPLE RESCUERS	SURF ARCCPR	BOT ARCCPR	OXYGEN GIVEN	FACE MASK	BLOOD PRESENT	GLOVES USED	BACK-BOARD	GUARDS INJURED	LO SKIN CANCER	IN-WATER HEIMLICH
I	TOTAL	5,033	997	73	85	55	243	6,486	123	85	2	4	12	5	183	195	123	106	1	5
	AVG	314.6	62.3	4.6	5.3	3.4	15.2	405.4	7.7	5.3	0.1	0.3	0.8	0.3	11.4	12.2	7.7	6.6	0.1	0.3
II	TOTAL	3,676	703	77	15	3	85	4,559	324	183	1	1	6	2	27	36	42	25	1	4
	AVG	282.8	54.1	5.9	1.2	0.2	6.5	350.7	24.9	14.1	0.1	0.1	0.5	0.2	2.1	2.8	3.2	1.9	0.1	0.3
III	TOTAL	3,383	1,449	81	38	13	156	5,120	138	94	1	3	8	4	74	91	75	105	2	6
	AVG	135.3	58.0	3.2	1.5	0.5	6.2	204.8	5.5	3.8	0.0	0.1	0.3	0.2	3.0	3.6	3.0	4.2	0.1	0.2
IV	TOTAL	1,602	411	15	37	1	29	2,095	90	37	1	0	4	1	13	33	42	34	0	2
	AVG	69.7	17.9	0.7	1.6	0.0	1.3	91.1	3.9	1.6	0.0	0.0	0.2	0.0	0.6	1.4	1.8	1.5	0.0	0.1
V	TOTAL	2,115	41	45	39	14	66	2,320	44	28	6	1	7	7	191	280	37	31	0	8
	AVG	68.2	1.3	1.5	1.3	0.5	2.1	74.8	1.4	0.9	0.2	0.0	0.2	0.2	6.2	9.0	1.2	1.0	0.0	0.3
VI	TOTAL	1,964	36	35	23	7	19	2,084	46	11	1	2	1	6	263	194	18	11	0	4
	AVG	51.7	0.9	0.9	0.6	0.2	0.5	54.8	1.2	0.3	0.0	0.1	0.0	0.2	6.9	5.1	0.5	0.3	0.0	0.1
VII	TOTAL	1,009	14	3	8	2	63	1,099	10	9	3	0	1	3	4	14	8	12	1	3
	AVG	33.6	0.5	0.1	0.3	0.1	2.1	36.6	0.3	0.3	0.1	0.0	0.0	0.1	0.1	0.5	0.3	0.4	0.0	0.1
VIII	TOTAL	565	12	5	13	8	0	603	9	5	0	1	1	0	6	6	5	3	0	1
	AVG	11.1	0.2	0.1	0.3	0.2	0.0	11.8	0.2	0.1	0.0	0.0	0.0	0.0	0.1	0.1	0.1	0.1	0.0	0.0
ALL	TOTAL	19,347	3,663	334	258	103	661	24,366	784	452	15	12	40	28	761	849	350	327	5	33
	AVG	86	16	1	1	0	3	108	3	2	0	0	0	0	3	4	2	1	0	0

FIGURE 17 Ellis & Associates 1995 NPWL Activity Report showing rescues by follow-up protocol and other data.

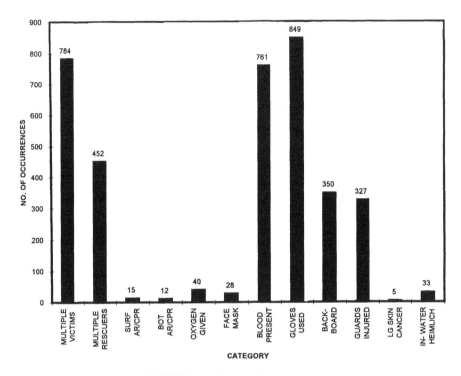

FIGURE 18   Graph of other data.

REFERENCES

1. Priest, L., "Lifeguarding in Waterparks," *Aquatics International*, 8/4, National Trade Publications, Latham, NY.
2. National Sporting Goods Association, 1995, *Sports Participation in 1995*, Mt. Prospect, IL.
3. Jeff Ellis & Associates, June 1996, *1995 Aquatic Accident and Rescue Statistical Report*.
4. Jeff Ellis & Associates, May 1996, *E&A News*.
5. Jeff Ellis & Associates, June 1996, *1995 Aquatic Accident and Rescue Statistical Report*.
6. National Safety Council, 1995 edition, *Accident Facts*.
7. Personal interviews, 1996.

16 Lifeguard Behaviors and Systematic Scanning Strategies

Tom Griffiths, Don Steel, and Hans Vogelsong

Penn State University has closely studied on-duty lifeguards for the past ten years. This chapter highlights the most significant findings of three comprehensive studies: the 1986 New Jersey Shore Study, the 1994 National Lifeguard Survey, and the 1995 National Survey.

THE 1986 NEW JERSEY SHORE STUDY

The examination of lifeguard behaviors by researchers at Penn State University began in 1986 with a study of New Jersey Ocean Lifeguards who were observed closely while on duty during the summer (Griffiths, 1987). Twelve well-trained ocean lifeguards were randomly selected and systematically observed for ten minutes each on busy beach days during the first two weeks in August between 1 P.M. and 2 P.M. Stopwatches were used to credit guards whose eyes were at least aimed toward the swimming area as defined on both sides by two red flags spaced approximately 200 feet apart on the beach. One watch ran continually for ten minutes, while the other watch was stopped only when the lifeguard's head was turned clearly away from the area of responsibility. This watch was used to measure "on-task" time during the ten-minute observations.

On average, lifeguards spent 5 minutes and 20 seconds looking at the swimming area for every 10 minutes they were observed. That meant 4 minutes and 40 seconds of every 10-minute interval were spent viewing other areas of interest. Friends, surfers on other beaches, and members of the opposite sex attracted almost as much attention from the lifeguards as the swimmers within their area of responsibility. This information was not reassuring for lifeguard supervisors or parents taking their children to guarded beaches for safety. Even though these lifeguards were well trained, there was only slightly better than a 50/50 chance the patrons in the water would be watched by them because 47% of the time the lifeguards were looking elsewhere. This lack of vigilant surveillance by well-trained lifeguards prompted further investigation into this specific area of water safety and lifeguard education.

THE 1994 NATIONAL LIFEGUARD SURVEY

In 1994, a 19-item questionnaire regarding lifeguard scanning and surveillance skills while on duty was completed by 763 lifeguards from 20 states and Canada (Griffiths, Steel, and Chambers, 1995). Of the lifeguards responding to the survey:

- 71%　worked at traditional swimming pools
- 20%　worked at water parks
- 6%　worked at lakes
- 2%　worked at ocean beaches

The findings were both interesting and informative and should help to better train future lifeguards. The majority of lifeguards in the study watched extremely large crowds and were responsible for large water surface areas. 25% of the sample watched zones greater than 5,000 sq ft while almost half of the sample was responsible for zones larger than 3,000 sq ft. 28% of the respondents watched more than 100 swimmers in their zones on busy days while 55% of the sample watched more than 75 swimmers in their zones.

Several state codes and some water safety texts suggest that each lifeguard should be responsible for an area not greater than 2,000 sq ft of water surface area. Based upon the data concerning the size of the zone in this study, the 2,000 sq ft suggestion seems to be unrealistic. New York State recently evaluated its state-run aquatic facilities and determined that its lifeguards could rescue victims in 30 seconds or less in zones that were no greater than 3,400 sq ft of water surface area. This type of research is not only valuable and practical but the 3,400 sq ft figure closely resembles the average figure reported by the nearly 800 lifeguards in this study.

Some states and agencies also prescribe specific lifeguard-to-swimmer ratios. Most recommended ratios are 25–50 swimmers per lifeguard. As the data reflects, the recommended ratios for lifeguards were not realistic. Lifeguard-to-swimmer ratios should probably be site specific, that is, determined at specific lifeguarding sites and environments for specific populations, activities, and environments, rather than generalized standards (Figure 1).

In order to stay alert while on duty, it was clear that most of the lifeguards wanted to be physically active; walking, talking and moving to new stations were all important in preventing boredom. Being interactive with fellow lifeguards and patrons also helped these lifeguards stay alert. Singing and listening to music was the leading way to prevent boredom in this survey. Lifeguards were quick to point out, however, that these diversions could take place *without* taking their eyes or attention from their zones. Lifeguards also reported that to stay alert they needed to watch high-risk patrons, high-risk activities, count swimmers, and effectively organize those in their zones. Ironically, the lifeguards in this study reported that they were more concerned about effective, efficient, and organized use of time rather than safety. Although lifeguards wanted to track their swimmers in an organized fashion, one third of the sample did not use any specific organizational techniques and 85% of the sample stated that they needed more information and training on scanning strategies.

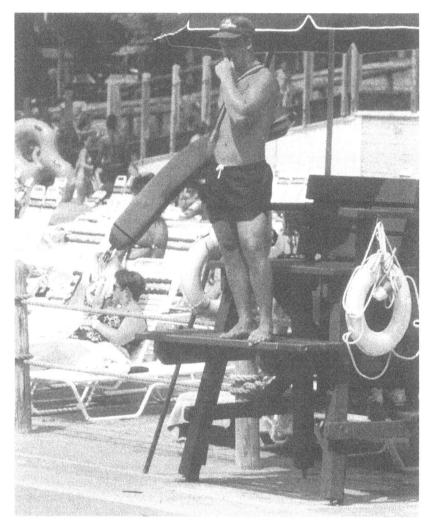

FIGURE 1   Standing lifeguards are more alert. (Photo courtesy of Paula Panton, Water Safety Products)

THE 1995 NATIONAL LIFEGUARD SURVEY

The lifeguarding sample in this follow-up study was quite large, with 2,769 lifeguards responding from 34 states and Puerto Rico (Figure 2). This large sample was also evenly divided along gender lines with 52% of the lifeguard sample male and 48% female. Those surveyed worked at the following facilities:

Swimming Pools	70%
Water Parks	18%
Ocean Beaches	8%
Lakes and Rivers	4%

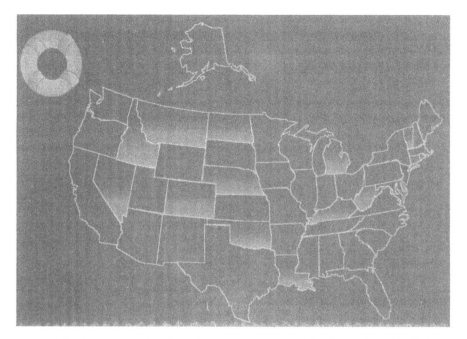

FIGURE 2   States shown in all black represent those participating in the 1995 National Lifeguard Survey.

The frequency distributions that resulted from the entire sample responding to the most applicable questions will be illustrated first. After reviewing the responses to the most pertinent questions in the survey, further analysis resulted in several significant differences regarding factors like gender, age, and experience. These important findings will be summarized after the appropriate percentages of responses are noted.

Age differences were examined in this survey. The age range of the entire lifeguard sample was wide, and while 50% of the sample was comprised of teenagers, 23% was older than 23 years:

- 16 years or younger   12%
- 17–19 years   38%
- 20–22 years   27%
- 23–25 years   11%
- 26 or older   12%

For the purposes of a more in-depth analysis, the sample was separated into two age categories. Teenagers were defined as those lifeguards 19 years or younger while adults were defined as those lifeguards 23 years of age or older. The data showed many significant differences between teens and adults. Responses from teens and adults follow.

More specifically, 55% of the adult lifeguards said they watched the water 100% of the time compared to 45% of the teens claiming that they watched their zones 100% of the time. It is important to note that in every water safety category surveyed, adult lifeguards responded more appropriately than teenage lifeguards.

Teens (19 and younger) considered themselves to:	Adults (23 and older) considered themselves to:
be babysitters	be educators/enforcers
be less confident	be more confident
not be as well trained	be better trained
watch smaller zones	watch larger zones
watch fewer people	watch more people
be supervised more often	be supervised less often

The lifeguard survey also examined experience levels of the lifeguards. Although half of all respondents worked at least three seasons, almost half of the entire sample were novice guards (less than three seasons):

- Less than one season   24%
- Between one and two seasons   16%
- Between two and three seasons   15%
- Between three and five seasons   20%
- More than five seasons   25%

The least experienced guards in the sample worked at water parks (35% of all water park lifeguards surveyed in 1995 worked less than one season). The most experienced lifeguards in the sample worked on ocean beaches. Nearly half of all lifeguards from ocean beaches worked a minimum of five seasons. Apparently, increased responsibilities and higher wages help to keep lifeguards working at ocean beaches longer. Swimming pool and water park managers may want to investigate exactly how ocean beaches are able to attract and retain older, more experienced lifeguards.

When asked how large the zone of coverage was for each lifeguard, the following results were tabulated. As one might expect, the most experienced lifeguards in the sample reported watching the largest areas while the least experienced lifeguards watched the smallest areas.

- Small (1,000 sq ft)   22%
- Medium (2,000–3,000 sq ft)   40%
- Large (3,000–4,000 sq ft)   18%
- Extra Large (4,000–5,000 sq ft)   6%
- Extreme (>5,000 sq ft)   14%

Note that 38% reported guarding more than 3,000 sq ft of surface area. This finding was similar to the 1994 National Lifeguard Study and the New York State study.

Not only did the lifeguards in the sample report watching very large water surface areas, swimmer ratios were reportedly high with 60% of the sample guarding more than 50 swimmers in their zone.

- 1–25 swimmers   14%
- 26–50 swimmers   26%
- 51–75 swimmers   20%
- 76–100 swimmers   15%
- More than 100 swimmers   25%

Additionally, more experienced guards reported watching larger numbers of swimmers than less experienced lifeguards, with ocean lifeguards watching the most swimmers followed by water park lifeguards and swimming pool lifeguards watching the smallest number.

When asked how much time the guards actually watched swimmers in their zones, respondents indicated that more than half of the lifeguards did not watch their swimmers 100% of the time:

- 25% time/watching   <1%
- 50% time/watching   4%
- 75% time/watching   9%
- 90% time/watching   40%
- 100% time/watching   47%

When this specific area was studied further in terms of lifeguard experience, there were no significant differences between levels of experience and percent of time watching the water. In fact, the least experienced lifeguards in this survey reported watching the water slightly more often than the most experienced lifeguards. This result may indicate that the least experienced lifeguards are trying to make a good impression on their employers or are still very concerned about their patrons whereas the most experienced lifeguards may have become complacent and over-confident with time.These findings indicate that even very experienced guards need to be supervised to ensure vigilant scanning. Very experienced guards may be overconfident when they are on duty or their scanning techniques may be more efficient and discerning than novice lifeguards.

Scan time is an important aspect of lifeguarding. As illustrated below, according to the responses of this sample, the time it took a lifeguard to complete one visual scan varied greatly:

- 1–5 seconds   14%
- 6–10 seconds   53%
- 11–15 seconds   22%
- 16–20 seconds   9%
- More than 20 seconds   2%

It is not surprising that the most popular scan time within the sample was 6–10 seconds because of the 10/20 rule advocated by Ellis & Associates and other training agencies. This rule suggests that every person in the zone of coverage should be visually checked every 10 seconds with an additional 20 seconds to rescue a distressed patron. While this concept is good for teaching lifeguards the importance of *constant* scanning, there was much variation in scan times in the sample. Upon further examination however, it does not seem appropriate to assign a ten-second scan to all aquatic facilities and zones considering the wide range of lifeguarding zones and environments that exist. Certainly a conscientious lifeguard scanning an ocean beach or a large wave pool would require more time than a lifeguard scanning a small, conventional swimming pool. Many lifeguards are taught to check for facial details and this would be impossible to do so in ten seconds in large, crowded zones. Individual aquatic facilities, therefore, should probably determine ideal scan times for the particular zones of coverage.

Questioned as to whether or not they were aware of any specific scanning techniques used by lifeguards, more than a quarter of the lifeguard sample were not familiar with any techniques:

- Yes   74%
- No   26%

When asked if they thought additional training and information on systematic scanning for lifeguards would help to be more effective on duty, their responses were:

- Yes   66%
- No   34%

In response to the question "How often does a supervisor check on you to make sure you are carefully watching the swimmers in your zone?" more than half the lifeguards reported that they were supervised only sometimes, rarely, or never.

- Never   3%
- Rarely   15%
- Sometimes   41%
- Often   33%
- Always   8%

Further analysis indicated that older, more experienced lifeguards were supervised the least, but ocean lifeguards were supervised more often than water park or swimming pool lifeguards.

When the lifeguards were asked how they prevented boredom on duty, they responded in the following fashion:

- Sing/listen to music   20%
- Change my posture or position   46%
- Talk to others   4%
- Count swimmers   18%
- Other   12%

Most of the time while on duty at waterside, the lifeguards in this survey preferred sitting to standing or walking, although more preferred to walk rather than to stand:

- Sit   63%
- Stand   16%
- Walk   19%
- Other   2%

When responding to the question "How would you best characterize your responsibilities," the lifeguards answered as follows:

- Babysitter   7%
- Enforcer   14%
- Preventer   66%
- Rescuer   9%
- Educator   4%

Although most lifeguards viewed themselves as "preventers," females characterized themselves as "enforcers," while males described themselves as "rescuers." Ocean guards, most of whom were male, also described themselves as "rescuers." Only older, more experienced lifeguards considered themselves to be "educators" in this study. Perhaps this characteristic should be imparted to younger, less experienced lifeguards.

To the question "How confident are you in your abilities to make a successful water rescue?" the majority of lifeguards responded that they were very confident:

- Very Confident   70%
- Fairly Confident   25%
- Not Sure   2%
- Not Very Confident   <1%
- Very Unconfident   03%

The responses of older, more experienced lifeguards and ocean guards indicated they were the most confident of all lifeguarding groups.

Responses to the question "Considering your lifeguarding course and your on-the-job training, how well are you trained to guard your facility?" were as follows:

- Very well trained   75%
- Fairly well trained 22%
- Not sure   2%
- Not very well trained <1%
- Not well trained at all <1%

Older, more experienced lifeguards reported they were better trained when responding to this question.

Some significant gender differences were found to exist in the lifeguard sample. Males reported being significantly more confident of their abilities to make a water rescue than females. Males also reported that they watched larger zones, greater numbers of swimmers, and thought they were better trained than their female counterparts. The large sample size should be truly reflective of the actual situation in the United States. But before searching for socio-psychological factors to explain these differences, it appears that these findings are more reflective of differences in age and experience than differences in gender. Upon further analysis, it appears that women simply leave the lifeguard profession much earlier than men. The data revealed that male lifeguards in this study were significantly older and more experienced than the female guards in the sample. Because the sample was composed of younger, less experienced females and older, more experienced males, it is only reasonable to expect that males would feel more confident. What appears to be significant gender differences in the lifeguarding profession at first glance, can be explained easily by age and experience factors.

There were also significant differences between males and females in regard to the type of aquatic facility where they were employed. Ocean lifeguards were composed of 87% males while only 13% of ocean lifeguards were females. Conversely, more women (76%) worked at conventional swimming pools than men (63%). When the lifeguards were asked to best characterize their responsibilities while on duty, men were more likely to describe themselves as "rescuers" while women described themselves as "enforcers."

The major purpose of this study was to reveal how lifeguards actually spend their time on duty rather than to speculate what the lifeguards *should* be doing while on duty. Additional information was gleaned from the data when age, gender, and experience factors were compared. Some timely information was illustrated by the study. Further discussion and future investigations should be aware of the following survey findings:

- Half of the lifeguard sample was made up of teenagers; our aquatic health care professionals are quite young. Also, 40% of the lifeguard force surveyed worked two seasons or less, indicating that many of our lifeguards have little experience.
- One third of the lifeguards guarded more than 3,000 sq ft of water surface area and 60% of the sample guarded more than 50 swimmers in their zone. These numbers are quite large.
- More than half the lifeguarding sample watched their swimmers less than 100% of the time. A significant number of lifeguards did not know how to scan, thought that they were less than "very well trained," and were not supervised often.
- Finally, based on this sample, it appears that several general characteristics hold true for lifeguards in the United States. Female lifeguards are younger and less experienced while male lifeguards are older and more experienced. This may simply suggest that females do not chose to remain in

the lifeguarding profession as long as males. Additionally, very few females guard at our oceans. Consistently throughout the survey, older, more experienced lifeguards reported themselves as being better trained, more confident and in general more challenged when on duty than younger, less experienced lifeguards. This is important information for those hiring, training, and supervising lifeguards. If one can assume that ocean situations require the most experienced guards, then perhaps pools and water parks should follow incentives for lifeguards developed by our nation's beach patrols.

Although lifeguarding education, training, and supervision have improved during recent years, lifeguards are actually working in situations that are not within the guidelines of some water safety agencies and experts. If the information provided by this survey is accurate and reliable, even more intensive site-specific lifeguard training may be required in the future, and water safety experts and agencies should become more cognizant of actual working conditions for lifeguards.

It is important to note that the National Lifeguard Studies conducted at Penn State University do not collect data on the actual vision capabilities of lifeguards on duty. This work, in our opinion, should be left to optometrists and ophthalmologists. A recent survey by Barry L. Seller, M.D., indicated that 10% of the lifeguards tested had sub-par vision (less than 20/30), and 17% of the lifeguards who participated had prescription lenses at home but did not use them while on duty.

Based on the results of the previous surveys and interviews of hundreds of lifeguards as well as experts in vision and surveillance, a systematic scanning strategy was developed for lifeguards. **The Five Minute Scanning Strategy** was developed by Griffiths, Chambers, and Steel. Although this technique is quite simple to learn, it is one of the first attempts to organize lifeguarding visual search patterns into an organized strategy that can be used by lifeguards working in a variety of environments. This scanning technique can in fact be adapted for any person engaged in surveillance or supervision. Basically, the Five Minute Scanning Strategy consists of alternating visual scanning patterns which last for five minutes. Each five-minute observational pattern is followed by a safety check or an accounting of people swimming in the lifeguard's zone of responsibility.

First an explanation is needed for why the visual scanning patterns were broken down into five-minute segments. Numerous vision experts consulted agreed that five minutes was approximately the maximum amount of time a subject could remain alert performing a visual task before either boredom or eye fatigue developed. Additionally, based on the data the authors collected from more than 8,000 lifeguards during the past several years, all lifeguard station rotations took place on a five-minute increment, that is, lifeguards changed their stations every 15, 20, 30, or 45 minutes. Considering all these factors, five-minute scanning patterns were practiced during a pilot project at Penn State University. The lifeguards enjoyed the flexibility of choosing their own visual search pattern and were

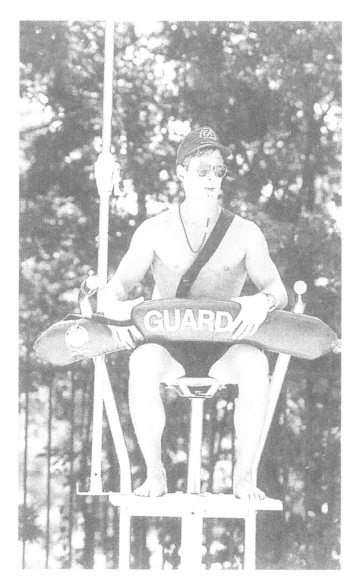

FIGURE 4   Remaining rescue-ready.

E&A clients include primarily water parks and flat-water pools in university, park, and recreation settings. The report data included here does not totally differentiate by type of facility, although some divisions are obvious.

RESCUES BY AREA

The chart and diagram of rescues by area show some interesting and perhaps unexpected facts. The wave pool, considered by many to be the "danger spot," has a high level of rescues, with almost as many in the slide and activity pools. Slide comfortable using one pattern for five minutes prior to summing up the in-water situation before changing to a different visual pattern.

The visual search patterns that are the most popular are horizontal, vertical, circular, and figure eight although other patterns are acceptable. For the purposes of this study, scanning and sweeping are defined differently. Scanning is the process of systematically observing the zone for a five-minute period. Sweeping refers to one visual pass through the lifeguard's zone, which typically takes 5–15 seconds. While sweeping through the zone, the eyes should stop every 10–15° to pick up details; details like facial expressions cannot be detected when the eyes are continually moving (Figure 3).

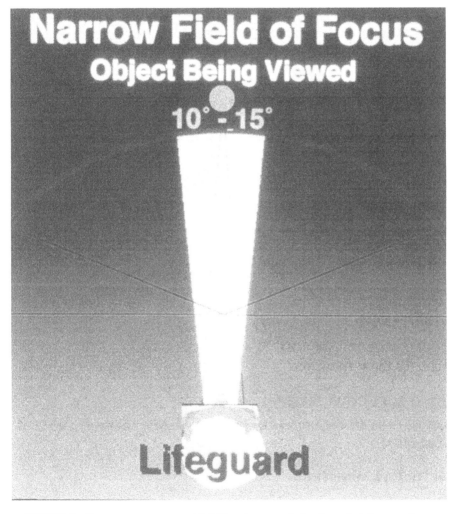

FIGURE 3   Eyes must stop every 10–15° to detect such details as facial expressions.

As the eyes successively sweep through the zone, different individuals in the water should be visually focused on so that, within five minutes, each patron is visually observed or "touched." It is imperative that both the head and eyes move during the process of scanning. Head movement is as essential as eye movement because it reduces eye fatigue and, more importantly, allows the lifeguard supervisor to detect active scanning from *behind* the lifeguard without the lifeguard detecting the supervisor. After each five-minute scan, the lifeguard should quickly count the patrons in the zone, and then change posture (sitting, standing, walking). It is also a good idea to mentally practice a rescue scenario on a patron in the zone who appears to be difficult to rescue. Also recommended is the monitoring of high-risk areas, activities, and people. Other lifeguards at the facility should be notified that all is "O.K." in a zone before scanning is continued. Younger, less experienced lifeguards should be mentored by older, more experienced lifeguards who are familiar with the specific risks and clientele of the facility at which they are employed. Management and lifeguards should determine roughly how many seconds are required to visually sweep each zone. The beauty of this technique is that lifeguards can now visually sweep and scan their zones with objective strategies that result in better accountability of the people in their zone. A safety check is completed after each five minutes to more accurately and objectively indicate to the lifeguard the status of the swimmers in his or her zone. A summary of the Five Minute Scanning Strategy is:

THE FIVE MINUTE SCANNING STRATEGY

(By Tom Griffiths, Ed.D., Virgil Chambers, and Don Steel, Ph.D.)

FIRST SWEEP

GENERALLY ASSESS THOSE IN THE ZONE

SECOND SWEEP

GROUP AND CATEGORIZE SWIMMERS INTO CLUSTERS OR QUADRANTS

THIRD SWEEP

BRIEFLY CENTER ON A FOCAL PERSON WITHIN EACH GROUP;
LOOK FOR FACIAL EXPRESSIONS

EACH SUCCESSIVE SWEEP

CHANGE FOCAL PERSONS UNTIL EVERYONE IN YOUR ZONE IS OBSERVED IN DETAIL AT LEAST ONCE

AFTER FIVE MINUTES

MAKE A SAFETY CHECK

REFERENCES

1. Griffiths, Tom, July 19, 1987, "Do Lifeguards Do What They Get Paid to Do?" *The New York Times*, p. 22.
2. Griffiths, Tom, Steel, Don, and Chambers, Virgil, Winter 1995, "The Five Minute Scanning Strategy," *NRPA Aquatic News*, pp. 6–7.
3. Griffiths, Tom, Steel, Don, and Vogelsong, Hans, February 1995, "Systematic Scanning for Lifeguards." *Parks and Recreation*, pp. 40–47.
4. Griffiths, Tom, Steel, Don, and Vogelsong, Hans, February 1996, "Lifeguarding Behaviors," *Parks and Recreation*, pp. 54–59.
5. Personal Conversation with Bob Burhans, January 1995, New York State Department of Health.
6. Seller, Barry L., M.D., February 1996, "Lifeguard Vision Project," *Parks and Recreation*, pp. 62–63.

17 Toward a Predictive Model for Rip Currents and Their Impact on Public Safety with Emphasis on Physical, Demographic, and Cultural Considerations

James B. Lushine, John R. Fletemeyer, and Robert G. Dean

The objective of this chapter is to determine within certain physical, demographic, and cultural parameters how rip currents impact public safety on surf beaches.

WHAT ARE RIP CURRENTS?

Several well-defined and fairly ubiquitous nearshore and/or beach phenomena have to date defied development of a sufficient understanding of their formation and underlying physics to garner consensus among the interested scientific and engineering communities. These include beach cusps, longshore bars, and rip currents, the latter being the subject of this chapter. Some or all of these phenomena may have multiple causes of formation and/or maintenance. Interest in developing improved understanding of these phenomena ranges from scientific curiosity to the water safety aspects associated with rip currents to the hope that an understanding of these somewhat esoteric features will strengthen our overall understanding of the physics of complex nearshore processes to allow a more effective attack on other areas of insufficient understanding. Indeed, a knowledge of the causes of rip currents could lead to a predictive capability and thus a means to minimize loss of life and provide a general increase in the safety of the nation's beach resource system.

Rip currents, also known as "sea pusses," "run outs," and "rip tides," are fairly strong seaward-directed flows of water that are quite pervasive. Despite their scientific, water safety, and engineering relevance, these features have not been studied extensively and at present their causes are poorly understood. A better understanding of rip currents would contribute to the general knowledge of surf zone processes and, in particular, to coupling with the offshore waters. Additionally, rip currents are known to occur over wide (several hundred kilometers) regions simultaneously, thereby posing broad water safety hazards. A capability to interpret the storm (wave) sequence and/or beach profile state conducive to the initiation of rip currents would facilitate improved planning for more effective allocation of water safety resources, resulting in fewer related drownings. Finally, in the design of segmented, submerged, or emergent breakwaters, there may be a design rationale in the spacing of break-waters to mimic the natural spacing of rip currents.

Our present knowledge of rip currents is based on a combination of observed characteristics and proposed mechanisms of generation and maintenance.

OBSERVED CHARACTERISTICS OF RIP CURRENTS

Shepard, Emery, and LaFond (1941), in a comprehensive field study of rip currents along the beaches near La Jolla, California, were apparently the first to describe rip currents as seaward-flowing features that originated near locations of wave divergence. This wonderfully descriptive article clarified many of the physical characteristics of rip currents, primarily along the southern California beaches; however, many of the results presented are general. The currents are the return flow of landward-directed, weaker flows that have occurred over a much greater shore parallel dimension than is occupied by the rip current. The terminology shown in Figure 1 was advanced with the shore parallel flows toward the rip termed "feeder" currents, the rapid seaward flow, the "neck," and the flows in the offshore region where the rip decreases in velocity, the "head." Several features identified were: (1) Rip normal to the shoreline; (2) The offshore distance to which the rips extended was approximately 300–800 m; (3) The widths of the rips ranged from 20–30 m; and (4) Rips usually occur off small indentations in the shoreline. Based in part on discussions with many lifeguards, the following were noted as possible visual indicators of the presence of rip currents: (1) Sediment-laden water; (2) Green water at the ends of the rip heads (due to the greater depths in the scour channels); (3) Foam belts on the outer edges of the rip head; (4) "Agitated" water at the outer boundaries of the rip heads; (5) Gaps in the advancing waves, with the waves breaking much closer to shore; and (6) Seaward movement of floating objects. Based on observations and recordings conducted at Scripps Pier in California it was found that the incidence of rips was much greater during periods of large waves. The trajectories and velocities associated with rips were explored by tracking drogues that had large drag elements below the water surface. The maximum currents were on the order of 1 m/s.

Of particular relevance to this chapter were the following three features evident in the work of Shepard et al. (1941): (1) Reference was made that Nicholls (1936) had observed rips to be present in the absence of a rip channel although such channels were always present in the cases reported by Shepard et al.; (2) There was no mention of the longshore *periodicity* of the rips; and (3) No note was made of *migrating* rip currents, which tends to suggest that rip channels are usually present. These channels would tend to "lock" the rip in place.

Shepard and Inman (1950a) described a comprehensive program of field meas-urements of nearshore currents and the forcing agents in the vicinity of the Scripps

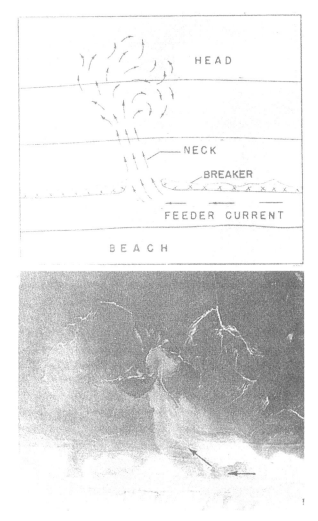

FIGURE 1 Characteristics and adopted rip current terminology. From Shepard, Emery, and LaFond (1941).

beaches in southern California. Methods employed included dye, drogues, and wave and tsunami gages. The general characteristics of nearshore circulation were defined as well as the patterns associated with rip currents. The correlation between rip currents and long period "even-crested" waves was noted as was the pulsating nature of rips and the relation of the period of pulsation with that of the surf beat caused by groups of waves. As in the previous paper, there was no mention of longshore periodicity of rips or of the tendency for migration of these features.

In a second paper, Shepard and Inman (1950b) extended their rip current studies to include comparisons of the relative frequencies of seaward and longshore bottom and surface currents and to attempt to predict the velocities of longshore currents and to examine rip currents from Oregon, Washington, and Hawaii. Incidence of

seaward and longshore surface bottom currents were determined by observing floating kelp and a weighted volleyball, respectively. Based on three locations in southern
California, it was found that slightly more than 50% of the surface currents were
offshore compared to those in the longshore direction. For the near-bottom currents,
the incidence of offshore bottom currents was slightly less than 80%, indicative of
the return flow associated with wave mass transport. Field observations of the spacing
of rip currents carried out in Oregon, Washington, and Hawaii demonstrated that,
in Oregon and southern Washington, the average rip spacing was found to be 400 m
with a standard deviation of 145 m. The observations on the island of Kauai, Hawaii
were conducted within a reefed embayment where extreme gradients in wave height
were found within fairly short distances. At one location, within 400 m, the wave
height decreased from 5.5 m to 1.5 m. These gradients caused rips at the locations
of lower waves. The momentum approach of calculating longshore currents of
Putnam, Munk, and Traylor (1949) was compared with field data. It was found that
although the equation appeared to predict the general features of the currents, it was
necessary to include a representation of the friction coefficient — which decreased
significantly with current velocity — in order to obtain reasonable agreement. The
role of natural or constructed obstructions such as headlands, jetties, and piers in
causing rip currents was noted.

McKenzie (1958) has reported on a six-year program of rip current observation
along the beaches of New South Wales, Australia, where the beaches are reasonably
straight and unobstructed for a distance of 1100 km. Five factors relating to rip
current characteristics are discussed: (1) The size and regularity of waves — Small
waves tend to be associated with more numerous, smaller, and less intense rip
currents. The strength of the rips is directly related to the strength of the waves;
(2) Tide — Lower tide stages tend to concentrate rips, and subsidiary rips may
develop at lower stages of tides to provide additional relief as the cross-sectional
area of the main channels are reduced by the lower tide levels; (3) Wave Direction —
In those cases where rips were caused by waves approaching the shoreline obliquely,
it was found that within the surf zone, the rip channels tended to be oriented into
the waves; however, outside the surf zone, the channels tended to bend away from
the waves; (4) Coastal configuration — At those locations where there was structural
control, such as a headland, the rips were often found on both sides of the control.
In some pocket beaches, in contrast to the observed results of Shepard and Inman
on the southern California beaches, the rips were found to occur at locations of the
higher waves; and (5) Slope and regularity of the nearshore — Although the range
of beach slopes along the New South Wales shoreline did not permit direct observations, McKenzie stated that due to the amount of water transported landward on
mildly sloping beaches, the incidence and strength of rip currents should be greater
than on steeper beaches.

PROPOSED MECHANISMS FOR THE GENERATION AND MAINTENANCE OF RIP CURRENTS

Several explanations have been given for the mechanisms which govern rip
currents, including: (1) Instabilities between the channels and topographic control
(Hino [1974] and Diegaard [1990]); (2) Interaction between synchronous edge waves

and incident waves (Bowen [1969] and Bowen and Inman [1969]); (3) Interaction between waves and rip currents (Dalrymple and Lozano [1978]); (4) Intersecting wave trains (Dalrymple [1975], Dalrymple and Lanan [1976], and Hammack et al. [1989]); and (5) Structural controls by natural and/or constructed features such as headlands, piers, jetties, etc. It is possible that several mechanisms are responsible for the formation and maintenance of rip currents. For example, it is generally agreed that structural controls can position rip currents. In addition to these uncertainties that exist regarding the mechanisms, several characteristics of rip currents have been questioned that are relevant to this chapter, including: (1) Whether or not *substantial* migrating rip currents can occur; (2) Whether substantial rip currents can occur without the presence of a rip channel; and (3) Whether the interaction between rips and incident waves causes increased or decreased wave heights in the vicinity of the rip. Answers to these questions would clarify the mechanisms governing rip currents. The paragraphs below review briefly the various hypotheses of rip current mechanisms.

Instabilities between Hydrodynamic and Sedimentary Systems

Hino (1974) and Diegaard (1990) have posed this problem as a two-dimensional hydrodynamic system on which a small cellular perturbation is imposed and have incorporated sediment transport and continuity equations. The stability of the overall system is considered, and the modes (rip spacings) with the greatest tendency for growth are identified. This is the only proposed mechanism that considers a positive feedback between cellular circulation and the sedimentary system, but in practice requires specification of an "initial" condition, which tends to include a two-dimensional bar and may not be well defined.

Interaction between Synchronous Waves and Edge Waves

The superposition of normally incident and edge waves was considered by Bowen (1969) and Bowen and Inman (1969). The edge waves can be standing or propagating, with migrating rips occurring in the latter case. At a fixed distance offshore, and at a particular time, the two wave systems superimpose alternately positively and negatively in the longshore direction. It is reasoned that since the onshore wave setup drives longshore currents and, through the radiation stresses, the wave setup depends on the wave height, these longshore varying wave heights will drive a cellular current system. Laboratory and field measurements and observations were carried out and interpreted as supporting this mechanism.

Dalrymple and Lozano (1978) conducted a theoretical analysis of the interaction of combined incident waves and rip currents on a prismatic beach. The problem was posed in terms of a normal mode formulation and the mode (spacing) most conducive to growth was selected as the one representative of rip currents. It is stated that the work done by the waves on the rip currents results in a reduced wave height in the vicinity of the rip. This study embodies two of the significant questions raised above: (1) whether significant currents can exist on a prismatic profile; and (2) whether the wave/current interaction results in wave heights that are lower or higher at the rip channel. The work by Dalrymple and Lozano represented an extension of the earlier contribution of LeBlond and Tang (1974).

Intersecting Wave Trains

Dalrymple (1975) and Dalrymple and Lanan (1976) have shown both theoretically and experimentally that synchronous waves arriving from equal and opposite wave directions with respect to the beach normal will cause a stationary longshore periodic wave setup along the shoreline which, in turn, leads to spatially periodic rip currents. If the waves were not synchronous or the wave directions were not precisely opposite, the locations of wave setup would propagate in the longshore direction. Hammack et al. (1989) have demonstrated both analytically and experimentally that a particular type of hexagonal wave pattern will, upon breaking on the beach, produce rip currents.

Structural Controls

Natural or constructed features, including headlands, groins, jetties, piers, etc. along the shoreline, can cause rip currents. For the simplest case, these currents occur on the upwave side of the structure and are simply the seaward deflection of the longshore current induced in the surf zone by oblique waves. Currents can occur on the "downwave" side through wave sheltering and nonuniform wave heights and wave setup. These currents have been termed "diffraction" currents by Gourlay (1976). For waves propagating normal to shore, it can be shown that energy losses at a groin cause more momentum transfer in deeper water than would normally occur and thus less shoreline setup adjacent to the groins. This would tend to position seaward-directed currents adjacent to the groins, a feature observed in nature. A similar explanation may apply due to wave energy losses by pilings under piers.

The list of references included with this chapter contains several rip current citations not reviewed herein.

HUMAN FACTORS

Several sources are used to determine the number of drownings associated with rip currents, principally in Dade and Broward counties of southeast Florida. Groups of people who might be particularly at risk are identified. An association of rip currents to both local wind and tides is established.

Initially, medical examiner death records of Dade and Broward counties in southeast Florida for the ten-year period 1979–1988 were examined for ocean or surf drownings. A death record includes a police report and autopsy information. The death records for the approximately 210 drownings during this period were examined for information concerning the likelihood that the drowning was primarily rip current related. Discarded as unlikely to be rip current related were drownings from boating or diving accidents. Homicides and suicides were summarily dismissed, as were drownings that occurred in very shallow water. Drownings that

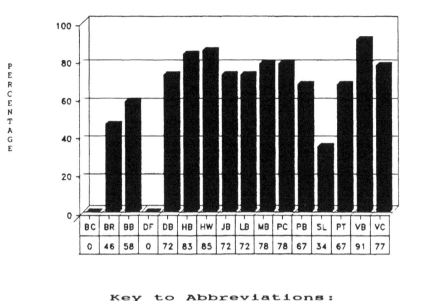

Key to Abbreviations:

BC = Brevard County   HB = Hallandale Beach   PC = Palm Beach County
BR = Boca Raton   HW = Hollywood Beach   PB = Pompano Beach
BB = Boyton Beach   JB = Jacksonville Beach SL = St. Lucie County
DF = Deerfield Beach   LB = Lantana Beach   TB = Town of Palm Beach
DB = Delray Beach   MB = Miami Beach   VB = Vero Beach
                                                VC = Volusia County

FIGURE 2   Relative percentage of rip current rescues vs. other rescues, compared by agency.

occurred where beach patrol observations indicated no rip currents existed were also excluded. To simplify any relationship between rip currents and meteorological and oceanographic elements, the approximately 15–20 drownings that occurred in conjunction with breakwaters and channels were not initially considered. This overall selection process reduced the 210 drownings to 148 potential rip current-related drownings.

In these 148 cases, the date, day, and local time of the drowning, the location of the drowning, and the age, sex, race, and home address (when available) of the victim were ascertained. Other pertinent facts, such as possible contributory causes to the death, including prior medical conditions and toxicology reports, were also tabulated.

In a study of near-drownings involving 249 cases from seven beach patrol agencies located in southeast Florida, 69.8% of the near-drownings were linked to rip currents. In a similar but more comprehensive study involving 17 beach patrol agencies and 4,579 cases, a total of 3,028 rescues (66%) were attributed by lifeguards to rip currents. Of particular interest in this study was the finding that there was considerable variation in the relative percentage of rip current rescues vs. other types of water rescues from beach to beach (Figure 2). Vero Beach, for example, reported that 91 of its rescues were due to rip currents while Deerfield Beach reported that none of its rescues were rip current related. This data is significant because it demonstrates that there is significant variability in rip currents from beach to beach, even among beaches located just a few miles apart.

The beach patrols for Miami Beach, Hollywood, Fort Lauderdale, and Dade County are responsible for "guarding" the ocean beaches of Dade and Broward counties. Each organization keeps a log of rescues performed, which usually indicates the location, date, and time of each rescue, the age, sex, and race of the victim, and the reason for the rescue. Rescue reports from January 1988 through July 1989 were tabulated. During this period there was a total of 541 beach patrol rescues involving 788 people on 119 days. As noted from the rescue reports, most of these rescues involved rip currents (usually denoted on the rescue form as a runout) or bathers who found themselves in water over their heads (denoted as a rescue from a hole). In addition, Haulover Beach in northern Dade County was closed or swimming restricted due to hazardous weather-related surf conditions 17 times in 1988.

PANAMA CITY, A CASE STUDY

A study conducted by Fletemeyer and Wolfe (1994), which surveyed 130 bathers on Panama City Beach, identified a number of demographic and culture factors that contributed to the relatively high drowning rate on this beach. The results of this study support much of the data just presented and include the following observations about the Panama City bather population, which contribute to the inordinate number of drownings on this beach.

- A relatively large bather population was from states lacking beaches.
- A relatively large number of bathers were categorized in this study as either "poor" or "fair" swimmers.
- A relatively large number of bathers lacked an understanding about the inherent dangers associated with rip currents.
- Panama City Beach is generally regarded as a summer beach and, therefore, bathing tends to be seasonal.

From the information gathered in this study, the authors concluded that, although some beaches, due to their physical characteristics, may be more likely to have rip currents than others, other cultural and demographic variables contribute to the high drowning rates experienced on some surf beaches.

Wind and tide measurements that were nearest in time to the rescues were collected to complete the database. This rescue information for 1988 was used to supplement the drowning information for that year. In addition, rescue reports for 1979–1987 were sampled on a selective basis at some of the beach patrol offices to help verify the likelihood of individual rip current drownings.

To attempt to normalize the number of rip current drownings and rescues with respect to the number of people at the beach, attendance totals at three Dade County public beaches and one Broward County beach were collected for portions of the period 1979–1988.

In addition to the rip current data in southeast Florida, clippings concerning surf drownings and near-drownings were collected from all major Florida newspapers from June 1989 through January 1995.

Initially, to determine the magnitude of the rip current drowning problem in southeast Florida, the 148 surf drownings from 1979 to 1988 that were identified as probably associated with rip currents through medical examiner records were examined in closer detail. A three-step approach was taken. First, the medical examiner records (principally the accompanying police reports), were examined for eyewitness accounts of the drowning. If eyewitnesses used such phrases as "current strong ... pulled into deeper water," "strong undertow," or "current was too strong to swim in against," the drowning was classified as likely to be rip current related. In this way, 42 of the 148 deaths were identified as likely rip current drownings. Next, the beach patrol rescue records for the day on which a drowning occurred were examined. If run outs were reported at any of the four southeast Florida beaches, it was assumed that rip currents could have been present along all the southeast Florida beaches, and that the drowning on that day was likely to be rip current related. This added another 30 cases, for a total of 72. Finally, after determining the wind and tide conditions with which rip currents were associated (see later sections for details), and comparing them to conditions on the day of the drowning, an additional 22 cases were presumed to be rip current related.

Thus, of the 148 potential rip current drownings in southeast Florida during the ten-year period 1979–1988, a total of 94 were determined to have been associated with rip currents. These drownings usually occurred at a rate of one per day and at infrequent intervals, but, on nine occasions, there were two drownings in one day, and six times the drownings occurred on two or three consecutive days. In addition to the likely rip current drownings, another 19 surf drownings were identified as otherwise likely related to weather conditions (see later sections for explanation). This brought the total number of weather-related surf drownings in Dade and Broward counties to 113. This total is far more than the combined number of other weather-related deaths — caused by lightning, hurricanes, tornadoes, and other types of hazardous weather — in these counties during this period. Lightning, for instance, accounts for an average of two deaths per year in Dade and Broward counties, with hurricanes and tornadoes accounting for even fewer. It may be questioned whether rip current deaths are directly weather related; however, since storm surge deaths in hurricanes are considered a direct consequence of weather, and because the relationship between wind and storm surge and wind and rip currents is analogous, rip current deaths should similarly be considered weather related.

Figure 3 shows a graph of the annual rip current surf drowings from 1979 to 1988 in southeast Florida. This shows 19 rip current drownings in 1979 followed by a decline to a minimum of 4 in 1982, then a slow increase through 1987, with a sharp increase to 18 in 1988. To determine if the reason for the yearly variation in rip current drownings could be accounted for by a varying number of beach-goers, attendance records from three Dade County beaches and from one Broward County beach were tabulated for portions of the same ten-year period. Of course, many of

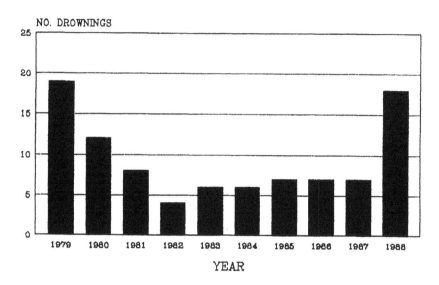

FIGURE 3   Annual number of rip current drownings in Dade and Broward counties of southeast Florida, 1979–1988.

the drownings occurred at unguarded beaches with unknown attendance figures. The number of rip current-related deaths normalized by the available attendance shows little change from the unnormalized data in terms of annual distribution. Another factor in the fluctuation of rip current drownings was speculated to be the "renourishment" of the beach. Renourishment is the process of pumping sand from offshore to the beach, thus widening it. The beaches of Dade County were renourished beginning in the mid-1970s and ending in the early 1980s. The number of drownings over the two-county area does not indicate any correlation with this renourishment, although it does not preclude local variations.

   Figure 4 presents a graph of the monthly frequency of weather-related surf drownings. The graph indicates 80 of the 113 (71%) weather-related drownings and 64 of the 94 (68%) rip current drownings occurred in the six-month period from March through August.

   To determine if the monthly distribution was related to the number of beach-goers, attendance at the guarded beaches was used to calculate the per capita monthly drownings. Comparing the per capita drownings to the actual drownings, the percentage for the period March through August was reduced from 68% to 57%.

   Although the beach attendance does not account entirely for the greater number of drownings during the period March through August, the number of people entering the surf zone may not be directly tied to the number of people attending the beach. Naturally, during the winter months, the air and sea temperatures are lower, so fewer people enter the water. An examination of the Miami Local Climatological Data (LCD) on each day on which a drowning occurred revealed, not surprisingly, that they occurred on days with a high percentage of possible sunshine and seasonal or above-normal air temperatures. During the winter the annual migration of stinging jellyfish also takes place,

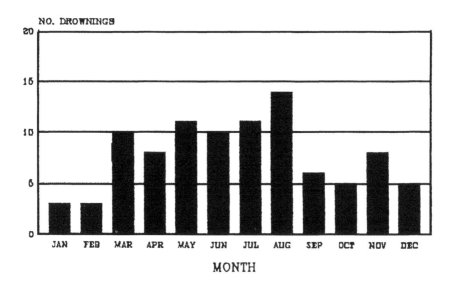

FIGURE 4   Monthly number of rip current drownings in Dade and Broward counties of southeast Florida, 1979–1988.

which undoubtedly discourages a number of people from entering the surf. The jellyfish are transported into the surf zone during periods of onshore winds — the same type of conditions under which rip currents may occur (as will be shown later in this chapter.)

Another factor to consider is a measure of the swimming ability of people entering the surf, which can be inferred by comparing the rip current drownings to the total number of weather-related drownings each month. As will be explained later, the weather-related drownings not associated with rip currents are the result of poor swimmers or nonswimmers being swept into deeper water under certain wind conditions. In the six-month period from March through August, 16 of 19 (84%) of the non-rip current, weather-related drownings occurred. It is assumed that a greater number of people entering the surf during that period were poorer swimmers, and this may account, in part, for the higher percentage of rip current drownings. Although rip currents are too powerful for even the strongest swimmer to overcome, stronger swimmers are, undoubtedly on the whole, more comfortable in the surf, which makes them less likely to panic if caught in a rip current.

Two other factors that are also worth considering with regard to the monthly distribution of weather-related drownings are the frequency and strength of rip currents. Detailed rescue records were only obtained during 1988, so the frequency of rip currents on a monthly basis and a possible measure of their strength over the entire ten-year period cannot be calculated directly; however, an attempt was made to infer their strength based on the 1988 data. In 1988, there were 64 days for which the presence of rip currents was inferred from either beach patrol rescue reports or from death records. The average number of deaths per "rip current day" was higher during the period September through February than

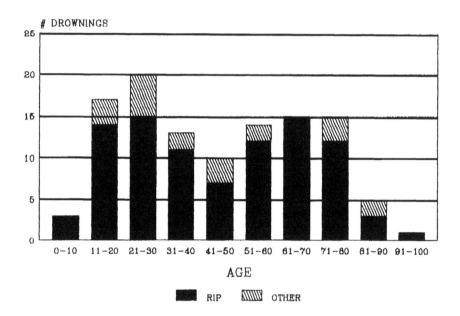

FIGURE 5   Frequency of rip current drownings by age at southeast Florida beaches, 1979–1988.

during the period March through August. This implies that rip currents are stronger during the fall and winter. This is supported by the Navy Climatological Data, which shows that the average easterly (onshore) wind speed along the southeast Florida coast is slightly greater during the September through February period. Later, it will be shown that there is a correlation between strong onshore wind flow and rip currents.

As might be expected, the largest number of weather-related surf drownings are on weekends, but a significant number of deaths also occur on weekdays. Most rip current drownings occur between 10 A.M. and 4 P.M. local time, which probably corresponds to the time of day when people are most frequently in the water, and could also be related to stronger rip currents aided by the daily onshore sea breeze.

Figure 5 shows the age distribution of weather-related drowning victims. A bimodal distribution shows one maximum in the age group 16–25 and the other in the age group 55–75. Tables 1 and 2 stratify weather-related drownings and weather-related rescues, respectively, by sex, race, and, in the case of drownings, residency. These statistics indicate a disproportionately high number of male victims. About 30% of the rip current drowning victims were tourists. It is unknown how many local residents were permanent or seasonal visitors. Considering only local residents, the racial make-up showed a higher percentage of black drowning victims than that of the local population. The reason for this racial difference could be due to a greater proportion of blacks going to the beach, but no figures are available to determine this.

TABLE 1
Demographics of weather-related surf drownings at south Florida beaches, 1979–1988.

Drowning Cause	Sex		Race		Residence	
	Male	Female	White	Black	Local	Tourist
Rip Current	82	12	77	17	57	32
Other	15	4	12	7	13	1
Total	97	16	89	24	70	33

TABLE 2
Demographics of weather-related surf rescues at south Florida beaches in 1988.

Rescue Cause	Sex		Race	
	Male	Female	White	Black
Rip Current	262	185	152	43
Other	24	24	9	33
Total	286	209	161	76

In an attempt to identify particular segments of the population who were at increased risk, several other comparisons were made. Figure 6, which depicts the age of local residents divided into racial groups, shows that a large number of older whites and younger blacks are represented. It is concluded that the three segments of the population most at risk to rip current drownings were tourists, local residents who were white and elderly (55 years or older), and local residents who were black and young (25 years or younger). The three groups comprised 70–75% of the drownings during the ten-year period.

Nine of the drowning victims were diagnosed by autopsy to have had some degree of artery or heart disease which may have contributed to the death. An additional seven of the drowning victims had blood alcohol or drug levels that might have impaired their ability to function normally in the water.

The rip current-related drownings enumerated above occurred at both guarded and unguarded southeast Florida beaches. Using the rescue reports from four of the guarded beaches in 1988, the daily and hourly distribution of rip current-related rescues and their demographics were ascertained. Rip current rescues in 1988 show a very large majority occurred between noon and 4 P.M., which, again, probably reflects the peak beach-going hours. Rescues related to the day of the week are interestingly distributed. As in the case of the drownings, most rescues were on Saturday. Unlike the drownings, about as many rescues occurred on Thursday and Friday as on Sunday. The fewest rescues were on Monday, Tuesday, and Wednesday, which was consistent with the drowning figures. No explanation for this distribution can be offered.

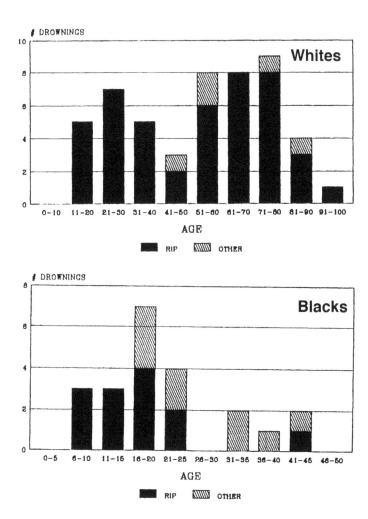

FIGURE 6   Frequency of rip current drownings by age for local white residents (top) and local black residents (bottom) at southeast Florida beaches, 1979–1988.

The average age of the rescued victims is much younger than the drowning victims, implying that older beach-goers tend to avoid the guarded and probably more crowded beaches. A total of 86% of the drowning victims were male while only 58% of the rescued victims were male. This indicates that either there is a greater percentage of females at guarded beaches or, possibly, that females are more likely to be rescued than males.

The rip current drownings were identified by county, with Dade having about twice the number as Broward. This is consistent with the difference in the overall morbidity rate between the two counties.

A newspaper clipping service for all major Florida newspapers shows the total number of rip current-related drownings in the state of Florida from January 1989 through December 1995 to be about 151 persons. Volusia County had the most drownings with 25. Bay County was second with 24. Other counties with more than 10 drownings included Dade with 17 and Escambia with 12. Due probably to a vigorous education campaign from 1989 to 1995, the number of current drownings in Dade and Broward counties of southeast Florida dropped from an average of nine per year from 1979 to 1989 to an average of less than three per year from 1990 to 1995.

PHYSICAL FACTORS

Along surf beaches that have rip currents, three factors are generally involved in their initiation and maintenance: wind waves, tides, and oceanic swells. National Data Buoy Center (NDBC) buoys off the east central and northeast coasts of Florida operationally measure wave heights, but no real-time wave measurements are available along the coasts of Dade and Broward counties. In the absence of swells there is a nearly direct relationship between wave height and wind speed. Because of the easy availability of wind observations, the local wind rather than the wind wave height was chosen to be compared to rip current initiation. Additionally, a close association between wind direction and wind speed and the incidence of rip currents in southeast Florida was supported by anecdotal information from beach patrol personnel.

To investigate the association between the wind and rip currents, wind observations during the ten-year period 1979–1988 were examined. The primary source of the wind observations was an NWS wind measuring instrument called a Device for Automatic Remote Data Collection (DARDC) located at the Miami Beach Patrol Office at Ocean Drive and 10th Street in Miami Beach, Florida. The site represented the wind measuring instrument closest to the ocean beaches in Dade and Broward counties that was routinely available during the ten-year period. The proximity of the anemometer to the beach was very important because of the sometimes large differences in wind between coastal and inland locations caused by mesoscale variations near the land-sea interface. The DARDC data is routinely collected each hour on the hour by the NWS's Weather Service Forecast Office (WSFO) in Miami, and the reading is archived locally.

A synoptic (large scale) windflow across southeast Florida was defined by using the geostrophic wind calculated from the National Hurricane Center (NHC) surface analysis closest in time to the event. Although the geostrophic approximation at the surface has certain limitations due principally to isobaric curvature and frictional and isallobaric effects, it was felt it represented reasonably well the large-scale wind flow. In addition, operational forecasts of the geostrophic wind can easily be made from numerical surface isobaric progs. The *Study of U.S. Navy Climate of the Caribbean Sea and Gulf of Mexico,* which includes the Florida coastal waters, was used for comparative purposes.

The time and height of high and low tide and the speed and direction of the tidal current for the ten-year period were obtained from *National Ocean Service's (NOS) Tide Tables — High and Low Water Predictions and from the Tidal Current*

Tables. Data for the Miami Harbor entrance, located about one mile south of the DARDC on Miami Beach, was used.

As surfers know, large, long-period swells are more frequent along the United States west coast and in Hawaii than along the east and Gulf coasts. These swells, which occur about a dozen times a year along the southern California coast, can cause strong rip currents. Intense extratropical storms in both hemispheres and occasional east Pacific hurricanes generate these swells, which sometimes propagate thousands of miles before impacting the surf zone. In the eastern United States, large swells, during the summer months when most people are at the beach, are caused by relatively infrequent tropical or subtropical cyclones. In southeast Florida large swells, except those from nearby tropical cyclones, are quite rare events anytime of the year due to the sheltering effects of the Bahama Islands and Cuba. Therefore, only a limited amount of data concerning the relationship of swells to rip currents was available in Florida, mainly along the northeast Florida coast. Relationships between rip currents and land swells generated by hurricanes Dean, Gabrielle, and Hugo in August and September 1989, tropical storm Gordon in 1994, and hurricane Luis in 1995 were made using ship and buoy observations and information from newspaper clippings.

To examine the association between wind speed and direction and the occurrence of rip currents, wind data from the Miami Beach DARDC and the calculated geostrophic wind were tabulated. The association between wind and rip current was made only on the 72 occasions from 1979 to 1988 when other sources of information, such as the medical examiner records or the beach patrol rescue logs, indicated the high likelihood that rip currents had occurred. The hourly observation of wind speed from the Miami Beach DARDC includes the latest one-minute average immediately prior to the polling and the peak wind recorded since the previous polling (both measured in knots). Unfortunately, the peak wind was not routinely recorded prior to 1985. The DARDC wind direction observation was made to the nearest ten degrees of the compass for the one-minute average speed after April 1984. Prior to April 1984, the wind direction was archived only to 16 points of the compass. The peak wind direction was not measured but was assumed to be the same as the one-minute average wind direction. This assumption is not always valid especially when convective activity is nearby.

The hourly DARDC wind observation closest in time to the rip current event was tabulated. Other DARDC wind observations, such as the average overnight wind, were noted for further evaluation. Since a wind at a single time and location may not be representative of conditions along a 30-mile stretch of coast, and since a geostrophic wind can be quickly calculated from a forecast of the surface pressure pattern, a geostrophic wind was calculated from a surface weather map. The map used was a hand-drawn pressure analysis done at the National Hurricane Center (NHC) at six-hour intervals. The analysis closest in time to the rip current was used for the geostrophic calculation. The geostrophic wind speed was calculated to the nearest three knots, and the direction to the nearest 16 points of the compass. Of course, geostrophy, especially at the surface, has errors which involve, among other things, isobaric curvature, friction, and isallobaric effects. The largest of these effects over the ocean is usually the curvature of the isobars, but since most of the cases examined here involved flow south of a strong subtropical ridge, the isobars usually had little curvature, and this limitation was for the most part minimal. In general, the geostrophic approximation gives an overestimate of surface wind. Gordon (1952) did an empirical study relating the geostrophic wind to the observed surface wind for ten-degree belts of latitude over all oceanic regions of the world. At the latitude of southeast Florida (25° north), the ratio of near-surface wind speed to calculated mean geostrophic wind speed is 0.87, while the directional deviation is 18°.

To obtain the best relationship between the local wind direction and speed and the incidence of rip currents, a number of factors was considered. The 72 drownings that were most likely to have been rip current related based on information from medical examiner reports and beach rescue logs were compared to the Miami Beach DARDC wind measurements closest in time to the drowning. Figure 7 is a wind rose constructed from this data, which shows the frequency of direction and the average scalar speed for the sustained wind and the peak wind. As noted previously, the peak and sustained wind directions were assumed to be the same. Also, there were fewer cases for the peak wind, because the peak wind information prior to 1985 was largely missing. It was noted that all of the wind directions were onshore. The southeast Florida coast is oriented nearly north-south, although certain sections are oriented about 20° clockwise to this direction. A large majority of the onshore winds were nearly normal to the coast. The average sustained wind speed closest in time to the drowning was 13 knots, and the average peak wind was 18 knots.

Looking more closely at the hourly DARDC wind data, it was observed that sometimes the wind was strong overnight, but it then weakened and veered (turned in a clockwise direction) during the following day. This occurred at the end of a several day episode of moderate to strong onshore windflows. Talks with beach patrol personnel indicated that rip currents that may have been ongoing because of the strong onshore winds for several days did not immediately cease when the wind decreased, but rather took several hours to completely terminate. The rip currents that occurred during the period of weaker winds following an episode of strong winds were designated as "residual" rip currents. If the cases during these residual events were deleted, an even greater relationship between strong onshore wind nearly normal to the coast and likely rip current drownings was noted. The average wind speed for this sample was 14 knots for the sustained wind and 20 knots for the peak wind.

When the residual rip current cases were studied in more detail, it was established that they occurred only during the 12-hour daylight period following the final night of a strong onshore wind episode. A wind rose was plotted for just these cases (Figure 8). A comparison of Figures 7 and 8 shows that the wind direction has veered and the speed is greatly reduced for these cases. The wind flow is still onshore but not perpendicular to the coast. The reason that rip currents may persist after the wind weakens and veers may be due to the fact that the ongoing closed cell circulation in the surf zone (Sonu, 1972), for waves normal to the coast, is maintained for a time by a wind that supports the feeder currents, but it is not totally disruptive to the outgoing rip current. Strong longshore currents are observed to disrupt the

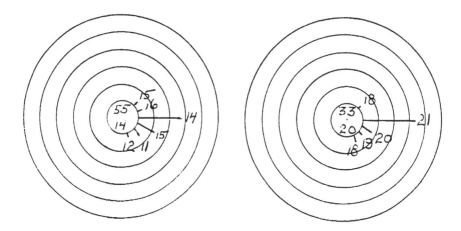

FIGURE 7   Wind rose for DARDC sustained wind, left, and peak wind, right, during rip current drownings on southeast Florida beaches 1979–1988, with residual events included.

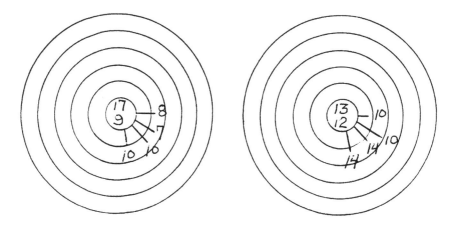

FIGURE 8   Wind rose for DARDC sustained wind (left) and peak wind (right) during rip current drownings on south Florida ocean beaches 1979–1988, for residual rip current drownings only.

outgoing rip currents. Residual rip current drownings accounted for 24 of the 94 deaths from 1979 to 1988.

Having shown that a good relationship existed between wind direction and speed and the incidence of rip currents, an attempt was made to quantify that relationship. In cases excluding the residual, a very strong relationship between rip currents and wind direction was established. *When rip current drownings or rescues took place, the wind direction was onshore 100% of the time.* Furthermore, the direction was onshore and within 30° of normal to the coastline about 90% of the time.

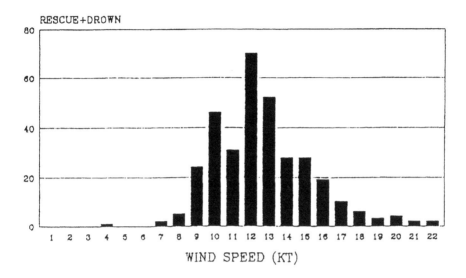

FIGURE 9 Frequency of DARDC sustained wind speed for combined rip current rescues and drownings on southeast Florida beaches, 1979–1988.

With respect to the wind speed, the relationship is not as strong as with the wind direction, but is still highly correlated. Using the DARDC one-minute sustained wind speeds and excluding residual cases, a frequency plot was drawn for all drowning and rescue reports from 1979 to 1988 (Figure 9). This plot shows 75% of the wind speeds were 10 knots or greater. Of the 25% below 10 knots, the age of the victim was 20 years or younger or 60 years or older, implying that these rip currents may have been weaker. For the DARDC peak wind values more than 95% occurred with peak winds of 17 knots or greater.

Having established that a strong onshore wind flow showed a consistent and reliable association with rip currents, the history of the wind during an episode in which rip currents were present was investigated. From the hour nearest to the rip current drowning or rescue, hourly winds from the Miami Beach DARDC were examined back in time to when the onshore wind first began and ahead in time to when the onshore wind weakened or ended. A total of 83 episodes in which rip current rescues or drownings occurred were identified during the period 1979–1988. Of course there were undoubtedly many more episodes during this ten-year period, but none that could be identified as having caused any drownings. An episode was loosely defined as beginning when the geostrophic wind direction became onshore and within 30° of normal to the coastline with a speed of at least 10 knots, and ending when the wind direction exceeded 60° normal to the coast or the wind speed decreased to five knots or less. Among the variables examined with respect to these episodes were their length, the time between them, and the time between the episode's beginning and the onset of the rip current. The length of the episodes ranged from a single day to 36 days, with a median length of 5–6 days. One or more drownings occurred during 67 of the total 83 episodes. The drownings took place from a minimum of three hours after an episode began to a maximum of 33 days after an episode began. The median time between the beginning of an episode and the first drowning was about three days. In eight of the episodes, the drowning took place on the first day. No obvious differences in wind speed or direction were noted for episodes when the drowning occurred on the first day and for those that occurred later in the episode. Days two and three of the episode were the days on which rip current drownings most frequently occurred. With reference to the very first drowning, when multiple drownings took place during an episode, the median time was midway between days two and three. When both drownings and rescues are included, the median was closer to day two. If a rip current was observed on the previous day, there was a great likelihood of a rip current on the subsequent day even if wind speeds were slightly lower. These statistics imply that the rip currents do not usually begin immediately at the onset of the onshore wind but build up with time. This may be analogous to the time it takes for waves on the open ocean to become fully developed.

The time between rip current episodes varied widely. The most frequent interval was 14 days; however, intervals of 2–10 days were also common. With respect to the time of year, slightly longer intervals occurred in the summer months, consistent with the generally weaker winds during that period. The average time between episodes is longer for those containing multiple drownings, as opposed to those with a single drowning which implies that (a) the rip current may be stronger given a longer time between episodes or perhaps (b) people become more cautious after the news of rip currents is publicized. The reason that the rip currents may be stronger after a long time between episodes is that the nearshore sand bar has reestablished itself, leading to a more drastic washout.

Periods during which weather-related drownings occurred that were **not** rip current related were also examined. These 15 occasions showed quite a different relationship to the beginning of the strong wind than did the rip current-related drownings. In 11 of these 15 cases, at least one of the drownings took place on the first day, usually within three–eight hours of the onset of stronger winds. The reason for this short interval between the beginning of strong winds and the drownings is unclear.

An investigation was made of the relationship between rip currents and both the time of high and low water and the tidal current speed and direction. After a cursory examination of rip currents and tidal heights, it was determined that the actual height of high and low water had little relationship to rip currents. This is not surprising because the range of tidal heights in southeast Florida, even during spring tides, is usually less than 3 ft. Episodes of perigean spring tides were not considered because of their relative low frequency. The National Ocean Service (NOS) derived times of high and low water levels, and the time, direction, and speed of tidal current were used to calculate the conditions at the time of the rip current. No attempt was made to correct the tide times, which were made at the Miami Harbor entrance (located from one to 31 miles south of the beaches of Dade and Broward counties), to the exact location of the incident since this would mean a maximum error of only about ten minutes. Another effect on the accuracy

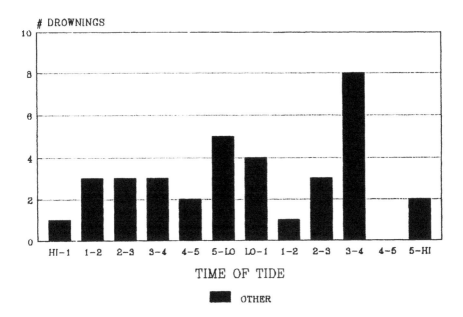

FIGURE 10 Number of rip current drownings on southeast Florida ocean beaches, 1979–1988, relative to times of high and low tide.

of the tidal time involved a resurvey of the tidal currents made during the mid-1980s, which was necessitated by the effects of dredging the Miami ship channel. However, the recomputed tidal current times showed only relatively small changes from earlier values.

Figure 10 shows a graph of drowning as related to tidal time. For ease in drawing the graph, the scale is not quite accurate in that a 12-hour tidal period is depicted rather than the average observed value of 12 hours and 22 minutes. This shortcoming was considered minimal in view of the accuracy of estimating the times of the drownings. This graph shows that 74% of the rip current drownings happened in the six-hour period from two hours before to four hours after low tide, and 55% occurred in the three-hour period from one hour before to two hours after low tide. A similar percentage was obtained when the rip current drowning and rescue data were combined. Komar (1976) noted a similar relationship between low tide and rip currents along the Oregon coast. The reason for this correlation may be due to either stronger rip currents, more people going into the surf during the time of low tide, or a combination of both.

An evaluation was made between tidal currents and rip currents but the correlation was not as strong as the one between rip currents and the time of low tide. However, in the absence of strong winds or large swells, and in locations with the right bathymetric conditions, tidal currents may be an important factor in rip current formation.

Rip currents generated by large oceanic swells, although relatively infrequent along the U.S. east and Gulf coasts, especially when compared to the U.S. west coast, Hawaii, or Puerto Rico, can be particularly hazardous because they may appear when local wind and sea conditions are relatively calm and catch the unsuspecting swimmer by surprise. As mentioned previously, swells along the southeast Florida coast are even rarer than elsewhere along the Florida east coast because of the sheltering effect of the Bahamas and Cuba. No rip current drownings or rescues in Dade and Broward counties can definitely be associated with swells during the period 1979–1988.

Along the east coast of Florida north of Palm Beach, large swells do occur, although infrequently. During the summer and fall when tropical cyclones, usually moving in a northward direction, pass east of the area, and in the winter months when strong extratropical lows often develop off the coast of the Carolinas, large northeast or east swells develop that can impact the United States east coast. In 1995 large swells generated by Hurricane Felix caused rip currents that drowned eight people along beaches from the Carolinas to New Jersey. Hurricane Emily in 1993 created rip currents that drowned three persons along the North Carolina and Virginia beaches and Hurricane Hugo caused swells that caused a deadly rip current at Daytona Beach, Florida, in 1989.

AWARENESS, PREDICTION, AND MITIGATION

To reduce the number of people impacted by rip currents, a three-pronged approach is suggested. Awareness programs can educate the beach-going public about the dangers of rip currents. Due to the increasingly violent nature of our society, it is recommended that explicitly graphic materials be developed that portray the consequences of being caught unprepared in a rip current. This could include corpses of drowning victims or perhaps dramatic reenactments of drownings. Use broadcast, cable, and closed-circuit television to air this material, including public service announcements, television "specials," educational videotapes, and written material.

Predictive efforts must include increased observations of oceanographic and meteorological variables. Direct wave height and wave direction measuring devices are needed at frequent intervals along the coasts. Some devices should be located near the beachfront itself to give current wave conditions while others should be located several miles offshore to allow for deeper water measurements. The observations then can be used in predictive models of the nearshore environment to predict the occurrence of rip currents. Although some models have already been developed, more sophisticated models with smaller space and time scales need to be established.

Mitigation efforts, such as physical barriers, theoretically have the potential for reducing high-energy wave activity that causes many rip currents. These barriers also have the potential for reducing beach erosion, and perhaps even providing some protection from the deadly storm surge of a hurricane. However, a balance will have to be struck between "protecting" the beach with these barriers and causing disruption of natural processes. Much research is needed before any implementation of these types of devices is justified.

REFERENCES

Commander Naval Oceanography Command, 1986, *U.S. Navy Climatic Study of the Caribbean Sea and Gulf of Mexico*, Vol. 3 (Florida Coastal Waters and Southwest Atlantic), Naval Oceanography Command Detachment, Asheville, NC.

Gordon, A. H., 1952, "The relation between mean vector surface wind and the mean vector pressure gradient over the ocean," *Geophys. Para. Appl.* 21, 49–51.

Komar, P. D., 1976, *Beach Processes and Sedimentation*, Prentice-Hall, Englewood, NJ, pp. 168–202.

National Oceanic and Atmospheric Administration, 1990, *50 Years of Population Change along the Nation's Coasts 1960–2010*. U.S. Department of Commerce, Washington, DC, U.S. Government Printing Office.

Sonu, C. J., 1972, "Currents," *J. Geophys. Res.*, 77, No. 181: 3232–47.

Index